Health and Disease Among Women: Biological and Environmental Influences

Edited by Roberta B. Ness
           Lewis H. Kuller

New York   Oxford
Oxford University Press
1999

Oxford University Press

Oxford   New York
Athens   Auckland   Bangkok   Bogotá   Buenos Aires   Calcutta
Cape Town   Chennai   Dar es Salaam   Delhi   Florence   Hong Kong   Istanbul
Karachi   Kuala Lumpur   Madrid   Melbourne   Mexico City   Mumbai
Nairobi   Paris   São Paulo   Singapore   Taipei   Tokyo   Toronto   Warsaw

and associated companies in
Berlin   Ibadan

Copyright ©1999 by Oxford University Press, Inc.

Published by Oxford University Press, Inc.
198 Madison Avenue, New York, New York 10016

Oxford is a registered trademark of Oxford University Press

All rights reserved. No part of this publication may be reproduced,
stored in a retrieval system, or transmitted, in any form or by any means,
electronic, mechanical, photocopying, recording, or otherwise,
without the prior permission of Oxford University Press.

Library of Congress Cataloging–in–Publication Data
Health and disease among women: biological and environmental influences/
edited by Roberta B. Ness, Lewis H. Kuller.
p.   cm.   Includes bibliographical references and index.
ISBN 0-19-511396-9
1. Women—Diseases.   2. Sex factors in disease.
3. Women—Health and hygiene.
I. Ness, Roberta B.   II. Kuller, Lewis H.
[DNLM: 1. Women's Health.   2. Estrogen Replacement Therapy.   3.
Sex Factors.   4. Genitalia, Female.   5. Reproduction.   6. Contraception.
WA 309 H433 1998]   RA564.85.H393   1998   616'.0082—dc21
DNLM/DLC for Library of Congress   98-5905

1 3 5 7 9 8 6 4 2

Printed in the United States of America
on acid-free paper

PREFACE

Women experience many diseases with a different frequency and/or severity than men. Gender differences in health and disease provide a classic natural experiment—that is, a natural phenomenon that can be observed and learned from. By observing the components of gender differences and the factors associated with them we can pose hypotheses about the underlying reasons for the differential distribution of disease. The theme of this book is that differences in the risk for some diseases between men and women and the determinants of higher risk for some diseases among subgroups of women are primarily determined by sex steroid hormone metabolism, reproduction, anatomy, and immune responses. These four factors are not sufficient to explain health and disease among women but they are major determinants interacting with lifestyle, environmental variables, physical and social environment, and genetic host susceptibility.

This book evaluates the biologic and psychosocial influences that help to explain why women are at greater or lesser risk for certain diseases and why some women may be at higher risk for disease than other women. This book also provides specific examples of how to link biologic and environmental mediation with epidemiologic observations. We believe that the interaction of biologic influences with behavioral, psychosocial, and lifestyle influences explains a good deal of the observed gender-specific variation in disease frequency between men and women. This approach has important implications: (*1*) it allows parallel research between different diseases to flourish; (*2*) it translates directly into health practice, as elements of mediation can be used to test for risk, modify behavior, and treat disease; and (*3*) it leads to an evaluation of competing risks from a range of health outcomes resulting from alteration of a given etiologic factor. That is, it provides a focus on risk factors, rather than outcomes, so that the risks and benefits can be assessed from a single risk related to many outcomes.

The chapters are grouped into parts on physiologic (hormonal, anatomic, immune-mediated, pregnancy-related), psychologic, and lifestyle influences on health and disease. The first chapters within each part provide background in basic physiology or demographics. The later chapters review specific areas of epidemiologic research and provide examples of how the current interest in women's health affords an opportunity to focus on the influences that mediate disease. The examples are not meant to be exhaustive but instead to illustrate this approach to the study of women's health. For example, within Part II on sex steroid hormones, the chapter on cardiovascular disease (Chapter 7) demonstrates the interactions between hormones and lifestyle in mediating disease; Chapter 8 on osteoporosis demonstrates the potential impact of hormone decline on an outcome; Chapter 9 on breast cancer demonstrates the potential impact of hormone excess at the tissue level on disease. Although each chapter focuses on a particular mediating influence, many chapters incorporate others.

Organizing research ideas by mediation of disease is unusual. The more traditional organization of clinical research and practice has been along disease-specific lines. With some exceptions, researchers usually have not thought about how etiologic factors may relate to several different disease states and about how what we learn from one disease may translate into knowledge about the mechanisms underlying a different disease state. This book not only presents a critical and up-to-date review of many aspects of women's health, but it also outlines the methodologic principles needed to approach them. Our hope in writing the book is to spark new research that will advance understanding of gender differences in health.

Pittsburgh, Pennsylvania   R.B.N.
March 1998

ACKNOWLEDGMENTS

Many thanks to my mom and dad for instilling that strong work ethic that was so necessary in completing the editing of this book; to my husband, David, for his support and patience when I thought I would never complete it; to my fabulous assistants, Thistle Elias and Lori Burleigh whose technical assistance were critical; to Deborah Brooks-Nelson for tackling the indexing, and to my children, Sara and Joel to whose good lifelong health and quality of life I dedicate this book.

RN

We would like to acknowledge support from the American Heart Association, Arthritis Foundation, Clinical Science Grant (SM, RRG), Lupus Foundation and Arthritis Foundation, Western Pennsylvania and Illinois Chapters (SM, RRG), and NIH grants AR44811 (SM), AR41607 (RRG) and AR30692 (RRG).

SM and RRG

I wish to thank Robert Jancart, M.D., Department of Pathology, Magee-Womens Hospital, Pittsburgh. Dr. Jancart located tissue of endometrial biopsies and took the photomicrographs of endometrial stages. In addition, I appreciate the helpful suggestions by Sarah Berga, M.D., and by Anthony J. Zeleznik, Ph.D. and for their critical reading of this manuscript.

KR

The preparation of this chapter has benefited from discussions with many individuals. I would like to thank faculty and students at the Graduate School of

Public Health who have listened to my presentations concerning this topic and responded with suggestions and critical questions. Both have helped to sharpen my thoughts. I would also like to thank two colleagues (Dr. David Plowchalk and Dr. Teresa Silvaggio) who have participated in discussions concerning these topics and have also assisted in the preparation of materials included in this chapter which have been published previously. Finally, I would like to thank the participants at the Medical Research Council, Institute for Environmental Health workshop on strategies in relation to population subgroups (Leicester UK, April 24–25, 1997) for their helpful questions and comments.

DM

CONTENTS

III   Anatomy of the Genital Tract and Immunology

IV Effects of Reproduction and Contraception on Women's Health

CONTRIBUTORS

Jibike Adegbile, M.D.
Department of Medicine
University of Alabama at Birmingham
School of Medicine
Birmingham, Alabama

Elaine J. Alpert, M.D., M.P.H.
Department of Social and Behavioral
    Sciences
Boston University
School of Public Health
Boston, Massachusetts

Joyce T. Bromberger, Ph.D.
Department of Epidemiology
University of Pittsburgh
Graduate School of Public Health
Pittsburgh, Pennsylvania

Kathryn L. Burgio, Ph.D.
Department of Medicine
University of Alabama at Birmingham
School of Medicine
Birmingham, Alabama

Annette Casoglos, M.P.H.
Department of Medicine
Wayne State University
School of Medicine
Detroit, Michigan

Willard Cates, Jr., M.D., M.P.H.
President
Family Health International
Research Triangle Park,
    North Carolina

Jane A. Cauley, Dr. P.H.
Department of Epidemiology
University of Pittsburgh
Graduate School of Public Health
Pittsburgh, Pennsylvania

Peggy A. Crowley-Nowick, Ph.D.
Department of Obstetrics, Gynecol-
    ogy and Reproductive Biology
Harvard Medical School
Boston, Massachusetts

Manning Feinleib, M.D., Dr. P.H.
Institute for Health Care Research
  and Policy
Georgetown University Medical Center
Washington, D.C.

LuAnn B. Gibson, M.P.H.
Department of Epidemiology
University of Pittsburgh
Graduate School of Public Health
Pittsburgh, Pennsylvania

Patricia S. Goode, M.D.
Department of Medicine
University of Alabama at Birmingham
School of Medicine
Birmingham, Alabama

Lillian M. Ingster, M.H.S.
Office of the Center Director
National Center for Health Statistics
Hyattsville, Maryland

Donna Kritz-Silverstein, Ph.D.
Department of Family and Preventive
  Medicine
University of California, San Diego
School of Medicine
La Jolla, California

Lewis H. Kuller, M.D., Dr. P.H. Uni-
  versity Professor
Department of Epidemiology
Graduate School of Public Health
University of Pittsburgh
Pittsburgh, Pennsylvania

Julie L. Locher, M.A.
Department of Medicine
University of Alabama at Birmingham
School of Medicine
Birmingham, Alabama

Frances Leslie Lucas, Ph.D.
Department of Medicine
Maine Medical Center
Portland, Maine

Susan Manzi, M.D., M.P.H.
Department of Medicine and Epi-
  demiology
University of Pittsburgh
School of Medicine
Pittsburgh, Pennsylvania

Donald R. Mattison, M.D.
Dean, Graduate School of Public
  Health
University of Pittsburgh
Pittsburgh, Pennsylvania

Elaine Meilahn, Dr.P.H.
Department of Epidemiology and
  Public Health
London School of Hygiene and Tropi-
  cal Medicine
London, England

Roberta B. Ness, M.D., M.P.H.
Department of Epidemiology
University of Pittsburgh
Graduate School of Public Health
Pittsburgh, Pennsylvania

Anne B. Newman, M.D., M.P.H.
Department of Medicine
University of Pittsburgh
School of Medicine
Pittsburgh, Pennsylvania

Rosalind Ramsey-Goldman, M.D.,
  Dr. P.H.
Department of Medicine
Northwestern University Medical
  School
Chicago, Illinois

Karen E. Remsberg, M.S.P.H.
Department of Medicine
University of Pittsburgh
Graduate School of Public Health
Pittsburgh, Pennsylvania

Kathleen D. Ryan, Ph.D.
Department of Cell Biology and
    Physiology
University of Pittsburgh
Magee-Womens Research Institute
Pittsburgh, Pennsylvania

Evelyn O. Talbott, Dr.P.H.
Department of Epidemiology
University of Pittsburgh
Graduate School of Public Health
Pittsburgh, Pennsylvania

Giuliana Trucco, M.D.
Department of Pathology
University of Pittsburgh, School of
    Medicine
Magee-Womens Hospital
Pittsburgh, Pennsylvania

Robert A. Wild, M.D.
Chief, Department of Obstetrics and
    Gynecology
University of Oklahoma
School of Medicine
Oklahoma City, Oklahoma

INTRODUCTION

Men and women differ with respect to morbidity and mortality. For example, in the United States in 1990, the life expectancy at birth was 72.7 years for white males and 79.4 years for white females, a difference of 6.7 years.[1] In that same year, the life expectancy at birth for black males was 64.5 years and for black females 73.6 years, a difference of 9.1 years. Despite the fact that life expectancy has been increasing over the past century, men continue to die at younger ages than women, and this has not changed over the past 80 years.

A refinement of this analysis is to combine the impact of disability with the rate of mortality so as to measure life's quality in addition to its duration. The metric for this, developed by the investigators involved in the Global Burden of Disease Study,[2] is the disability-adjusted life year (DALY), which represents the sum of the number of years of life *lost* as a consequence of premature mortality plus the number of years of life lived with a disability.[3,4] Disabilities can persist for varying periods of time and are of variable severity. Through the DALY the number of years of life impaired by a disability is adjusted by both the duration and severity of the disability.

These disability- or quality-adjusted life year metrics have stimulated considerable discussion because they imply that the burden of disease in human populations (including differences between men and women) is very different from what mortality statistics suggest. From this disability-modified, burden-of-disease perspective, the leading causes of disability throughout the world in 1990 were the following: unipolar major depression, iron deficiency, falls, alcohol use, chronic obstructive pulmonary disease, bipolar disorder, congenital anomalies, osteoarthritis, schizophrenia, and obsessive compulsive disorders.

Many of these conditions are more common among women. Thus, although women live longer than men, more of their years are clouded by disability and reduced quality of life. A nonexhaustive list of diseases that cause disability most commonly in women includes breast cancer, rheumatoid arthritis and systemic lupus, depression, incontinence, and osteoporosis.

This book focuses on the potential biologic and environmental influences that may mediate differences in health between men and women. *Health and Disease Among Women* promotes an approach to studying the epidemiology of women's health that combines an understanding of pathophysiology with observations about disease susceptibility; it then develops appropriate models that link pathophysiology to observations in epidemiological studies. This book also demonstrates the importance of trying to develop better interpretations of pathophysiology to explain known epidemiological or clinical observations. For example, recent epidemiologic studies have suggested that low bone mineral density in postmenopausal women may be related to a reduced risk of breast cancer, but to somewhat higher risks of cardiovascular disease and possibly colon cancer. These observations could be related to variations in sex steroid hormone metabolism or to concentrations of growth hormone and insulin-like growth factors. More detailed pathophysiological studies are needed to interpret associations between bone mineral density and other diseases among postmenopausal women.

Similarly, various lifestyle attributes have been related to disease without attempting to understand the underlying pathophysiology of observed associations. For example, if increased physical activity is associated with decreased risk of cardiovascular disease and breast cancer, then a critical question is whether there is a specific pathophysiological basis as well as a common association between physical activity and both diseases, such as hormone metabolism, hypothalamic pituitary physiology, or growth hormone action.

The study of women's health has been limited in the past by a focus on specific diseases or behavioral attributes. Some investigators, for example, have studied diet and women's health, such as the role of fat in the diet and its relationship to risk of coronary heart disease, while other investigators have studied dietary fat and risk of breast cancer, often without considering the similarities of the associations of fat in the diet with both coronary heart disease and breast cancer. *Health and Disease Among Women* also examines biologic and environmental influences that affect a variety of disease endpoints. For many exposures to such factors—and this is epitomized by hormone replacement therapy—both risks and benefits may result from a single exposure. Thus a focus on multiple outcomes allows for an overall evaluation of health effects.

The study of women's health can be subdivided into several categories; these are reflected in the different sections of this book. Part I deals with diseases in which certain lifestyles or psychological factors are more common

among women than men. These factors are associated with substantial variations in the risk and incidence of some diseases. For example, differences in oc-
cupation-related conditions may be related to differences in exposure to environmental toxins within specific occupations and/or to possible variations in
response to such exposure that are related to hormone metabolism, anatomy, or
immunology. Another example of a disease affected by psychosocial influences
is domestic violence, in which the victims are most often women and the perpetrators are more likely to be men. These differential rates may be due in part to
differences in social economic status, social roles, physiology, and alcohol and
drug use.

Part II examines diseases in which the differences in hormone metabolism
between men and women appear to play a critical role. Examples include breast
cancer, osteoporosis, cardiovascular disease, and polycystic ovary disease. The
interrelationships of common lifestyle factors (such as cigarette smoking, diet,
and weight gain) with hormone metabolism, reproductive history, and host susceptibility are important in understanding the epidemiology, etiology, and natural history of these diseases. For example, to understand the differences in risk
factors for cardiovascular disease in men and women, (including lifestyle and
host susceptibility factors), it is important to consider the older age of onset, on
average, among women than men.

Part III includes diseases that are primarily limited to women because of
women's unique anatomical attributes. It presents the anatomy and pathology of
the genital tract as the first step toward exploring the etiology, natural history,
and treatment of these diseases. Examples include incontinence and morbidity
from sexually transmitted diseases, as well as ovarian and uterine cancers and
other diseases of the uterus, such as fibroids and endometriosis. In this section,
we will also discuss immunologically mediated diseases. The much higher
prevalence of autoimmune diseases among women than men, especially among
premenopausal women, strongly indicates differences in immune response between the sexes. Thus an understanding of the etiology of these autoimmune
diseases depends on knowledge of the interrelationship between endocrinology
and immunology.

Part IV includes problems among women that are related to pregnancy and
contraception, including health conditions during pregnancy, sexually transmitted diseases, and thrombosis. Long-term health consequences of childbearing
may include altered cardiovascular risk and ovarian cancer risk. An understanding of the pharmacology of exogenous hormones and of the physiology of reproduction is critically important for comprehending the etiology of these
health outcomes.

Within these major parts we include diseases associated with greater life
expectancy among women than men, and consequently, increased long-term
disability and reduced quality of life among elderly women. The high frequency

of urinary incontinence in women is just one example of how the interrelation-ships between aging, anatomy, and hormone metabolism are of growing impor-tance in evaluating problems of aging among women.

Health problems of older women are clearly related to prior life experi-ences. Factors that determine health and disease among women, including edu-cational level, occupation, reproductive history, and environmental exposures, vary between older and more recent birth cohorts. Exposure to environmental factors that contribute to risk of disease may have occurred during the pre-menopausal years. For example, a long incubation period for cancer cells may link certain environmental exposures early in life with an increased risk of breast cancer. And oophorectomy prior to natural menopause may continue to be associated with increased risks of osteoporosis and coronary heart disease and perhaps with decreased risks of breast cancer among older women.

The study of women's health requires at least a basic knowledge of female anatomy, hormone and reproductive physiology, and immunology, as well as an understanding of the methodology of studying the determinants of health and disease, including the physical, biochemical, and social/behavioral risk factors, and how they interact with genetics or host susceptibility. Rather than providing a complete anthology of women's health, this book focuses on specific exam-ples that are related to the broad categories of women's health as described above and provides examples of hormone metabolism, anatomy, immunology, social/behavioral risk factors, and aging as they relate to the study of the epi-demiology of women's health.

REFERENCES

1. National Center for Health Statistics. Health United States, 1995. DHHS Pub. No. PHS 96-1232. Hyattsville, MD: Public Health Service, 1996.

2. World Development Report 1993, Investigating in Health, World Development Indicators. New York, Oxford University Press, 1993.

3. Murray CJL, Lopez AD. Global Burden of Disease, Vol. II: Global Health Statis-tics: A Compendium of Incidence Prevalence and Mortality Estimates for over 200 Con-ditions. Cambridge, MA: Harvard University Press, 1996.

4. Murray CJL, Lopez AD. Evidence-based health policy—lessons from the Global Burden of Disease Study. Science 1996;274:740–743.

I

PSYCHOSOCIAL AND LIFESTYLE ISSUES

I

SOCIOECONOMIC GRADIENTS IN HEALTH AMONG MEN AND WOMEN

Manning Feinleib and Lillian M. Ingster

This chapter provides background for understanding the effects on health and disease of the general social and economic condition of women and of age and race-specific subsets of women. The social and economic roles of men versus women have been changing over time, but remain quite different. We review evidence of positive and negative health effects from women's current aggregate social and economic situation and discuss mediators of the socioeconomic situation among women.

The role and socioeconomic status of women have fluctuated with the changing structure of society through the millennia. In the early known history of human hunter-gatherers, women were of equal necessity to the survival of the group and thus held equal status within it. Subsequently, during the agricultural evolution of society and later industrial eras, women were relegated to the home or to menial labor and were rendered subservient. Krieger and Fee[1] note that when science arose as the arbiter of truth, men sought to prove female inferiority by demonstrating the structural "weakness" of their bodies.[2] Mental frailty was ascribed to women's menstrual cycles, and tasks requiring mental prowess were considered beyond their ken.[3,4] In the early 20th century, the discovery of hormones[5] and chromosomes[6] solidified the social and cultural divisions based on gender,[7] and further inquiry into environmental causes was considered unnecessary. These notions became part of the medical research curriculum.[8] What was ignored was the way societal expectations translate into

---

* The opinions of the authors may not reflect the official positions of their respective institutions.

physiological health and its variation among women. Although there are real physiological differences between the sexes, these differences are manipulated by different cultures into very divergent sets of implications for behavior, social class standing, and civil and legal rights. As Verbrugge[9] writes, "Sex is constant across an individual's life . . . and fundamentally biological . . . (yet) it is both covertly and overtly involved in role training and rewards, the formation and maintenance of social ties, productive activities at home and elsewhere, and encounters with health risks and their physical outcomes." During the last two or three generations, contemporary Western culture has witnessed a renaissance of the role and status of women alongside that of men. This dramatic compression of the time required to observe such changes in socioeconomic status and activity provides the epidemiologist and social scientist an opportunity to research and test the various hypothesized relationships between social class indicators and their relationship to women's health.

METHODS IN SOCIOECONOMIC STUDY OF GENDER DIFFERENCES

Research on gender differences must be approached with caution, for the debate still rages over the extent of "nature versus nurture." While research has focused on issues of multiple role occupancy, workplace roles, and how roles are internalized and affect stress and coping behaviors, any explanation of gender differences in these areas that implies biological determinism may suffer from any of the following four fallacies.[10] *(1)* Developmental fallacies claim that gender differences during early childhood are carried over into adulthood. This line of thinking fails to acknowledge that early behavior may be affected by either innate biology or learned socialization. *(2)* Cross-cultural fallacies infer innate origins of gender differences from their widespread incidence. Gender differences consistent across societies may occur, however, because most societies face similar life conditions. *(3)* Cross-species fallacies presume biological determination from non-human primate studies, but there is no a priori reason why sex differences may be learned among humans but not among primates, or vice versa. *(4)* Evolutionary fallacies assume that behavior necessary for survival must be innate rather than learned. Natural selection, however, operates on behavioral traits and it is irrelevant whether those traits are acquired through learning or genetic programming.[11] Distributional evidence simply does not tell us as much as we would like. Furthermore, there may be qualitative differences that are not taken into account by social class theories. In other words, some differences may not be due to prevalent dominant/subordinate role theories but to differences in cognitive abilities, play styles, moral reasoning, and some physiologic responses from psychological and biological factors. Finally, it must be recognized that women of color experience the world differently from white women. Their social environment has undergone more dramatic change in the past 30 years than that of white women, and yet, less has been studied about their roles and health hazards.[12]

Social class may be defined as positions that social groups occupy relative to each other in the economic and social organization of society. People's social class is reflected in their work, their educational opportunities, their material resources, and the environments in which they live. While these attributes are not themselves synonymous with social class, they reflect the way social class structure concretely affects people's lives. Sociologists distinguish between two dimensions: (*1*) the structural dimension focuses on economic and demographic differences among groupings; and (*2*) the cultural dimension addresses behavior, habitat, and attitude characteristics of groupings.[13] Current study of social class has its roots in the writings of three prominent philosophers: Karl Marx, Max Weber, and Emile Durkheim. Karl Marx dichotomized society into two social classes—those who owned or controlled the means of production, and those who labored to produce commodities.[14] Although this juxtaposition of economic power was maintained as the only true basis for social class identity, Marx later modified his theory to allow for the unemployed and small businessmen. Max Weber expanded on the theories of Marx to create three axes of social class: class, prestige, and power.[15] The first is economic, as with Marx, and is measured by income or wealth. The second is an indication of social importance or honor conveyed by the community, such as that accorded to clerics and physicians. This is often a measure of life's "opportunities" based on social networks. The third axis is political power, or the ability to control societal decisions. Emile Durkheim added the context of social support and cultural identity to the social class paradigm, and the power of community identity. In the United States, most measures of social class are based on Weber's three axes. Current research utilizes three primary measures—occupation, education, and income—or a composite of these. Both occupation and education can apply to either of Weber's prestige or class categories; the third, income, falls into his class category.

The effects of socioeconomic status (SES) upon health have been modeled in various ways. One is that income grants access to good housing and healthier environments, reduces exposure to social stresses such as high crime rates, unemployment, and residential and marital instability; provides access to medical care and other amenities (including access to better nutrition for all family members); and presumably conveys more desirable working conditions. Another SES indicator of health is occupation, which controls for exposure to physically toxic or stressful environments and can offer related rewards. Choice of occupation also affects one's ability to exercise control[16] over one's work and work environment, job security, and access to housing and medical care. Finally, education influences healthy behaviors, value structures, and problem-solving abilities, all of which are related to lifestyle and the importance of good nutrition and exercise and other disease-preventive measures. Obviously, these three factors overlap, although studies have found that the correlation among them is low, indicating that these indices of social class are not interchangeable, and they measure different facets of social class.[17]

Liberatos et al.[18] discuss in detail numerous concerns over measurement that include both generic and index-specific issues. In general, there are several overarching issues: (1) whether the three primary measures capture the same conceptual issues or are separate but related facets of socioeconomic roles; (2) whether these measures are qualitative or quantitative, nominal, ordinal, or interval; (3) how one should conceptually identify exactly what one is measuring; (4) how one should account for temporal changes in these measures and their relative rankings; and (5) which measures of health outcomes should be used, for quite different relationships exist with prevalence versus incidence estimates, especially in inferring "causal" sequence.

The index-specific issues are many. Occupational measures may be nominal or ordered according to some ranking schema. Some of the better-known rankings of occupation[19] include the British Registrar General's Scale, which ranks occupations into social strata; Duncan's Socioeconomic Index, which ranks occupations by a prestige score based upon the male labor force; the Edward's Social-Economic Grouping used by the Census Bureau of the United States, which stratifies occupations within white-collar and blue-collar divisions; the Nam-Powers' Occupational Status Scores, which utilize separate education-based and income-based arrays for occupations; and Siegel's Prestige Scale and Treiman's Standard International Occupational Prestige Scale. There are numerous study-specific rankings of occupation that are not comparable across studies. The basic problem with occupational indices lies in the arbitrariness of the rankings; there is no accepted method to assign a hierarchical order that encompasses all occupations. These rankings inevitably reflect the biases of their creators. Second, some of these rankings, such as the British Registrar General's Scale, were created to produce a smooth mortality gradient, and thus any examination of status by mortality or morbidity is largely a tautology. Third, these rankings are constrained by the perspectives of their decade of origin. These perspectives can change dramatically over time and reflect gender stereotypes regarding predominantly male versus female occupations. Some indices are based solely upon the male labor force and thus are not useful for examining gender differences. Operationally, occupational data require obtaining a great deal of information from respondents and is often complex to code.

Education is a favorite index collected by researchers because of its ease of collection, relative ease of definition, and stability over time. Generally, one's educational level remains fixed over one's adult lifetime, although more recent trends of going back to school among the middle-aged population may change that view. A major problem with education is that there is a definite age-cohort relationship in educational attainment, where the older population has simply not had the educational opportunities of the younger population (a cohort effect). Some observers have also noted that younger cohorts are becoming more homogeneous in their educational attainment and that there are regional differences within the U.S. which persist. Finally, increments in education do not bestow the same gain in income or prestige for women as for men, or for minority groups as for whites.

Income as an index of social status also has difficulties associated with its use and interpretation. It is the most difficult of the three measures to collect, with the highest refusal rates among respondents, and groupings are seldom standardized across surveys. It is unreliable as a single indicator of social class because it varies considerably within occupations and can be wildly inconsistent with educational attainment. Income groupings also reflect time and regional constraints. Like education, increments of income are not associated with equal increments in prestige or status by gender or race/ethnicity. The instability of income over time and the inability to factor in opportunity costs can especially influence estimates of individual income versus family income. Naturally, income is age related, with lower levels occurring in early and late years and peaks in the middle years of life (an age effect as opposed to a cohort effect). Finally, there are unresolved concerns about comparability across time that are influenced by cost-of-living and definitions of households and household size.

Although a number of composite indices of occupation, income, and education exist, there are several concerns about using these measures. The first is that ranking by these measures can result in highly skewed distributions of occupations. Some indices are not sensitive to gender or race/ethnicity differences in social status. Other composites that base one rank (such as occupation) on the contributions of the two others and then create a composite of all three, give excess weight to the contribution made by the two variables through redundancy. As noted earlier, study-specific indices often lack comparability. Research techniques that utilize factor analysis or similar statistical approaches result in reducing these measures to a single dimension.

There are several specific concerns about using socioeconomic indices to ascertain women's social class. Early research in these areas classified women according to their husband's status,[20] believing the latter was of more value in determining risk. Current research indicates that the social status of husband and wife may differ if assessed individually. The combination of both spouses' employment alters the composite social status of the family, although the wife's employment generally has less effect than the husband's. A downward change in the status of the wife tends not to negatively affect the husband's social class, but the reverse is not true. As noted earlier, some index rankings were based solely upon the male labor force, and may not reflect female occupations accurately. The issue of how to rank young, unmarried women remains, as their status may not reflect their individual attainment but that of their parents from whom they may continue to receive support. In addition, the question of how to rank divorced and widowed spouses is still unresolved.

Several criteria have been cited[18] as relevant when considering which socioeconomic indices to use for study. Researchers must begin with some conceptual basis relating social class to health outcomes. The role of social class must be thought through, as not all measures will demonstrate an association simply because they are irrelevant to the outcome measure. The characteristics of the study population must be weighed against the applicability of the chosen measure. Is the chosen measure appropriate to the time frame under study? That is, are the inherent assumptions of the measure related to a particular era's perspectives? What is the evidence for reliability and validity of the chosen measure, particularly with respect to population subgroups? Contemporary research indicates that, if possible, it is better to use more than one measure so that related but different facets of social status will not be missed and flexibility is enhanced. This is especially true if the conceptual relationship is unclear. It is also important to decide conceptually whether the relationship relates to discrete categories of the index or continuous measures, such as in educational attainment. Finally, survey researchers in particular should weigh issues of respondent burden and refusal rate, complexity of coding, and comparability of results with other studies.

DIFFERENCES IN SES BETWEEN WOMEN AND MEN: EDUCATION, OCCUPATION, AND INCOME

In the previous discussion of social class and socioeconomic indices, the structural or mechanistic models of how SES affects health were discussed. To reiterate, for some scales and end points there may be a direct causal relation, such as between occupational hazards and injuries, or between occupational exposures and risk of cancer. But generally, SES is believed to operate in a more global, indirect manner. Loosely speaking, persons of higher social class are pictured as having more adequate nutrition and housing, cleaner and safer environments, and readier access to health care and preventive services. They are presumed to have higher self-esteem, broader social networks, and psychological support systems that ameliorate stressful situations. Through training or by adopting group norms, they are believed to have more healthful behaviors and more effective coping skills than people of a lower SES. To a large extent, these impressions are borne out by the available data. Reviews of the data available through 1991 have been presented recently by Feinstein[21] and Adler et al.[22] However, these reviews do not discuss gender differentials. To examine gender differences in health in relation to SES level, we have used data drawn from several large national surveys conducted in the United States during the last decade.

The social class indicators that are available from national surveys are based on education, income, occupation, and industry. Some surveys provide this information for each individual respondent while others characterize the entire family by a composite of these, e.g., total family income, or by the characteristic of the head of household or some other adult. The following analyses are based on single indicators, without any rankings employed. It is important to bear in mind that while data from national surveys excel at permitting generalizations about the overall population, they do not permit conclusions for small subsets of the population such as one would get from small area analyses.

Tables 1–1 and 1–2 show the distribution of the U.S. population by education and family income as determined in the National Health Interview Surveys (NHIS).[23] In these surveys, education of the "responsible adult" in the family is used to classify all of the family members; thus it is more appropriate to describe the data as the distribution of persons living in families where the "responsible adult" has the indicated level of education. By this definition, less than 1% of the population has unknown education. On the other hand, family income is not reported for approximately 15% of the families. Even though family indicators are used, there are differences in the distributions by gender, with women generally living in poorer, less educated families than men. This is probably due to the imbalance in families headed by single mothers. As discussed previously, a cohort effect can be seen in the higher proportion of people over age 65 (as compared to younger cohorts) with lower levels of education. The lower levels of income for the elderly is likely to result from both a cohort effect and an age effect, which cannot readily be separated from these national data. About 24% of women versus 13% of men over age 65 live in families with annual incomes of less than $10,000.

The distribution by occupation and industry of the large sample of the U.S. population contained in the Current Population Surveys used in the National Longitudinal Mortality Study[24] is shown in Table 1–3. In the broad groupings used by the Bureau of the Census, men and women are engaged in quite different occupations. Men tend to be craftsmen, managers or administrators, transport workers, laborers, and farmers, while women are concentrated in clerical and service jobs. These disparities may reflect older, cultural role identities. However, among the contemporary categories of professional and technical workers (e.g., nurses, teachers, scientists, writers) and operatives (e.g., assem-

Table 1–1. Distribution of U.S. Noninstitutionalized
Population by Education, Age, and Sex, 1990

AGE AND EDUCATION	FEMALE		MALE	
	NUMBER[a]	PERCENT	NUMBER[a]	PERCENT
All ages				
All education levels	125496	100.0	118010	100.0
Less than 12 years	18496	14.7	15264	12.9
12 to 15 years	74023	59.0	69650	59.0
16 years or more	32213	25.7	32423	27.5
Unknown	764	0.6	673	0.6
Under 18 years				
All education levels	31286	100.0	32788	100.0
Less than 12 years	4347	13.9	4522	13.8
12 to 15 years	18791	60.1	19655	59.9
16 years or more	7967	25.5	8435	25.7
Unknown	181	0.6	176	0.5
18–44 years				
All education levels	53101	100.0	51013	100.0
Less than 12 years	4917	9.3	4484	8.8
12 to 15 years	32519	61.2	31212	61.2
16 years or more	15385	29.0	15064	29.5
Unknown	280	0.5	253	0.5
45–64 years				
All education levels	24032	100.0	22059	100.0
Less than 12 years	3631	15.1	2883	13.1
12 to 15 years	14114	58.7	12507	56.7
16 years or more	6137	25.5	6519	29.6
Unknown	150	0.6	150	0.7
65 years and over				
All education levels	17077	100.0	12150	100.0
Less than 12 years	5600	32.8	3376	27.8
12 to 15 years	8598	50.3	6276	51.7
16 years or more	2725	16.0	2404	19.8
Unknown	154	0.9	94	0.8

[a]In thousands.

[*Source:* Collins and LeClere, 1996[23]]

blers, dress makers, packers, laundry workers), men and women are equally represented. The disparities by industry of employment are not as striking, with men tending to dominate in manufacturing (e.g., steel, radio/tv, aircraft, bakery) and construction industries and women dominating among personal (e.g., beauticians, hotel staff, laundry) and professional (e.g., health, education, welfare, religious) services. However, the specific segments of these industries occupied by men and women may be quite different.

Table 1–2. Distribution of U.S. Noninstitutionalized
Population by Family Income, Age, and Sex, 1990

AGE AND FAMILY INCOME	FEMALE		MALE	
	NUMBER[a]	PERCENT	NUMBER[a]	PERCENT
All ages				
All family incomes	125496	100.0	118010	100.0
Under $10,000	15644	12.5	10636	9.0
$10,000 to $19,999	21770	17.3	19208	16.3
$20,000 to $34,999	28424	22.6	28029	23.8
$35,000 or more	39477	31.5	41722	35.4
Unknown	20181	16.1	18415	15.6
Under 18 years				
All family incomes	31286	100.0	32788	100.0
Under $10,000	3612	11.5	3701	11.3
$10,000 to $19,999	5224	16.7	5434	16.6
$20,000 to $34,999	7666	24.5	8022	24.5
$35,000 or more	10673	34.1	11229	34.2
Unknown	4111	13.1	4402	13.4
18–44 years				
All family incomes	53101	100.0	51013	100.0
Under $10,000	5886	11.1	4145	8.1
$10,000 to $19,999	8404	15.8	7714	15.1
$20,000 to $34,999	12795	24.1	12764	25.0
$35,000 or more	18629	35.1	18932	37.1
Unknown	7387	13.9	7458	14.6
45–64 years				
All family incomes	24032	100.0	22059	100.0
Under $10,000	2115	8.8	1203	5.5
$10,000 to $19,999	3824	15.9	2632	11.9
$20,000 to $34,999	5219	21.7	4694	21.3
$35,000 or more	8314	34.6	9627	43.6
Unknown	4560	19.0	3903	17.7
65 years and over				
All family incomes	17077	100.0	12150	100.0
Under $10,000	4032	23.6	1586	13.1
$10,000 to $19,999	4318	25.3	3428	28.2
$20,000 to $34,999	2744	16.1	2550	21.0
$35,000 or more	1860	10.9	1935	15.9
Unknown	4123	24.1	2651	21.8

[a]In thousands.

[*Source:* Collins and LeClere, 1996[23]]

Table 1–3. Distribution of the Current Population Survey Samples Ages 25–64
Used in the National Longitudinal Mortality Study by Occupation and Industry

MAJOR OCCUPATION	MALE (%)	FEMALE (%)	MAJOR INDUSTRY	MALE (%)	FEMALE (%)
Professional–Technical	16.6	18.1	Agriculture	4.9	1.9
Manager-Administrator	16.4	8.2	Mining	1.9	0.3
Sales	5.8	5.8	Construction	10.8	1.3
Clerical	5.7	32.9	Manufacturing	26.8	17.1
Craftsmen	22.4	1.9	Transportation	9.4	4.0
Operative	10.6	11.1	Wholesale/Retail	15.8	19.4
Transport	6.1	0.8	Finance	4.5	7.5
Laborers	5.5	1.2	Business	4.5	3.3
Farmers	2.8	0.5	Personal Services	1.6	6.8
Farm Laborer	1.2	1.1	Entertainment	0.9	0.9
Service	7.0	16.5	Professional Services	12.0	32.4
Private household	0.0	2.1	Public Administration	6.8	5.1
TOTAL	100.0	100.0	TOTAL	100.0	100.0

[*Source:* Rogot et al., 1992[24]]

SES AND RISK FACTORS

National surveys have shown rather clear-cut gradients in behaviors and physiologic risk factors for certain socioeconomic characteristics. For example, although cigarette smoking has dropped significantly among both men and women during the last two decades and although a larger proportion of men are current cigarette smokers than women,[25] the gap seems to be narrowing, as shown in Table 1–4. For both genders, there is a marked inverse gradient in the proportion smoking with number of years of schooling. Whereas 41% of men and 31% of women with less than high school education are current smokers, less than 15% of either sex who have completed college continue to smoke. The decline in the proportion smoking has also been greatest for those with more years of education, falling by about 50% for college-educated people of either sex during the past 20 years, although it is especially marked among college women compared to less-educated women.

For many risk factors, race and ethnic background are also important confounders of the inverse relationship between risk factors and socioeconomic level. Some representative data for level of education are shown[25] in Table 1–5. The decline in smoking among more educated women is most pronounced in

Table 1–4. Age-Adjusted Prevalence (percent) of Current Cigarette Smoking by Persons 25 Years of Age and Over According to Sex and Education, U.S., 1974–1993

YEARS OF EDUCATION	1974	1979	1985	1990	1993	CHANGE 1993 vs. 1974 (%)
Males	43.0	37.6	32.9	28.3	27.2	−36.7
<12 years	52.4	48.1	46.0	41.8	41.0	−21.8
12 years	42.6	39.1	35.6	33.2	30.5	−28.4
13–15 years	41.6	36.5	33.0	25.9	27.4	−34.1
16 or more years	28.6	23.1	19.7	14.6	14.6	−49.0
Females	32.2	29.6	27.8	23.2	22.7	−29.5
<12 years	36.8	35.0	36.7	32.1	31.0	−15.8
12 years	32.5	29.9	29.6	26.3	26.7	−17.8
13–15 years	30.2	30.0	26.7	21.1	21.8	−27.8
16 or more years	26.1	22.5	17.4	13.6	12.4	−52.5

[*Source:* National Center for Health Statistics, 1996[25]]

Table 1–5. Prevalence of Selected Risk Factors Among Women 25 Years of Age and Older by Race, Hispanic Origin, and Level of Education

RACE/ETHNICITY	LEVEL OF EDUCATION		
	LESS THAN HIGH SCHOOL	HIGH SCHOOL	MORE THAN HIGH SCHOOL
Current cigarette smokers (percent)			
Non-Hispanic White	40.0	29.3	18.4
Non-Hispanic Black	31.9	24.9	22.5
Hispanic	13.9	18.5	11.6
Prevalence of sedentary lifestyle (percent)			
Non-Hispanic White	40.9	29.4	20.0
Non-Hispanic Black	49.0	37.6	29.0
Hispanic	51.9	33.8	28.4

[*Source:* National Center for Health Statistics, 1996[25]]

non-Hispanic whites but appears minimal in Hispanic women. In contrast, sedentary lifestyle declines with greater education rather consistently among all three groups.

SES AND MORBIDITY

The measure of morbidity that will be used in this discussion is self-reported restricted activity days per person as gathered in the National Health Interview Sur-

Table 1–6. Restricted Activity Days per Person per Year by Sex and Age

	MALE	FEMALE	RATIO F/M
All ages	13.0	16.7	1.28
Under 18 years	9.4	9.8	1.04
18–44 years	9.9	13.5	1.36
45–64 years	17.2	21.0	1.22
65 years and over	28.1	33.4	1.19

[*Source:* Collins and LaClere, 1996[23]]

Table 1–7. Restricted Activity Days per Person per Year (PPPY) by Sex, Age, and Education Level

AGE AND EDUCATION	MALE RESTRICTED ACTIVITY DAYS PPPY	RATIO[a]	FEMALE RESTRICTED ACTIVITY DAYS PPPY	RATIO[a]	RATIO F/M
All ages					
Less than 12 years	20.3	2.16	27.1	2.28	1.33
12 to 15 years	13.0	1.38	16.1	1.35	1.24
16 years or more	9.4	1.00	11.9	1.00	1.27
Under 18 years					
Less than 12 years	8.9	0.97	10.4	1.14	1.17
12 to 15 years	9.6	1.04	10.0	1.10	1.04
16 years or more	9.2	1.00	9.1	1.00	0.99
18–44 years					
Less than 12 years	13.3	1.93	18.2	1.77	1.37
12 to 15 years	10.8	1.57	14.3	1.39	1.32
16 years or more	6.9	1.00	10.3	1.00	1.49
45–64 years					
Less than 12 years	31.4	3.02	39.2	2.90	1.25
12 to 15 years	17.5	1.68	19.6	1.45	1.12
16 years or more	10.4	1.00	13.5	1.00	1.30
65 years and over					
Less than 12 years	35.4	1.56	39.9	1.52	1.13
12 to 15 years	25.9	1.14	31.1	1.18	1.20
16 years or more	22.7	1.00	26.3	1.00	1.16

[a]Relative to the 16 years or more education category.

[*Source:* Collins and LaClere, 1996[23]]

vey.[23] The rates of restricted activity increase with age for both sexes. Boys and girls under the age of 18 report approximately the same rates of restricted disability days but among adults, women report approximately 25% more disability days than do men (Table 1–6). The largest disparity occurs at ages 18 to 44, which may be due in part to childbearing and child-rearing roles of women. However, because the discrepancy persists in all subsequent age-groups, child responsibilities probably do not fully explain these morbidity differences by gender.

For each age-group over 18, there is a marked inverse relation between education level and rates of restricted activity for both sexes (Table 1–7). The measures of social class are based on the characteristics of the family as described in the NHIS i.e., family income and education of the "responsible adult." The effect of education seems to be greatest among adults ages 45 to 64 with both men and women in families with college education having one-third the rates of restricted activity as those with less than a high school education. Overall, the impact of education on restricted activity days is similar for men and women.

The inverse gradients of morbidity by family income are even more marked (Table 1–8). For adults aged 45 to 64, those in families with incomes of $35,000 or more had only about one-fifth the rate of restricted activity as did those in the poorest families with incomes of less than $10,000. The gradients with income are greater for men than for women so that within each age-group over age 18, men in families with higher incomes had lower disability rates than did women in such families. For families with incomes of less than $20,000, the restricted activity rates for men and women tended to be more similar.

SES AND MORTALITY

The classic study by Kitagawa and Hauser[26] of differential mortality in the United States, based upon a sample from the 1960 census, reported virtually no differentials in mortality by education among men over the age of 65, but there was a marked inverse relationship between education and mortality among women and younger men.[26] The differentials have been maintained among women, and during the latter part of the century, male mortality has also shown a marked inverse gradient with education.[27,28] Recent data from a large national study highlight the SES differentials in mortality. The National Longitudinal Mortality Study (NLMS) has followed several large representative samples of the U.S. population during the period 1979 to 1989.[29] These samples were drawn from several Current Population Survey cohorts and contain detailed information on family income, individual education levels, and industry and occupation of each respondent. The SES indicators of family income and level of education show a marked and regular effect on mortality rates among both men and women.

Table 1–8. Restricted Activity Days per Person per Year (PPPY) by Sex, Age, and Family Income

AGE AND FAMILY INCOME	MALES			FEMALES			RATIO F/M
	RESTRICTED ACTIVITY DAYS PPPY	RISK RATIO 1[a]	RISK RATIO 2[b]	RESTRICTED ACTIVITY DAYS PPPY	RISK RATIO 1[a]	RISK RATIO 2[b]	
All ages							
Under $10,000	22.9	2.63	1.00	29.4	2.58	1.00	1.28
$10,000 to $19,999	17.7	2.03	0.77	19.2	1.68	0.65	1.08
$20,000 to $34,999	11.6	1.33	0.51	14.3	1.25	0.49	1.23
$35,000 or more	8.7	1.00	0.38	11.4	1.00	0.39	1.31
Under 18 years							
Under $10,000	11.0	1.20	1.00	11.7	1.24	1.00	1.06
$10,000 to $19,999	9.5	1.03	0.86	10.5	1.12	0.90	1.11
$20,000 to $34,999	9.2	1.00	0.84	9.5	1.01	0.81	1.03
$35,000 or more	9.2	1.00	0.84	9.4	1.00	0.80	1.02

18–44 years							
Under $10,000	17.3	2.51	1.00	20.9	1.97	1.00	1.21
$10,000 to $19,999	13.7	1.99	0.79	16.0	1.51	0.77	1.17
$20,000 to $34,999	9.6	1.39	0.55	13.0	1.23	0.62	1.35
$35,000 or more	6.9	1.00	0.40	10.6	1.00	0.51	1.54
45–64 years							
Under $10,000	54.8	5.83	1.00	56.6	4.42	1.00	1.03
$10,000 to $19,999	30.8	3.28	0.56	25.2	1.97	0.45	0.82
$20,000 to $34,999	16.3	1.73	0.30	18.4	1.44	0.33	1.13
$35,000 or more	9.4	1.00	0.17	12.8	1.00	0.23	1.36
65 years and over							
Under $10,000	41.4	2.19	1.00	43.4	1.74	1.00	1.05
$10,000 to $19,999	29.8	1.58	0.72	30.6	1.22	0.71	1.03
$20,000 to $34,999	20.8	1.10	0.50	26.4	1.06	0.61	1.27
$35,000 or more	18.9	1.00	0.46	25.0	1.00	0.58	1.32

[a]Relative to the $35,000 or more income category.

[b]Relative to the under $10,000 income category.

[Source: Collins and LaClere, 1996[23]]

Family income is a powerful predictor of mortality. Using a family income of less than $5000 (1980 dollars) as the reference group, there is a marked inverse relation of all-cause mortality with family income for all persons under the age of 65 and for men over the age of 65[29] (Table 1–9). For those under age 65 with family incomes in excess of $50,000, the age-adjusted mortality rates are only 27% to 43% of those with the lowest incomes. Only for women over the age of 65 does there seem to be little effect of family income on total mortality. We can see that the effect of family income appears to convey more benefit to men than to women. These recent NLMS data illustrate gradients that are much steeper than those observed by Kitagawa and Hauser, although the patterns are similar.

Table 1–9. Adjusted Mortality Ratios by Family Income: National Longitudinal Mortality Study, 1979 Through 1989 Follow-up

AGE GROUP	FAMILY INCOME (1980 $)	MEN		WOMEN	
		AARR	MARR	AARR	MARR
25–44	<$5k	1.00	1.00	1.00	1.00
	$5k−	0.76	1.00	0.63	0.74
	$10k−	0.60	0.97	0.52	0.68
	$15k−	0.44	0.80	0.47	0.65
	$20k−	0.35	0.70	0.42	0.60
	$25k−	0.34	0.76	0.39	0.60
	$50k+	0.27	0.67	0.38	0.62
45–64	<$5k	1.00	1.00	1.00	1.00
	$5k−	0.84	0.96	0.77	0.95
	$10k−	0.65	0.88	0.67	0.92
	$15k−	0.54	0.80	0.58	0.84
	$20k−	0.47	0.75	0.52	0.78
	$25k−	0.41	0.71	0.47	0.75
	$50k+	0.32	0.63	0.43	0.69
65 years and over	<$5k	1.00	1.00	1.00	1.00
	$5k−	0.94	0.98	0.99	1.00
	$10k−	0.84	0.90	0.94	0.94
	$15k−	0.78	0.86	0.95	0.94
	$20k−	0.75	0.84	0.92	0.89
	$25k−	0.73	0.84	0.96	0.91
	$50k+	0.66	0.84	0.93	0.90

AARR, age- and race-adjusted relative risk; MARR, multivariate-adjusted relative risk with adjustment for age, race, employment status, marital status, and household size.

[*Source:* Sorlie et al., 1995[29]]

Education is also a powerful determinant of deaths from all causes. Among those with less than high school education (less than 12 years of schooling), the death rates are approximately the same for any given educational level[29] (Table 1–10). But for those completing high school there is improvement in the relative mortality with each subsequent level of education completed. The effect varies with age, being most pronounced for younger individuals. For college graduates within the 45- to 64-year-old age group (but to a lesser extent for the 25- to 44-year-old age group), men derive more benefit from their greater education than do women. Analysis of trends in mortality by education level from 1960 through the 1990s indicates that women have displayed an education-re-

Table 1–10. Adjusted Mortality Ratios by Years of Education, Using 9–11 Years as Reference Group: National Longitudinal Mortality Study, 1979 Through 1989 Follow-up

AGE GROUP	EDUCATION (YEARS)	MEN AARR	MEN MARR	WOMEN AARR	WOMEN MARR
25–44 years old	0–4	1.12	0.65	0.97	0.61
	5–7	1.00	0.86	0.66	0.60
	8	1.02	0.92	1.08	0.99
	9–11	1.00	1.00	1.00	1.00
	12	0.72	0.85	0.66	0.76
	13–15	0.67	0.80	0.56	0.65
	16	0.43	0.56	0.46	0.54
	17+	0.35	0.46	0.42	0.48
45–64 years old	0–4	0.96	0.76	1.05	0.83
	5–7	1.14	1.00	1.16	1.06
	8	1.01	0.96	1.05	1.03
	9–11	1.00	1.00	1.00	1.00
	12	0.83	0.93	0.78	0.88
	13–15	0.75	0.90	0.78	0.92
	16	0.58	0.75	0.66	0.82
	17+	0.50	0.67	0.63	0.82
65 years and older	0–4	0.96	0.89	1.01	0.94
	5–7	1.01	0.97	1.04	1.00
	8	1.04	1.03	1.03	1.02
	9–11	1.00	1.00	1.00	1.00
	12	0.90	0.94	0.94	0.95
	13–15	0.87	0.93	0.91	0.92
	16	0.81	0.91	0.92	0.94
	17+	0.68	0.80	0.77	0.79

AARR, age- and race-adjusted relative risk; MARR, multivariate-adjusted relative risk with adjustment for age, race, employment status, marital status, and household size.

[*Source:* Sorlie et al., 1995[29]]

lated disparity in mortality during the entire period while for men it seems to be a more recent phenomenon.[26,27] The differential mortality rates by education were particularly striking for deaths from heart disease.[28] It is speculated that the secular trends in heart disease mortality may have shown an inversion during the course of the century, being considerably higher among the higher social classes during the early part of the century, and then becoming lower during the latter part of the century among the more affluent and better educated. This phenomenon, however, apparently applied only to men whose habits related to such cardiovascular risk factors as smoking, high-fat diets, and less physical exercise. It is presumed that these habits were more adverse during the years prior to World War II and then improved during later years. The improvement in these lifestyle behaviors is thought to have been influenced in large measure by educational attainment.

SES AND USE OF HEALTH CARE SERVICES

The relationship between SES and the use of health care services is rather complex and varies with the type of care considered, the index of SES, and the population group studied. Since there is an inverse relation between morbidity and SES, one might expect an inverse relation with use of health services. However, because of the uneven distribution of health insurance, various barriers to access to health care, and diverse propensities to seek health care when appropriate, the relation of various measures of health care use to SES does not have a simple pattern.

Table 1–11 uses data from the National Health Interview Survey[23] to examine two indices of use of health services—percent of persons with physician contacts during the past year and percent of persons with short-term hospital episodes during the past year—in relation to two SES measures—family income and education of the responsible adult. For physician contacts (an index of acute ambulatory care), females tend to show more frequent use than males, particularly at younger ages. For short-term hospital episodes, the gender differences vary markedly by age. At the childbearing ages, the proportion of women with hospital episodes is more than double that for men. Over the age of 45, however, a greater proportion of men require hospitalization than women. The durations of hospital stays (not shown) tend to be somewhat longer for men than for women, which suggests that the increased hospitalization among men is due to more serious illnesses.

The trends by SES level within sex groups also vary by the type of health care utilized. Generally speaking, the proportion of persons in lower SES levels who have been hospitalized is greater than among those in higher SES levels for both sexes (Table 1–11). However, the variation in acute ambulatory care (percent with physician contacts) with SES level is slight. These trends pertain to both indices of SES level. Other studies have emphasized that people of lower SES tend to make less use of preventive health services, which may lead to more advanced disease when diagnoses are eventually made and thus lead to more frequent hospitalizations.[30]

The complexities of these relations make interpretations unclear, given that there are a variety of confounders that may be involved. For example, persons with insurance may tend to overuse health services and definitely use such services more frequently than those without insurance, even after adjusting for frequency and severity of illness.[31–33] Those using physicians may tend to have more conditions diagnosed and treated than those who see physicians less frequently. Serious illness requiring frequent use of health services, especially hospitalization, may lower the patient's income and/or render them unemployable. However, there seems to be a clear tendency for those of lower SES to be hospitalized more frequently than those of high SES; the presumption is that this parallels more serious morbidity and may reflect limited access to primary care.

OCCUPATION, INDUSTRY, AND MORTALITY

Occupation and industry have a rather complex relation to mortality. Returning to data from the National Longitudinal Mortality Study,[24] mortality rates for several major occupation categories are shown in Table 1–12. Occupation is recorded as the current occupation of the respondent at the time of the interview, and deaths are accumulated over the follow-up period from 1979 to 1985. These are descriptive categories of occupation and involve no ranking, thus any interpretation of social class status is implicit. The number of expected deaths is calculated by multiplying the proportion of total deaths observed among respondents in a specific age–race–sex group by the number of people with the characteristic of interest in that age–race–sex group. Although some of the observed-to-expected (O/E) ratios stand out because of the small number of deaths in a particular category, others are worth noting. In professional/technical occupations, the observed numbers of deaths were well below the expected numbers of deaths, about equally so for men and women. For men, the occupations designated transport equipment operatives, laborers, and service workers showed observed deaths to be substantially higher than expected. This was not so clear for women. Women's "excess" deaths appeared to be in occupations in private households, which traditionally involve very few men. The "big" picture, when we look at a regression of the O/E ratio for women in relation to that for men, is illustrated in Figure 1–1 (the numbers refer to occupations in Table 1–12). For the most part, there is a weak relationship between the results for women and those for men, indicating discrepancies in the mortality experience between the genders, but overall agreement that certain occupations carry greater risks for both genders than other occupations. The only large difference appears to be in

Table 1-11. Percent of Persons with Physician Contact in the Past Year and Percent with Short-Term Hospital Episode in the Past Year, by Sex, Age, Family Income, and Education of Responsible Adult Family Member

AGE / FAMILY INCOME	PERSONS WITH PHYSICIAN CONTACT					PERSONS WITH SHORT-TERM HOSPITAL EPISODE				
	PERCENT		RISK RATIO			PERCENT		RISK RATIO		
	FEMALE	MALE	F/M	FEMALE	MALE	FEMALE	MALE	F/M	FEMALE	MALE
18–44 years										
Under $10,000	81.1	62.1	1.31	1.00	1.00	15.3	6.6	2.32	1.00	1.00
$10,000 to $19,999	79.0	58.8	1.34	0.97	0.95	13.3	5.6	2.38	0.87	0.85
$20,000 to $34,999	81.2	62.3	1.30	1.00	1.00	12.1	4.3	2.81	0.79	0.65
$35,000 or more	83.4	64.6	1.29	1.03	1.04	10.0	3.5	2.86	0.65	0.53
45–64 years										
Under $10,000	79.5	70.9	1.12	1.00	1.00	14.7	16.7	0.88	1.00	1.00
$10,000 to $19,999	77.6	69.6	1.11	0.98	0.98	9.9	12.4	0.80	0.67	0.74
$20,000 to $34,999	80.4	70.3	1.14	1.01	0.99	8.2	9.8	0.84	0.56	0.59
$35,000 or more	82.7	73.1	1.13	1.04	1.03	6.7	7.0	0.96	0.46	0.42
65 years and over										
Under $10,000	87.3	80.1	1.09	1.00	1.00	19.0	21.2	0.90	1.00	1.00
$10,000 to $19,999	87.6	84.1	1.04	1.00	1.05	15.1	19.5	0.77	0.79	0.92
$20,000 to $34,999	87.3	85.5	1.02	1.00	1.07	13.3	16.7	0.80	0.70	0.79
$35,000 or more	89.0	86.7	1.03	1.02	1.08	14.5	15.8	0.92	0.76	0.75

EDUCATION OF

AGE	EDUCATION OF RESPONSIBLE ADULT									
18–44 years	Less than 12 years	73.7	51.7	1.43	1.00	1.00	15.8	5.1	3.10	1.00	1.00
	12 to 15 years	80.1	61.1	1.31	1.09	1.18	11.8	4.7	2.51	0.75	0.92
	16 years or more	85.2	65.7	1.30	1.16	1.27	10.3	3.2	3.22	0.65	0.63
45–64 years	Less than 12 years	78.7	68.4	1.15	1.00	1.00	12.7	12.8	0.99	1.00	1.00
	12 to 15 years	79.1	69.7	1.13	1.01	1.02	8.5	9.4	0.90	0.67	0.73
	16 years or more	83.2	74.1	1.12	1.06	1.08	6.3	7.0	0.90	0.50	0.55
65 years and over	Less than 12 years	87.3	81.9	1.07	1.00	1.00	17.4	20.5	0.85	1.00	1.00
	12 to 15 years	86.7	83.5	1.04	0.99	1.02	15.3	17.5	0.87	0.88	0.85
	16 years or more	89.1	86.9	1.03	1.02	1.06	13.8	16.6	0.83	0.79	0.81

[Source: Collins and LeClere, 1996[23]]

Table 1-12. Deaths from all Causes, Ages 25-64, by Major Occupation and Sex

MAJOR OCCUPATION	OBSERVED DEATHS		EXPECTED DEATHS		O/E	O/E
	MALE	FEMALE	MALE	FEMALE	MALE	FEMALE
1. Professional, technical, and kindred workers	679	262	884.7	321.8	77	81
2. Managers and administrators, except farm	996	182	1079.7	169.5	92	107
3. Sales workers	377	119	359.4	145.0	105	82
4. Clerical and kindred workers	408	685	386.1	679.2	106	101
5. Craftsmen and kindred workers	1467	35	1418.2	40.2	103	87
6. Operatives, except transport	689	292	656.9	285.0	105	102
7. Transport equipment operatives	438	14	387.3	13.8	113	101
8. Laborers, except farm	410	24	339.0	23.1	121	104
9. Farmers and farm managers	178	15	244.4	12.1	73	124
10. Farm laborers and farm foremen	79	17	77.3	28.7	102	59
11. Service workers, excluding private household workers	590	437	475.5	399.3	124	109
12. Private household workers	0	116	2.4	80.5	0	144
TOTAL	6311	2198	6310.9	2198.2		

[*Source:* NIH Publication 92-3297, Rogot et al., 1992[24]]

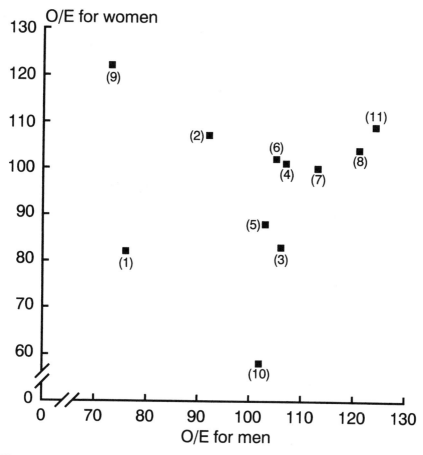

Figure 1–1. Correlation of O/E mortality by major occupation for men and women [Modified and reproduced from Rogot et al., 1992, thanks to the National Heart, Lung, and Blood Institute[24]]

the agricultural occupations. The differences in risks experienced by the two genders in some of these occupations may be due to differences in physiology, coping skills, competing stresses, and differences in the work environment according to gender.

In contrast, Table 1–13 presents the data for mortality by industry, a more common analysis. There appears to be more agreement between the O/E ratios for men and for women. For men, the largest ratios were observed in the mining, business, and personal services industries; excess deaths were also observed for women in these industries. Observed deaths were less than expected among men in agriculture, finance, and public administration, and among women, in transportation. A regression of the O/E ratio for women in relation to

Table 1–13. Deaths from all Causes, Ages 25–64, by Major Industry and Sex

| MAJOR INDUSTRY | OBSERVED DEATHS | | EXPECTED DEATHS | | O/E | |
	MALE	FEMALE	MALE	FEMALE	MALE	FEMALE
1. Agriculture, forestry, and fisheries	306	42	367.7	45.8	83	92
2. Mining	121	6	100.1	5.1	121	118
3. Construction	722	25	642.1	23.9	112	105
4. Manufacturing	1751	401	1764.8	393.7	99	102
5. Transportation, communication, public utilities	604	58	595.9	72.1	101	80
6. Wholesale and retail trade	1034	459	964.6	441.0	107	104
7. Finance, insurance, and real estate	248	145	291.8	142.2	85	102
8. Business and repair services	282	68	242.1	59.6	116	114
9. Personal services	133	221	112.5	191.0	118	116
10. Entertainment and recreation services	54	18	47.5	16.2	114	111
11. Professional and related services	651	632	724.0	693.2	90	91
12. Public administration	405	125	457.8	116.2	88	108
TOTAL	6311	2200	6310.9	2200.0		

[**Soruce:** NIH Publication 92-3297, Rogot et al., 1992[24]]

that for men, as shown in Figure 1–2 (the numbers refer to industries in Table 1–13), shows that except for public administration, finance, and transportation, the mortality experience of each gender in the various industries is essentially equivalent.

Because it is difficult to conceptualize the role that occupation plays in mortality analyses (with the exception of work-related deaths), researchers frequently use work-related injuries within occupation or industry categories to determine work-related risk. For example, one study that examined gender differences in work-related risks among electric utility workers[34] found that gender-specific injury rates were higher for male workers than for female workers, but when the data were adjusted for occupation, job experience, and age, it was found that the women had considerably elevated injury rates compared to men.

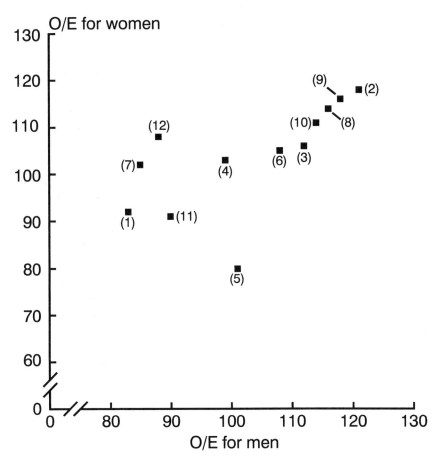

Figure 1–2. Correlation of O/E mortality by major industry for men and women [Modified and reproduced from Rogot et al., 1992, thanks to the National Heart, Lung, and Blood Institute[24]]

ECOLOGICAL STUDIES

No chapter on socioeconomic gradients in health would be complete without a brief discussion of some ecological studies. These are inherently more difficult to interpret than studies based on individuals because of the risk of the "ecological fallacy" resulting from ascribing the same risks to all persons within a category. Yet this should not preclude gaining some insight from these observations, particularly when there is strong conceptual support for the results. Evidence bearing out gender differences in health comes from three recent studies using postcode sectors in Scotland, boroughs in Amsterdam, and neighborhoods in Barcelona. Each documented inverse relations between mortality and a variety of socioeconomic measures. The study of mortality differentials in Scotland[35] between 1981 and 1991 grouped postcode sectors by Carstairs composites of various socioeconomic census variables. The results support an inverse relationship between socioeconomic status and mortality, with widening of the relative discrepancy across the social strata over time and some evidence that the disparities among women are greater than among men.

Similar support for differentials between poor and affluent localities come from a study of mortality differentials by borough in Amsterdam, The Netherlands.[36] In characterizing the rather homogeneous boroughs within a heterogeneous city, the authors were able to demonstrate that young men in poorer neighborhoods suffer most from excess mortality due to external causes, whereas women in such areas tend to die from smoking-related causes. Another urban study from Barcelona, Spain,[37] created a more unusual SES neighborhood index, including such factors as telephone use, powerful cars, and a rating for buildings and land. Their data also support the inverse relationship between affluence and mortality, finding the strongest relationship for variables such as percent illiterate and/or unemployed. Both illiteracy and unemployment were more frequent among women. However, the improvement in mortality with increasing affluence was greater among men than among women. The authors caution against use of their indicators for studying inequalities among women because these indicators are a much better reflection of the SES status of men in their society than of women. They concur that illiteracy is a variable that is usually determined early in life and is more strongly associated with health behaviors than other indicators, whereas occupation is not correlated as such and has the additional drawbacks of yielding a value only for employed persons, and generally women are tabulated according to their husbands' occupation.

Synthesis

Virtually all studies addressing the issue of socioeconomic level and measures of morbidity and mortality have shown remarkable concordance in the direction of the association and reasonable agreement in the magnitude of the trends. For most measures, women show higher levels of morbidity than men at all adult ages, with the absolute level of morbidity decreasing for both sexes as the SES level increases and the relative disparities between men and women tending to increase as the SES level goes up. Thus men seem to be affected more favorably than women by improving their SES level.

Women have lower mortality rates than men at all ages and the absolute mortality rates decrease for both sexes as the SES level increases. However, contrary to the trends for morbidity data, the relative disparities between men and women decrease as the SES level improves. Thus again, men seem to be more favorably affected by an improving SES level than are women. These relations are shown in diagrammatic form in Figure 1–3. Although we have described the trends in terms of improving SES levels, the description can be portrayed mutatis mutandis in terms of worsening SES level, i.e., men are affected more severely by worsening SES class than are women. Still another way of describing the effect of SES level on morbidity and mortality is to note that the disparity between the higher SES groups and the lower SES groups is wider for men than for women.

Any explanation for these differentials in the effect of SES level on health must be construed as being conjectural, yet some speculation is warranted. As noted early in this chapter, the debate over nature versus nurture is far from settled. The general social and economic conditions of women have changed in recent decades, but the specific aspects that would alter their health risks relative to men have not been documented. Changes in health-related behaviors or in

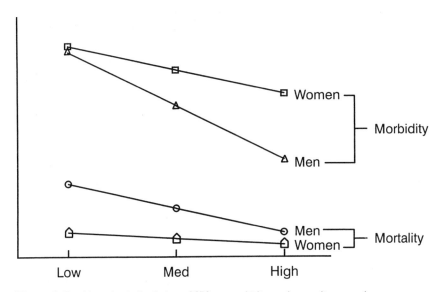

Figure 1–3. Hypothetical relation of SES to morbidity and mortality rates, by sex

physiologic characteristics according to SES level among women have not been well documented. One possible explanation is that women's risks may be dominated by endogenous factors, such as hormonal make-up or other physiologic factors that might be relatively insensitive to SES factors, whereas among men, exogenous factors, such as smoking, exercise, and nutrition, which vary considerably by SES level, are dominant risk factors. A somewhat different explanation is based on the observation often mentioned in the popular and research literature that not only do women have educational and job levels that are not equivalent to those of men, but even within presumably equivalent situations, women do not accrue the same benefits as men. That is, they do not acquire the same job opportunities as men, do not receive equivalent salaries and/or equivalent job control (i.e., decision-making power) for equivalent work, do not experience the same job mobility, job stress, or promotion potential as their male peers, and do not receive the comparable respect and recognition from their peers. Furthermore, women do not shed other responsibilities with increasing affluence to the extent that their male counterparts accomplish, i.e., they still maintain most of the childbearing, child-rearing, and household maintenance responsibilities which are not distributed equally among men and women, regardless of outside occupation. These exogenous factors may explain the smaller impact of increasing affluence on women's mortality than that on men. Conversely, at the other end of the SES spectrum, most social welfare programs shield women from the extremes of poverty to a greater extent than men. This combination could explain the smaller discrepancies in the impact of SES for women than for men.

A major methodological issue that has been raised in the international literature is that many socioeconomic factors as defined in this chapter were chosen precisely because of their ability to explicate relations between men's health and economic status. A different set of factors (as yet undefined) may prove to be more discriminating among women and have better correlation with health behaviors and health status indicators. As stated at the beginning of this chapter, although there are real physiological and psychological differences between the sexes, and differences in cognitive abilities, play styles, and moral reasoning, the differences are manipulated by different cultures into very divergent sets of implications for behavior, social class, and civil and legal rights. These are both covertly and overtly involved in role training and rewards, in the formation and maintenance of social ties, in productive activities at home and elsewhere, and in encounters with health risks and their outcomes.[9]

REFERENCES

1. Krieger N, Fee E. Man-made medicine and women's health: the biopolitics of sex/gender and race/ethnicity. In: Krieger N, Fee E, eds. Womens Health, Politics, and

Power: Essays on Sex/Gender, Medicine, and Public Health. Amityville, NY: Baywood Publishing Co, 1994, pp. 11–29.

2. Gould SJ. The Mismeasure of Man. New York: W.W. Norton, 1981.

3. Haller JS, Haller RM. The Physician and Sexuality in Victorian America. Urbana, IL: University of Illinois Press, 1974.

4. Apple RD, ed. Women, Health, and Medicine in America: A Historical Handbook. New Brunswick, NJ: Rutgers University Press, 1990.

5. Oudshoorn N. Endocrinologists and the conceptualization of sex. J Hist Biol 1990;23:163–187.

6. Brush S, Nettie M. Stevens and the discovery of sex determination by chromosomes. Isis 1978;69:163–172.

7. Long DL. Biology, sex hormones and sexism in the 1920s. Philos Forum 1974;5:81–96.

8. Fee E, Acheson RM, eds. A History of Education in Public Health: Health that Mocks the Doctors' Rules. New York: Oxford University Press, 1991.

9. Verbrugge LM. Gender, aging, and health. In: Markides KS, ed. Aging and Health: Perspectives on Gender, Race, Ethnicity, and Class. Newbury Park, CA: Sage Publications, 1989, pp. 23–78.

10. Ember CR. A cross-cultural perspective on sex differences. In: Munroe RH, Munroe RL, Whiting BB, eds. Handbook of Cross-Cultural Development. New York: Garland STPM Press, 1981, pp. 531–580.

11. Giele JZ. Gender and sex roles. In: Smelser NJ, ed. Handbook of Sociology. Newbury Park, CA: Sage Publications, 1988, pp. 292–323.

12. Lillie-Blanton M, Martinez RM, Taylor AK, Robinson BG. Latina and African American women: continuing disparities in health. In: Krieger N, Fee E eds. Women's Health, Politics, and Power: Essays on Sex/Gender, Medicine, and Public Health. Amityville, NY: Baywood Publishing Co, 1994, pp. 31–59.

13. Susser M, Watson W, Hopper K, et al. Theories and indices of social class. In: Sociology in Medicine. New York: Oxford University Press, 1985, pp. 188–212.

14. Turner JH, Beeghley L. The Emergence of Sociological Theory. Homewood, IL: The Dorsey Press, 1981, pp. 170–190.

15. Turner JH, Beeghley L. The Emergence of Sociological Theory. Homewood, IL: The Dorsey Press, 1981, pp. 247–259.

16. Williams DR. Socioeconomic differentials in health: a review and redirection. Soc Psychol Q 1990;53:81–99.

17. Abramson JH, Gofin R, Habib J, Pridan H, Gofin J. Indicators of social class. A comparative appraisal of measures for use in epidemiologic studies. Soc Sci Med 1982;16:1739–1746.

18. Liberatos P, Link BG, Kelsey JL. The measurement of social class in epidemiology. Epidemiol Rev 1988;10:87–121.

19. Miller DC. Handbook of Research Design and Social Measurement, 5th ed. Newbury Park, CA: Sage Publications, 1991.

20. Marmot MG. Social/economic status and disease. Annu Rev Public Health 1987;8:111–134.

21. Feinstein JS. The relationship between socioeconomic status and health: a review of the literature. Milbank Q 1993;71(2):279–322.

22. Adler NE, Boyce WT, Chesney MA, Folkman S, Syme SL. Socioeconomic inequalities in health. No easy solution. JAMA 1993;269:3140–3145.

23. Collins JG, LeClere FB. Health and selected socioeconomic characteristics of the family: United States, 1988–1990. National Center for Health Statistics. Vital Health Stat 1996;10(195).

24. Rogot E, Sorlie PD, Johnson NJ, Schmitt C. A Mortality Study of 1.3 Million Persons by Demographic, Social, and Economic Factors: 1979–1985 Follow-up. Bethesda, MD: National Institutes of Health, 1992, NIH 92-3297.

25. National Center for Health Statistics. Health United States 1995. Hyattsville, MD: Public Health Service, 1996, DHHS #96-1232.

26. Kitagawa M, Hauser M. Differential Mortality in the United States: a Study in Socioeconomic Epidemiology. Cambridge, MA: Harvard University Press, 1973.

27. Feldman JJ, Makuc DM, Kleinman JC, Cornoni-Huntley J. National trends in education differentials in mortality. Am J Epidemiol 1989;128:919–933.

28. Feldman JJ, Makuc DM. Socioeconomic factors in ischemic heart disease morbidity and mortality. Report of the Conference on Socioeconomic Status and Cardiovascular Health and Disease. Bethesda, MD: National Heart, Lung, and Blood Institute, 1995, pp. 27–33.

29. Sorlie PD, Backlund E, Keller JB. U.S. mortality by economic, demographic, and social characteristics: The National Longitudinal Mortality Study. Am J Public Health 1995;85:949–956.

30. Hayward RA, Shapiro MF, Freeman HE, Corey CR. Who gets screened for cervical and breast cancer? Results from a new national survey. Arch Intern Med 1988;148:1177–1181.

31. Brook RH, Ware JE Jr, Rogers WH, et al. Does free care improve adults' health? New Engl J Med 1983;309(23):1426–1434.

32. Rask KJ, Williams MV, Parker RM, McNagny SE. Obstacles predicting lack of a regular provider and delays in seeking care for patients at an urban public hospital. JAMA 1994;271(24):1931–1933.

33. Hafner-Eaton C. Physician utilization disparities between the uninsured and insured: comparisons of the chronically ill, acutely ill, and well nonelderly populations. JAMA 1993;269(6):787–792.

34. Kelsh MA, Sahl JD. Sex differences in work-related injury rates among electric utility workers. Am J Epidemiol 1996;143:1050–1058.

35. McLoone P, Boddy FA. Deprivation and mortality in Scotland, 1981 and 1991. Br Med J 1994;309:1465–1470.

36. Reijneveld SA. Causes of death contributing to urban socioeconomic mortality differences in Amsterdam. Int J Epidemiol 1995;24(4):740–749.

37. Borrell C, Arias A. Socioeconomic factors and mortality in urban settings: the case of Barcelona, Spain. J Epidemiol Community Health 1995;49:460–465.

2

GENDER DIFFERENCES IN RESPONSE TO DRUGS AND ENVIRONMENTAL TOXICANTS

Donald R. Mattison

The role of gender differences in the disposition of, and response to drugs (pharmacokinetics and pharmacodynamics) and environmental toxicants (toxicokinetics and toxicodynamics) is in some dispute. Indeed, there is little in contemporary textbooks of toxicology or environmental or occupational medicine to alert readers to the potential importance of gender differences. Regarding the influence of gender on pharmacokinetics, some argue that there are few gender-related differences[1-3] while others suggest that women have been underrepresented in clinical trials[4,5] and as a consequence we don't fully understand the extent of gender differences. In fact, women appear to have a higher frequency of adverse reactions to drugs, suggesting significant gender differences in disposition and dynamics.[6] Recently, Calabrese[7-9] suggested that gender differences in several toxicokinetic factors could be observed in humans and Fletcher et al.[10] have made similar observations about some drugs.

Women are assuming an increasing role in the workforce outside the home and now account for 46% of those employed.[11] The comparative distribution of women among different employment sectors is shown in Table 2–1.[12] The similarities and differences between men and women raise concerns about our lack of knowledge of occupational hazards among women. The organizers of a National Cancer Institute conference on this problem stated that ". . . inclusion of women is an important but typically overlooked component in occupational cancer research. . . ." They suggested that this could be remedied if ". . . studies of occupational cancer among women . . . [were] conducted with sophisticated exposure assessment methods that are . . . used in studies of men."[11]

Table 2–1. Proportion of Working Men and Women Employed
Within Major Employment Sectors in the United States

EMPLOYMENT SECTOR	PERCENT OF WORKING MEN	PERCENT OF WORKING WOMEN
Service	24	48
Public administration	5	4
Agriculture	4	1
Construction	10	1
Mining	1	0
Manufacturing	21	12
Transportation, communication, and public utilities	10	4
Wholesale and retail trade	20	21
Finance, insurance, and real estate	5	9

[Modified and reproduced from Stellman, 1994, derived from the U.S. Department of Labor survey of employment and earnings, pages 814–825, 1992[12]]

Men and women have many basic biologic similarities, such as the nature of DNA and the control of gene expression. From this vantage point, a chapter on the differences between men and women makes little sense. Although men, on average, have a larger body size and there is a strong relationship between body size and various anatomic, physiologic, metabolic, pharmacokinetic parameters, we can readily adjust studies for body size. From this perspective, differences between men and women are likely to be similar to those observed among men or among women—they are simply population differences. Despite their obvious similarities, however, men and women have major differences, (see, for example, Table 2–2) and it is important to try to understand when these are biologically relevant and when they are not.[13,14]

A growing body of data demonstrates biological differences between males and females in both humans and experimental animals.[7,8] One common example is that there are substantial gender differences between male and female experimental animals in response to some toxicants and toxins.[7–9] Interestingly, these gender differences are not consistent across species. For example, among some species the males are most sensitive to toxicants while among others the females are most sensitive. How do these differences arise in experimental animals? What do gender differences in the response of experimental animals mean with respect to identifying gender differences in humans? Do these gender differences represent body size differences, interindividual variation, or are they biologically important differences that require attention in public health, medicine, and policy?[5,6]

This chapter evaluates potential gender differences related to environmental and occupational toxicants. It has been divided into sections to explore gen-

Table 2–2. Pharmacokinetic, Toxicokinetic, and Toxic Factors
and Similarities and/or Differences Between Men and Women

COMPOUND	DIFFERENCE
Aflatoxin	Liver cancer: M > F (2.5- to 5-fold)
Benzene	$T_{1/2}$: F > M
Lead	Hematological changes (FEP, ALA): F > M
Lithium	Thyroid toxicity: F > M (5-fold)
Lorazepam	$T_{1/2}$ M > F (1.3-fold)
Nortriptyline	Plasma: F > M (1.3-fold)
Oxazepam	$T_{1/2}$: F > M (1.3-fold)
Propoxyphine	V_d: M > F: (0.2-fold)
Rifampicin	Rate of absorption: F > M (1.1-fold)
Cigarette smoke	Lung cancer: F > M (after adjusting for cumulative dose)
Testosterone	Metabolism: F > M
Trichloroethylene	Acid metabolite: F > M
	Alcohol metabolite: M > F

[Reprinted from British Journal of Industrial Medicine, Calabrese, pages 577–579, 1985, 1986, 1996[7–9]]

der differences in environment (i.e., exposure), host (i.e., pharmacokinetics and toxicokinetics), and response.

ENVIRONMENT

To some extent, men and women inhabit different environments (Table 2–3).[15,16] To help measure these differences, the index of sexual dimorphism (ISD) is used, which is defined as the ratio of male to female mean value for a parameter of interest. Women are at home more than men (119 vs. 103 hr, ISD = 0.87), whereas men spend more time away from home (52 vs. 38 hr, ISD = 1.37) and traveling (12 vs. 10 hr, ISD = 1.20). Men spend more time in job-related activities than women, while women spend more time in house, yard, child-care, services, and shopping-related activities. Time spent in other activities, such as social interactions, entertainment, and leisure, is similar.

In the work environment, employment of men and women varies between different sectors (Table 2–1).[12] Women are more likely to be employed in the service, finance, insurance, and real-estate sectors, and less likely to be employed in agricultural, construction, mining, and manufacturing sectors.

Among women who work in the chemical industries there is a paucity of data concerning exposures to toxic substances. Recently, Stewart and Blair[17] evaluated relative exposures to formaldehyde among men and women working in industries that produce or use formaldehyde. In these industries, male exposures, on their first jobs, were about 20% greater than those of women. However, by their last jobs the exposure differential was reduced to 8%. In jobs with

Table 2–3.   Time and Activity Patterns of Men and Women in the United States

ACTIVITY	HOURS PER WEEK		ISD (M:F)
	MEN	WOMEN	
Job related	35.8	18.0	1.99
House/yard	8.5	20.0	0.43
Child care	1.2	3.9	0.31
Services/shopping	3.9	6.3	0.62
Personal care (sleep)	77.3	79.0	0.98
Education	2.3	1.1	2.09
Organizations	2.5	3.2	0.78
Social/entertainment	8.0	8.9	0.90
Active leisure	5.9	5.2	1.13
Passive leisure	22.8	22.7	1.00
Total	168.2	168.3	1.00
Time spent at home	103	119	0.87
Time spent away from home	52	38	1.37
Time spent traveling	12	10	1.20

[Modified and reproduced from the U.S. EPA, Exposure Factors Handbook, August 1996[15] and American Industrial Health Council Exposure Factor Source Book, May 1994[16]]

the highest exposure to formaldehyde, the exposure for men was about 15% higher than for women. To the extent that these data can be generalized to other work settings, they suggest that when women and men work in the same environment, their experience concerning exposures may be quite different.

While there appear to be fewer women working in agriculture, many women are exposed to pesticides through subsistence farming or gardening. The pesticides used in agricultural and domestic settings are designed to be toxic to a range of species—and consequently are frequently human toxicants as well. In a study conducted by the U.S. EPA, the ratio of adipose tissue concentrations in males versus females for a group of organochlorine pesticides and their metabolites in human males and females ranged from 0.91 to 1.33. This suggests that chronic environmental exposures are similar for men and women.[18]

Environmental exposures may not be totally congruent for men and women, however, and this may lead to differences in skin responses to contact allergens.[19–23] Women are seen more frequently with complaints of contact dermatitis and are more likely to have positive patch tests.[20,22] The responses to many of these test agents are related to exposures that may be more common among women than men. When tested with an agent to which they were naive (dinitrochlorobenzene) women had a more intense response (greater skin thickness and steeper slope on the dose–response curve). In contrast, response to poison ivy (contacted with equal frequency) is similar among women and men.[23]

Other potential differences in exposures may result from gender differences in dietary intake. For example, fluid intake is described by a lognormal distribution with substantial overlap between men and women older than 18 (Fig. 2–1).[15,16] Among men, mean total fluid intakes range from 1.8 to 2.2 liters/day, whereas among women, fluid intake ranges from 1.5 to 1.6 liters/day. The total fluid intake among women between the ages of 15 and 49 varies with pregnancy and lactation. The greatest fluid consumption is among women who are lactating. These differences in fluid consumption may be important in predicting risk from chemical or biological hazards in drinking water.

Food consumption patterns also vary by gender and ethnicity (Table 2–4).[15,16,24] Based on the total population, women eat more fruit but less fish and vegetables than men (ISD = 0.95, 1.27, 1.25, respectively). Meat, dairy, and

DIFFERENCES IN EXPOSURE

Dietary Patterns

Total Liquid Intake in Adults 18 - 55 +

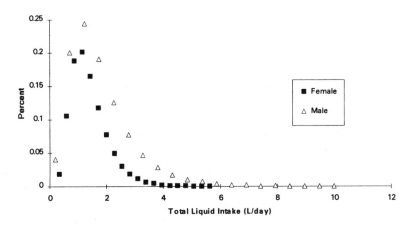

Total liquid intake (L/day)									
	Male				**Female**				
Age	Mean	SD	10%	90%	Mean	SD		10%	90%
18 - 30	2.18	1.26	1.12	3.49	1.54	0.73		0.93	2.3
31 - 54	2.11	1.19	1.15	3.27	1.6	0.5		0.95	2.36
55+	1.83	0.99	1.03	2.77	1.48	0.76		0.84	2.17
18 - 55	2.04	1.14			1.55	0.67			

Figure 2–1. Fluid ingestion in the United States [Reprinted from U.S. EPA Exposure Factors Handbook, August 1996[15] and AIHC Exposure Factors Source Book, May 1994[16]]

Table 2–4. Food Consumption by Gender and Pregnancy Status

FOOD GENDER AND AGE	PER CAPITA[a] (GM/DAY)	PERCENT CONSUMING IN 1 DAY	INTAKE AMONG EATERS (GM/DAY)
Fruit			
Male 20+	133.00	46.50	286.00
Female 20+	140.00	52.70	266.00
ISD (M:F)	0.95	0.88	1.08
Vegetables			
Males 20+	232.00	85.00	273.00
Females 20+	183.00	82.90	221.00
ISD (M:F)	1.27	1.03	1.24
Fish			
Male 20+	15.00	10.90	138.00
Female 20+	12.00	10.90	110.00
ISD (M:F)	1.25	1.00	1.25

Mean Number of Local Fish Meals Consumed per Year

	ALL RESPONDENTS			CONSUMERS ONLY		
	PREGNANCY	< 1 YEAR	> 1 YEAR	PREGNANCY	< 1 YEAR	> 1 YEAR
Mohawk	3.9	9.2	23.4	4.6	10.9	27.6
Anglo	7.3	10.7	10.9	15.5	23.0	23.0

[a]Per capita intake is calculated for total population including those who do not consume the food.
[Reprinted from Fitzgerald et al., 1995,[24] U.S. EPA, Exposure Factors Handbook, August 1996[15] and American Industrial Health Council Exposure Factors Source Book, May 1994[16]]

grain consumption is, in general, greater among males. Consumption of fish is especially interesting because one source of this food is subsistence fishing. In general, indigenous populations are most likely to consume fish in the United States, and much of this fish is obtained by subsistence fishing. For example, Mohawk women in upstate New York consume about 30 meals of fish each year (note the difference between consumers and all surveyed). Unfortunately, the waters from which these fish are harvested are contaminated with polychlorinated biphenyls. The resultant fish advisories, warning pregnant and lactating women to stop or substantially decrease their consumption of these fish, led to a general reduction in fish consumption by Mohawk women of reproductive age.

HOST

The data reviewed in the section on gender differences in environmental exposures suggest the need to explore more explicitly the role of gender in disease.

An analysis of host factors will further strengthen that assertion. One of the obvious ways that men and women differ is in anatomical and physiological parameters (Table 2–5).[25,26] Important differences include body weight, body composition, surface area, blood volumes, organ and tissue volumes, metabolism, cardiovascular, pulmonary, and gastrointestinal and renal structure and function.[16,27] While men differ among themselves, on average they also differ from women, weighing more, being taller, and having a larger surface area.[28,29]

Other physical factors that differ between men and women include joint motion,[30] skeletal sizes,[31,32] optic sizes,[33] resting metabolic rate,[34] and brain anatomy and function.[35] Body composition also differs between men and women. Women have more adipose tissue than men (32% vs. 21%), less skeletal muscle (29% vs. 40% of body weight), and lower skin weight (3.1% vs. 3.7%).[27]

Total body water is approximately 40% more in men than in nonpregnant women, although during pregnancy there is an increase in maternal body water (29 to 33 liters). Similarly, extracellular and intracellular water volumes are smallest in nonpregnant women, larger in pregnant women, but smaller than those observed in men. Pulmonary function also differs between men and women. Pregnant women have the largest per-minute volume of air and as a result, the greatest volume of air exchanged in an 8-hour period.

Anatomical, physiological, and toxicokinetic characteristics of men and nonpregnant and pregnant women are compared in this chapter, where data allow. The following section explores absorption, distribution, metabolism, and elimination.

Table 2–5. Anatomic and Physiologic Parameters for Men and Nonpregnant and Pregnant Women

PARAMETER	REFERENCE ADULT MALE	REFERENCE ADULT FEMALE	ISD (M:F)	PREGNANT FEMALE	ISD (M:PF)
Body weight (kg)	70	58	1.21	62.5	1.12
Body length (cm)	170	160	1.06	160	1.06
Body surface area (cm²)	18,000	16,000	1.13	16,500	1.09
Total body water (L)	42.0	29.0	1.45	33.0	1.27
Extracellular water (L)	18.2	11.6	1.57	15.0	1.21
Intracellular water (L)	23.8	17.4	1.37	18.8	1.27
Minute volume (L/min)	7.5	6.0	1.25	10.5	0.71
Respiratory rate (breaths/min)	15	15	1.00	16	0.94
Volume of air exchanged in 8 hr (L)	3600	2900	1.24	5000	0.72

[Fundamental and Applied Toxicology, Mattison et al., pages 215–218, 1991[27]]

Absorption

Absorption is the process by which chemicals or drugs cross body surfaces, such as the gastrointestinal, respiratory, or skin surfaces, and enter the bloodstream. Table 2–6[26] summarizes processes important for absorption, and differences between men and women. Examples of gender differences in absorption include rifampicin (women absorb the drug more efficiently),[7,8,10] benzylamine (following transdermal absorption women excrete three times more than men), and intramuscular (IM) cephradine (which has a slower rate of absorption and lower bioavailability in women).

For some exposures the rate and extent of transdermal absorption are important determinants of systemic effects.[36] As the epidermal surface area exposed to the chemical increases, the amount transferred per unit time increases. Since the total body surface area is, on average, greater for males, transdermal absorption may also be greater[37] (Fig. 2–2).[15,16] As the thickness of the epithelial surface decreases, the rate of transport increases. Differences in the thickness of the epidermis, in particular, the stratum corneum, may therefore affect transdermal absorption. Depending on the location, there are variations in epidermal thickness between males and females. For example, in the arms and fingers, the epidermis is slightly thicker in males,[38] which may decrease transdermal absorption in the workplace.

Increasing the hydration state of the stratum corneum increases transdermal absorption of many polar molecules. While gender-specific differences in the hydration state of the epidermis have not been investigated, inferences may be made from data on the extracellular and intracellular body water content in males and females. Total body water, intracellular body water, and extracellular body water are greater in pregnant than nonpregnant women, and even greater

Table 2–6. Physiological Parameters that Influence Absorption

PARAMETER	PHYSIOLOGIC DIFFERENCE	TOXICOKINETIC IMPACT
Gastric juice pH	Acidity M > F > pregnant F	Altered absorption of acid/bases
Gastric juice flow	M > F	Change in absorption
Intestinal motility	M > F > pregnant F	Absorption increased
Gastric emptying	M > F > pregnant F	Absorption, gastric metabolism increased
Dermal hydration	Increased in pregnant F	Altered absorption in pregnant F
Dermal thickness	M > F	Absorption decreased
Body surface area	M > pregnant F > F	Absorption increased
Skin blood flow	Increased in pregnant F	Absorption increased
Pulmonary function	M > pregnant F > F	Pulmonary exposure increased
Cardiac output	M > pregnant F > F	Absorption increased

[Reprinted from Fundamental and Applied Toxicology, Mattison et al., pages 215–218, 1991[27] and Silvaggio and Mattison, pages 825–834, 1992[50]]

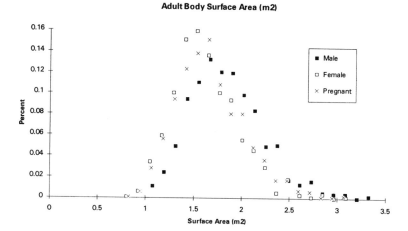

ADULT BODY PARAMETERS

	Min	**5%**	**15%**	**50%**	**85%**	**95%**	**Max**
Body Surface Area (m²)							
M	1.5	1.66	1.76	*1.94*	2.14	2.28	2.3
F	1.4	1.45	1.53	*1.69*	1.91	2.09	2.1

Figure 2–2. Total body surface area available for transdermal absorption [Reprinted from U.S. EPA Exposure Factors Handbook, August 1996[15] and AIHC Exposure Factors Source Book, May 1994[16]]

in males.[39] Pregnant women may thus have increased transdermal absorption of certain toxicants, compared with nonpregnant women, based on the hydration state of the stratum corneum.

Blood flow to the skin may also affect transdermal absorption of toxicants. According to Williams and Leggett,[40] the percentage of cardiac output to the skin (5%) and blood perfusion rates (120 ml/kg/min) do not differ between males and females. However, there are changes in blood flow to different regions of the skin during pregnancy. While there are only small increases in blood flow to the forearm and leg during pregnancy, blood flow to the hand increases approximately sixfold, and blood flow to the foot doubles.[41] These alterations in dermal blood flow during pregnancy may have a significant impact on transdermal absorption of xenobiotics.

Pulmonary volumes and respiratory rates are important toxicokinetic parameters, especially when the route of exposure is via inhalation (Table 2–7).[26,39] In addition, absorption, metabolism, and excretion may all be related to pulmonary function. Gender differences in pulmonary function can alter the toxicoki-

Table 2–7. Pulmonary Parameters per Adult Men and Women

	TOTAL LUNG CAPACITY (L)	FUNCTIONAL RESIDUAL CAPACITY (L)	VENTILATORY CAPACITY (L)	VOLUME OF DISTRIBUTION (ML)	TOTAL VOLUME (ML/BREATH)	VOLUME (L/MIN)	REGULAR RESPIRATION BREATHS (MIN)	VOLUME/8 HR REST (L)
Men	5.6	3.1	4.3	160	750	7.5	15	3600
Nonpregnant women	5.0	2.8	3.3	130	487	6.0	15	2900
ISD (M:W)	1.12	1.11	1.30	1.23	1.54	1.25	1.00	1.24
Pregnant women	4.7	2.3	3.3	—	678	10.5	16	5000
ISD (M:Pregnant F)	1.19	1.35	1.30	—	1.11	0.71	0.94	0.72

[Reprinted from Drug and Chemical Action in Pregnancy, Mattison, pages 37–102, 1986,[26] and Silvaggio and Mattison, pages 25–36, 1992[48]]

netics of certain chemicals. Lung volumes correlate with total body weight and surface area; therefore, one would expect higher volumes in men. On average, total lung capacity, functional residual capacity, vital capacity, and dead space are all higher in men than women. However, if we calculate vital capacity (and the lower 10% and upper 90% bounds) for 18-year-old men and women, then the mean vital capacities are 4469 (4260 to 4672) mL and 4162 (4003 to 4339) mL, suggesting considerable overlap.

Pulmonary function changes during pregnancy. Although the respiratory rate is unaltered, the tidal volume is increased by 39%. Increases in minute ventilation parallel increases in tidal volume. As a result, the amount of inhaled toxicants may be significantly greater during pregnancy. During an 8-hour exposure, the largest pulmonary dose would be delivered to the pregnant woman. The increases in tidal and minute volumes also suggest an increase in pulmonary distribution and alveolar mixing of gases, lessening the time to reach alveolar steady state. Gas transfer, however, appears to be decreased because of interstitial changes in the lungs during pregnancy. For example, the pulmonary diffusion capacity of carbon monoxide is reduced from 26.5 to 22.5/min/mm Hg.[42]

Pulmonary function increases with exertion (Table 2–8),[15] probably in response to increasing CO_2.[43] This ventilatory response to increasing carbon dioxide differs by gender. Women in general have a shallower ventilatory response to hypercapnia than men (ISD ~1.3). Genetic and body size effects on the ventilatory response to carbon dioxide are less clearly defined. It is clear, however, that progesterone modulates the sensitivity to increasing CO_2, with lowest resting Pa_{CO2} seen during the luteal phase. Men treated with progesterone also demonstrate increased sensitivity to CO_2. This suggests that the ventilatory response to exertion will be shallower in women than men, increasing toward the male values during the luteal phases of the menstrual cycle.

Cardiac output and regional distribution of blood flow are two important parameters that affect toxicokinetics, especially absorption. Williams and Leggett[40] have proposed reference values for resting blood flow to organs and

Table 2–8. Minute Ventilation Means (Ranges) by Gender and Activity Level

SUBJECT	WT (KG)	VENTILATION (L/MIN)			
		RESTING	LIGHT	MODERATE	HEAVY
Male[a]	70.0	5	20	35	90
		(2.3–18.8)	(2.3–27.6)	(14.4–78.0)	(34.6–183.4)
Nonpregnant female	65.4	5	14	20	70
		(4.2–11.66)	(4.2–29.4)	(20.7–34.2)	(23.4–114.8)

[Reprinted from U.S. EPA, Exposure Factors Handbook, pages 3–14, 1989[41a]]

tissues for typical 35-year-old males and females. There are significant differences in resting blood flow as a percentage of cardiac output to skeletal muscle (greater for men) and adipose tissue (greater for women). These may reflect gender-based differences in the percentage of total body mass represented by each tissue.[40]

Cardiac output increases approximately 50% during pregnancy.[41] This occurs via an increase in both stroke volume and heart rate. The increase in cardiac output occurs by the end of the first trimester and remains elevated over the remainder of pregnancy. Blood flow to the skin and kidney is also increased, and there are no significant changes "reported" in cerebral or hepatic blood flows. During pregnancy the increased cardiac output is distributed to the uterus (increase in uterine blood flow is 150 ml/kg/min at term).[44,45] This value is comparable to uterine blood flows determined in experimental animals. Renal blood flow is increased by approximately 50% very early in pregnancy, and blood flow to the skin and kidney is also increased. No significant changes are reported in cerebral or hepatic blood flows, however, there is a paucity of information regarding regional blood flow changes during pregnancy.[46]

Cardiac output (CO) and regional distribution of flow are important for toxicokinetics. Because cardiac output is related to body size, it is best normalized to surface area. As such, men and women have similar mean cardiac indices of 3.5 L/min/m². Cardiac output is commonly standardized and reported as the cardiac index (CI):

$$CI = \frac{CO \ (L/min)}{BSA(m^2)}$$

where BSA is the body surface area. When standardized for BSA, CI is nearly identical for both sexes from ages 18 to 44.[27] Among men and women the distribution of CO, or regional blood flow, differs for some body sites. Distribution of CO is similar for men and women for some organs (adrenal 0.3% CO, bone 5% CO, brain 12% CO, lung 2.5% CO, skin 5% CO, and thyroid 1.5% CO) and different for others (adipose M = 5% CO, F = 8.5% CO; heart M = 4% CO, F = 5% CO; kidney M = 19% CO, F = 17% CO; liver M = 25% CO, F = 27% CO; and muscle M = 17% CO, F = 12% CO). Note, for example, that blood flow to skeletal muscle is greater for men, and flow to adipose tissue is greater for women, reflecting the gender-based differences in body composition.[27]

Absorption occurs at different sites along the gastrointestinal tract, including the stomach, the small intestine, and the large intestine. The rate of absorption is influenced by multiple factors including gut transit times, lipid solubility of the agent, pH at the site of absorption, and ionization and molecular weight of the agent. Gut mobility, and as a consequence, transit times are different in men and women.[47] Mean transit times are shorter in men (44.8 hr vs. 91.7 hr in women). As fiber ingested increases, the transit time decreases, but female gut transit times are consistently longer. Gastric fluid differs between men and women in several ways. Gastric juice is more acidic in males than females (pH ≈ 1.92 vs. 2.59). Basal and maximal flow of gastric juice and acid secretion is also higher in men than in women. During pregnancy, gastric acid secretion is further reduced by 30%. This decline in gastric secretion increases the pH of the gastrointestinal tract, resulting in decreased absorption of weak acids and increased absorption of weak bases.

Iron and ethanol have significant differences across gender in gastrointestinal absorption. In experiments measuring incorporation of iron into red blood cells by pre-adolescent males and females, tracer doses of iron were administered. In these experiments, 45% of the ingested iron was incorporated into erythrocytes by females, compared with 35% among males (ISD ≈ 0.78). While there are several pharmacokinetic factors that separate males from females in the disposition of ethanol, one is related to absorption. Ethanol ingested by men is metabolized more rapidly in the gut. As a result, less ethanol is available for absorption.

Distribution

Distribution is the process by which a xenobiotic is translocated from sites of absorption or metabolism to tissues and organs throughout the body. The total amount of chemical in the body is the *body burden*, and the apparent volume of distribution is integral to determining the body burden of a xenobiotic. Body composition parameters are especially important in regard to volume of distribution (Table 2–9).[26,39,48] Gender- and gestation-specific differences in these parameters may account for differences in the concentration of a xenobiotic at the target site and result in varying responses.

Table 2–9.   Body Composition Parameters that Influence Distribution

PARAMETER	PHYSIOLOGIC DIFFERENCE	TOXICOKINETIC IMPACT
Plasma volume	Pregnant F > M > F	Decreased concentration
Total body water	M > pregnant F > F	Decreased concentration
Plasma proteins	M, F > pregnant F	Concentration ±
Body fat	Pregnant F > F > M	Increased body burden of lipid-soluble xenobiotics
Cardiac output	M > pregnant F > F	Increased rate of distribution

[Reprinted from Mattison, pages 37–102, 1986,[26] Silvaggio and Mattison, pages 25–36, 1992,[48] 1994[39]]

On average, total body water, extracellular water, intracellular water, total blood volume, plasma volume, and red blood cell volume are greater for men than nonpregnant women. Therefore, if an average male and an average female are exposed to the same dose of a water-soluble xenobiotic, the greater total body water, extracellular water, intracellular water, and plasma volume will increase the volume of distribution and thus decrease the concentration of the xenobiotic in the male. As noted previously, however, there is important variation in height and weight among men and women and these result in considerable overlap. For example, consider the pharmacokinetic data for ethanol (Table 2–10).[10] These data illustrate the smaller volume of distribution for ethanol in women than men, producing higher peak concentrations from the same dose.

During pregnancy, changes in body weight, plasma proteins, plasma volume, extracellular fluid volume, total body water, and body fat may alter xenobiotic distribution.[25,26,36,49] Maternal weight increases from 50 kg at the start of pregnancy to approximately 63 kg at 40 weeks of pregnancy. Total body water increases from 25 liters to 33 liters over the course of pregnancy but remains less than the adult reference male (42 liters). Maternal extracellular fluid volume increases from 11 to 15 liters over the pregnancy, compared to 18.2 liters in the adult reference male. In contrast, plasma volume increases from 2.5 liters to 3.8 liters in the pregnant female at term, which is greater than the 3 liters in the adult reference male. These volume measurements in the pregnant female exceed all nonpregnant female values and also exceed total blood, plasma, and red blood cell volume for the adult male. These differences may be important, especially for xenobiotics distributed into plasma.

In many toxicokinetic models, maternal volume of distribution increases continuously during gestation; however, it does not increase for all xenobiotics. At times, it is inferred that an increase in volume of distribution has occurred because of a decrease in plasma concentration. However, other factors such as an increase in the rate of elimination, a decrease in a binding protein, or a decrease in the rate of absorption may also reduce serum concentrations. Decreases in plasma-binding proteins, such as albumin, may increase the amount of free xenobiotic available for extravascular distribution, delivery to target tissues, and elimination. Total protein and serum albumin concentrations do not significantly differ between males and nonpregnant females.[50] However, total protein content of serum decreases during pregnancy, mainly because of a decrease in albumin.

Body fat composition also affects toxicokinetics. The body can be divided into fat-containing and fat-free tissues. Body fat as a percentage of total body weight is higher in women than men and increases by age in both sexes.[51] The total body fat for an adult reference male is 13.5 kg. Maternal body fat increases by about 25% during pregnancy, from 16.5 kg in the nonpregnant female to 19.8 kg at 40 weeks gestation.[26,52,53] The larger proportions of body fat in women and

Table 2–10. Pharmacokinetic Parameters

DRUG	PHARMACOKINETIC PARAMETER	MALE	FEMALE	COMMENTS
Aspirin	Half-life (min)	20.6	16.2	Aspirin is cleared more rapidly from the blood of women than from men, suggesting need for different schedule of administration
Salicylic acid	12-hour urinary recovery of metabolites			Male and female metabolic patterns for salicylic acid are different
	% salicyluric acid	6.53%	18.9%	
	% glucuronidation	43.6%	24.4%	
Theophylline	Half-life (hours)			Half-life of theophylline is shorter in women than in men (either smokers or nonsmokers), suggesting need for different schedule of administration
	Non-smokers	9.3	6.0	
	Smokers	6.9	4.6	
Acebutolol	Area under the concentration–time curve (ng hr/ml)	4861	6410	Concentration–time profile is larger in women than men, suggesting greater therapeutic and potential side-effects
Propranolol	Clearance (ml/min/kg)			Propranolol is cleared more rapidly in men than in women; this is also reflected in the higher clearance of metabolites. Women have greater potential for therapeutic and adverse effects
	Total clearance	65.7	40.2	
	Clearance (glucuronidation)	8.5	5.6	
	Clearance (side-chain oxidation)	12.1	5.1	
Ethanol	Volume of distribution (L/kg)	0.62	0.45	When ethanol is ingested, men metabolize more in first-pass metabolism than women, and volume of distribution is smaller in women than in men. These suggest the potential for greater blood concentrations among women than in men.
	Clearance (mg/hr/kg)	78.6	88.6	
	First-pass metabolism (nmol/L hr)	5.2	1.2	
Iron	Absorption measured as % of dose incorporated into red blood cells	35.2%	45.0%	More ingested iron is absorbed by females than males

[Reprinted from Journal of Adolescent Health, Fletcher et al., pages 619–629, 1994[10]] the increase in body fat during pregnancy may increase the body burden of lipid-soluble, slowly metabolized toxicants, especially during gestation.

Metabolism

Metabolism is a major factor in determining response to xenobiotics (Table 2–11).[26,39,48] Biotransformation occurs predominantly in the liver, but there are also extrahepatic sites of metabolism, such as the lung, kidney, intestinal tract, and skin. Biotransformation can also occur in the placenta and in fetal tissues. Many factors affect the rate of biotransformation of xenobiotics. Factors that affect uptake of xenobiotics by target tissues are also important in metabolism, as the toxicant must reach cellular sites of biotransformation. Thus, lipid solubility, protein binding, dose, and route of exposure all affect the rate of biotransformation. In addition, individuals show large variation in metabolism of xenobiotics. However, when pharmacokinetic parameters are evaluated for most drugs, correcting for height, weight, surface area, and body composition eliminates most gender-dependent differences. In humans, gender-dependent differences in biotransformation have been observed for a few specific xenobiotics, such as nicotine, chlordiazepoxide, flurazepam, acetylsalicylic acid, and heparin.[54]

Metabolism of chemicals may be estimated by basal metabolic rates. For all ages, on average, men have a higher basal metabolic rate than women. This rate incorporates a number of cellular functions from different cell types. Since the metabolism of adipose tissue differs from that of muscle tissue, some of the differences between men and women are attributed to body composition.[55] Cunningham[56] reviewed multiple studies and concluded that the lower basal meta-

Table 2–11. Physiological Parameters that May Influence Differences in Metabolism

PARAMETER	PHYSIOLOGIC DIFFERENCE	TOXICOKINETIC IMPACT
Hepatic	Higher BMR in M ± hepatic metabolism in pregnant F	Increased metabolism
Extrahepatic	Metabolism by fetus/placenta	± metabolism
Plasma proteins	Decreased in pregnant F	± metabolism
Renal blood flow GFR	Pregnant F > M > F	Increased renal elimination
Pulmonary function	M >pregnant F > F	Increased pulmonary elimination
Plasma proteins	Decreased in pregnant F	± elimination

[Reprinted from Mattison, pages 37–102, 1986,[26] Silvaggio and Mattison, pages 25–36, 1992,[48] and Journal of Occupational Medicine, pages 849–854, 1994[39]]

bolic rate per unit body surface area in women reflects the reduction in lean body mass due to a smaller skeletal muscle component. The altered hormonal milieu of pregnancy is associated with changes in hepatic and extrahepatic xenobiotic metabolism.[26,57,58]

Elimination

Xenobiotics are generally eliminated from the body by renal, hepatic, or pulmonary routes.[10] Toxicants may also be excreted via bodily secretions such as sweat, tears, and milk.[59] Renal function is important for elimination. Chemicals can be excreted into the urine through glomerular filtration, passive diffusion, and active secretion. Increases in renal blood flow and glomerular filtration will increase the elimination rate of xenobiotics cleared by the kidneys. When standardized for body surface area, renal blood flow, glomerular filtration, tubular secretion, and tubular reabsorption are all greater in men than nonpregnant women.[48] During gestation, changes in renal blood flow, glomerular filtration rates, hepatic blood flow, bile flow, and pulmonary function may alter maternal elimination of a xenobiotic. Maternal renal plasma flow increases from 500 to 700 ml/min/1.73 m^2, a 1.44-fold increase over the nonpregnant female value and a 1.1-fold increase over the male value. Glomerular filtration also increases during pregnancy. At the beginning of gestation, glomerular filtration is approximately 100 ml/min/1.73 m^2. By 20 weeks' gestation, the glomerular filtration rate has increased to approximately 150 ml/min/1.73 m^2, a 1.5-fold increase over the nonpregnant female value and a 1.2-fold increase over the male value.[60]

Volume of distribution and elimination rates interact to modify the concentration of a toxicant in the maternal organism during gestation. There is a paucity of data regarding the impact of changes in pulmonary and hepatic function on elimination. As a result of the increase in minute volume, the amount of inhaled toxicants significantly increases. These same increases in pulmonary function during pregnancy may also increase pulmonary elimination. However, it is unknown whether these postulated increases in pulmonary elimination are sufficient to override the increase in pulmonary absorption.

RESPONSE

Although reasons for excluding women from clinical trials have included fear of pregnancy and menstrual cycle variations in pharmacokinetics, both appear generally unfounded.[5] Drugs that have clear variations in pharmacokinetics during the menstrual cycle include antipyrine, metaqualone, and theophylline. Those that appear invariant include paracetamol, nitrazepam, salicylate, alprazolam, ethanol, and propranolol.[61]

Having data on gender differences in absorption, distribution, metabolism, and elimination allows exploration of gender differences in disposition and response to chemicals and drugs. Several examples will be reviewed to illustrate the relevance of the data.

Methylprednisolone is eliminated more rapidly in women than men.[62] Women are also more sensitive to cortisol suppression, perhaps because they are more sensitive to the effects of cortisol on basophils and helper T lymphocytes. These data are interesting because the gender differences in pharmacokinetics and pharmacodynamics are not significant, which suggests that men and women should receive the same dose and treatment schedule.

Propranolol is cleared more rapidly from men than women because men have higher rates of clearance of the metabolites produced by both side-chain oxidation and glucuronidation. However, volume of distribution and other metabolic pathways (ring-oxidation) do not differ by gender.[63] The differences between types of oxidation appear to be due to responses in sex hormones. Both side-chain oxidation and glucuronidation are increased by testosterone in men (and perhaps women), whereas ring oxidation is not.[64,65] There appears to be little influence of circulating endogenous hormone levels on propranolol disposition among women, although synthetic hormones (oral contraceptives) appear to alter disposition. There is little gender difference or variation during the menstrual cycle on protein binding of propranolol.[64,65] In contrast, there is a significant decrease in protein binding among women treated with oral contraceptives.

Caffeine is a drug found in a broad variety of foods and beverages and is frequently consumed by adults. Because high concentrations of caffeine produce toxicity (restlessness, anxiety, palpitations, etc.), the dose ingested may be titrated by physical and/or mental status. For example, during pregnancy, there are alterations in both volume of distribution (increasing from 25 to 33 liters) and half-life (increasing from 3.5 to 10.5 hr) of caffeine. As a result, the dose needed during pregnancy to produce the same blood concentration profile falls by more than half.[26] The metabolism of caffeine, which occurs along several pathways, is generally slower in women than men, although it can be stimulated by common habits like cigarette smoking.[66]

Ethanol, a water-soluble chemical, is predominantly distributed into body water.[67] Given that body water volumes are smaller in women than men, it would be expected that peak concentrations would be higher (Tables 2–9, 2–10).[10,26,39,48] However, other pharmacokinetic processes must also be considered.[68,69] For example, both the stomach and liver participate in ethanol metabolism at what appears to be a lower rate in women than men. Following absorption, women appear to clear alcohol from their blood more rapidly than men. It has been suggested that the slower clearance in men is a consequence of higher testosterone levels, as testosterone inhibits alcohol dehydrogenase. Interestingly, the pharmacodynamics of ethanol appear different in men and women, as women are more sensitive to sedation than men.

Arsenic has been demonstrated to produce human lung, bladder, and kidney cancers.[70,71] Because arsenic is found in the drinking water of some communities, and in some instances, in quite high concentrations, it is possible to explore a range of health or biological effects across populations. These population-based studies can illuminate gender differences in response. For example, in a study by Chen and colleagues,[70] residents in 42 villages along the southwestern coast of Taiwan were studied to determine the cancer potency index for lung, liver, bladder, and kidney cancer in men and women. Lung cancer in association with arsenic appears to be independent of gender, although women appear somewhat more likely to develop bladder and kidney cancer than men. The mechanism for this gender difference, if true, remains undefined. Gender differences that may be relevant include greater inhibition of lymphocyte replication in women,[72] similar sensitivity to sister-chromatid exchange,[73] increased micronuclei formation in females exposed to a broad range of pesticides,[74] immunocompetence,[75] and cytogenetic end points.[76]

Another pulmonary toxicant of significant public health concern is ozone (O_3), because of its toxic effects on pulmonary function.[77,78] While some authors have suggested gender differences in decrements of forced expiratory flow and airway resistance (with males exhibiting an increased sensitivity), others have suggested that increased sensitivity is an artifact of tissue surface area calculation within the lung.[77] Pulmonary hyper-responsiveness may also influence response to environmental toxicants.[79]

One agent, or more correctly, complex exposure, associated with human cancer is cigarette smoking. The temporal relationship between onset of smoking and risk of lung cancer is well known. Indeed, as increasing numbers of women have begun to smoke, their risk of lung cancer has also increased. Smoking also decreases fertility and age at menopause.[80] The data on smoking and cancer in men and women may illuminate the relationships among gender, mixture of carcinogenic and toxic agents found in direct and indirect smoking, and risk for disease. Studies that have explored the risk for lung cancer have suggested that women appear to be two to three times more sensitive to cigarette smoke as a risk factor than men, and have demonstrated that postmenopausal estrogen may also increase the risk of lung cancer among smokers. Through an analysis of the sensitivity of lymphocytes to mutagens, some authors[81] suggest that men and women do not appear to differ in risk. Others,[82] however, suggest that an increased sensitivity may be due to differences in p53 mutational spectra and c-erbB-2 expression between men and women. Women with lung cancer are more likely to have GC→TA mutations than men. In addition, women have higher carcinogen adduct formation and more of the tumors

contain c-erbB-2 staining than observed in men. It is not clear if there are gender differences in the expression of the enzymes responsible for activation or
inactivation of these carcinogens.[83]

This two- to threefold difference in the incidence of lung cancer (M >F)
stands in direct contrast to a two- to fivefold difference in sensitivity (F >M)
and suggests that the observed gender difference in the incidence of lung cancer
may represent substantial differences in exposures. For most countries, there is
a two- to tenfold greater incidence of stomach and lung cancers among men
than women. However, when mortality rates for all cancers (ICD 140–239) except lung (ICD 162) and stomach (ICD 151) are compared, there are only slight
excesses in rates among males.[84]

It is interesting to observe that similar enhanced female sensitivity to cigarette smoke and an enhanced interaction with ethanol have also been observed
in association with oral cancers. In this analysis, smoking was characterized by
two different metrics—pack years or cumulative tar. In either case, women were
between one and three times more likely to develop oral cancer than men. The
interaction between smoking and alcohol intake increases the risk more than
fivefold for oral cancers among women. This suggests that women have less
first-pass metabolism of ethanol than men and smaller volume of distributions
(Table 2–10),[10] which act to increase the circulating concentration and consequent biological effect.

ANIMAL DATA

If there are gender differences in diseases among humans, it is also interesting
to explore the gender differences in the spontaneous occurrence of disease
among experimental animals. Unfortunately, there is not a large body of data
tracking the spontaneous occurrence of disease in experimental animals. One
potential data source is the control animals used in various pharmacological
and/or toxicological experiments. Because of federal regulatory interest in identification of chemical carcinogens, the National Toxicology Program (NTP) has
been involved in testing about 140 chemicals for their ability to induce cancers
in mice and rats. The control animals from these experiments represent resources for describing the spontaneous appearance of disease in laboratory animals. Consider, for example, the spontaneous tumor rates in rats and mice at selected sites.[85] Liver cancer occurs more frequently in mice than rats, and within
those rodents, more frequently in males. It is important to point out, however,
that the ISD is greater in rats than mice. Lymphoma/leukemia occurs at the
same rate in female rats and mice but with substantial differences among males.
It is also interesting to note the gender reversal in ISD for lymphoma/leukemia
from rats to mice. Pituitary tumors are much more common in rats and occur

more frequently in females (ISD < 1). Lung tumors are more common in mice and males (ISD > 1). Breast, uterine, and testicular tumors are more common in rats, whereas ovarian tumors are more common in mice. Across these different sites there are clear gender differences in tumor rates, much like the gender differences observed in humans.

Because pesticides are specifically designed for toxicity to biological systems of some sort, it seems reasonable to evaluate the analysis of gender differences in the testing of pesticides. For this analysis, all three volumes of a current reference source on the toxicity of pesticides were reviewed.[86] For ease of comparison, and because the rat was the most frequently used experimental animal for pesticide toxicity testing, information from the acute toxicity experiments conducted to determine the LD_{50} (dose that killed 50% of study animals) in rats was identified and summarized. In general, over the 122 acute toxicity experiments conducted with pesticides in rats, the female LD_{50} was smaller than the male LD_{50} ($P < 0.001$). The mean M:F ratio of LD_{50}s (i.e., the ISD) was 1.4, which suggests that the LD_{50} for females was about 60% of that for males. Note that in these experiments, dosing is typically adjusted for body size and the LD_{50}s are calculated and reported in mg/kg body weight. While this group of chemicals is designed to be toxic, their structures and mode of action are very diverse. Despite the structural and mechanistic diversity of these chemicals, the female rat was generally more sensitive than the male rat to acute toxicity.

CONCLUSION

In this review of gender differences in agents, environments, and host responses, the data discussed do suggest gender differences. Men and women differ in the environments they inhabit, the agents they encounter, and their responses to those agents. We need to explicitly consider gender in clinical trials, studies of occupational exposures and their health effects, and most importantly, in the development of health policy.

REFERENCES

1. Kato R. Sex related differences in drug metabolism. Drug Metab Rev 1974; 3:1–31.

2. Guidicelli JF, Tillement JP. Influence of sex on drug kinetics in man. Clin Pharmacokinet 1977;2:157–166.

3. Bonate PL. Gender related differences in xenobiotic metabolism. J Clin Pharmacol 1991;31:684–690.

4. Schmucker DL, Vessell ES. Under representation of women in clinical drug trials. Clin Pharmacol Ther 1993;54:1–15.

5. Mastroianni AC, Faden R, Federman D, eds. Women and Health Research, Ethical and Legal Issues Including Women in Clinical Studies. Washington, DC: Institute of Medicine, National Academy Press, 1994.

6. American College of Clinical Pharmacy White Paper: Women as research subjects. Pharmacotherapy 1993;13:534–542.

7. Calabrese EJ. Toxic Susceptibility, Male/Female Differences. New York: Wiley-Interscience, John Wiley & Sons, 1985.

8. Calabrese EJ. Sex differences in susceptibility to toxic industrial chemicals. Br J Ind Med 1986;43:577–579.

9. Calabrese EJ. Gender Differences in Response to Toxic Substances Report submitted to the Office of Prevention, Pesticides and Toxic Substances, United States Environmental Protection Agency, Washington DC, 1996.

10. Fletcher CV, Acosta EP, Strykowski JM. Gender Differences in human pharmacokinetics and pharmacodynamics. J Adolesc Health 1994;15:619–629.

11. Pottern LM, Zahm SH, Sieber SS, et al. Occupational cancer among women: A conference overview. J Occup Med 1994;36:809–812.

12. Stellman JM. Where women work and the hazards they may face on the job. J Occup Med 1994;36:814–825.

13. Baker LC. Differences in earnings between male and female physicians. N Engl J Med 1996;334:960–964.

14. Kaplan SH, Sullivan LM, Dukes KA, Phillips CF, Kelch RP, Schaller JG. Sex differences in academic advancement—results of a national study of pediatricians. N Engl J Med 1996;335:1282–1289.

15. U.S. EPA. Exposure Factors Handbook, Vol. I: General Factors; Vol. II: Food Ingestion Factors; Vol. III: Activity Factors. Washington DC: Office of Research and Development, National Center for Environmental Assessment, August 1996.

16. American Industrial Health Council (AIHC) Exposure Factors Source Book. Washington DC: AIHC, May 1994.

17. Stewart PA, Blair A. Women in the formaldehyde industry: Their exposures and their jobs. J Occup Med 1994;36:918–923.

18. Levine R. Recognized and possible effects of pesticides in humans. In: Hayes Jr WJ, Laws Jr ER, eds. Handbook of Pesticide Toxicology, Vol. 1. New York: Academic Press, 1991, pp. 275–360.

19. Bjornberg A. Skin reactions to primary irritants in men and women. Acta Derm Venerol 1975;55:191–194.

20. Jordan WP, King SE. Delayed hypersensitivity in females. The development of allergic contact dermatitis during the comparison of twelve predictive patch tests. J Med 1977;3:19–26.

21. Leyden JL, Kligman AM. Allergic contact dermatitis: Sex differences. Contact Dermatitis 1977;3:333–336.

22. Rees JL, Friedmann PS, Matthews JNS. Sex differences in susceptibility to development of contact hypersensitivity to dinitrochlorobenzend (DNCB). Br J Dermatol 1989;120:371–374.

23. Kwangsukstith C, Maibach HI. Effect of age and sex on the induction and elicitation of allergic contact dermatitis. Conatac Dermatitis 1995;33:289–298.

24. Fitzgerald EF, Hwang SA, Brix KA, Bush B, Cook K, Worsick P. Fish PCB concentrations and consumption patterns among Mohawk women at Akwesasne. J Expo Anal Environ Epidemiol 1995;5(1):1–19.

25. Mattison DR, Blann E, Malek A. Physiological alterations during pregnancy: Impact on toxicokinetics. Fundam Appl Toxicol 1991;16:215–218.

26. Mattison DR. Physiological variations in pharmacokinetics during pregnancy. In: Fabro S, Scialli AR, eds. Drug and Chemical Action in Pregnancy. New York: Marcel Dekker, 1986, pp. 37–102.

27. International Life Science Institute, Risk Science Institute (ILSD). Physiological Parameter Values for PBPK Models. Washington DC: ILSI, December 1994.

28. Hattis D. Use of biological markers and pharmacokinetics in human health risk assessment. Environ Health Perspect 1991;90:229–238.

29. Renwick A, Hattis D. Introduction to the workshop on variability in toxic response human and environmental. Rapporteur's summary. Environmental Toxicol Pharm 1996;2:79–84.

30. Grimston SK, Nigg BM, Hanley DA, Engsberg JR. Differences in ankle joint motion as a function of age. Foot Ankle 1993;14:215–222.

31. International Commission on Radiological Protection. Basic anatomical and physiological data for use in radiological protection: The skeleton. Ann ICRP 1995; 70:1–79.

32. Langton CM, Langton DK. Male and female normative data for ultrasound measurement of the calcaneus within the UK adult population. Br J Radiol 1997;70:580–585.

33. Miglior S, Brigatti L, Velati P, et al. Relationship between morphometric optic disc parameters, sex and axial length. Curr Eye Res 1994;13:119–124.

34. Garrel DR, Jobin N, DeJonge LHM. Should we still use the Harris and Benedict equations? Nutr Clin Pract 1996;11:99–103.

35. Swaab DF, Hoffman MA, Lucassen PJ, Purba JS, Raadsheer FC, Van de Nes JAP. Functional neuroanatomy and neuropathology of the human hypothalamus. Anat Embryol 1993;187:317–330.

36. Mattison DR. Transdermal drug absorption during pregnancy. Clin Obstet Gynecol 1990;33:718–727.

37. Burmaster DE. LogNormal distributions for skin area as a function of body weight. Risk Anal 1998;18(1):27–32.

38. Southwood WFW. The thickness of the skin. Plast Reconst Surg 1975;15:423–429. Cited in: Annals of the International Commission on Radiological Protection, ICRP 1975;23:49.

39. Silvaggio T, Mattison DR. Setting occupational health standards: Toxicokinetic differences among and between men and women. J Occup Med 1994;36:849–854.

40. Williams LR. Leggett RW. References values for resting blood flow to organs of man. Clin Phys Phsiol Meas 1989:187–217.

41. deSwiet M. The cardiovascular system. In: Hytten FE, Chamberlain G, eds. Clinical Physiology in Obstetrics. Oxford: Blackwell, 1980, pp. 3–42.

41a. U.S. EPA. Exposure Factors Handbook. Washington, DC: U.S. Environmental Protection Agency, 1989, 3–14.

42. deSwiet M. The respiratory system. In: Hytten FE, Chamberlain G, eds. Clinical Physiology in Obstetrics. Oxford: Blackwell, 1980, pp. 79–100.

43. McGurk SP, Blanksby BA, Anderson MJ. The relationship of hypercapnic ventilatory responses to age, gender and atheleticism. Sports Med 1995;19:173–183.

44. Moawad AH, Lindheimer MD, eds. Uterine and Placental Blood Flow. New York: Masson, 1982, pp. 19–199.

45. Metcalf J, Stock MK, Banon DH. Maternal physiology during gestation. In: Knobil E, Neill J, eds. The Physiology of Reproduction. New York: Raven Press, 1988, pp. 2145–2176.

46. Brinkman CR. Biologic adaptation to pregnancy. In: Maternal Fetal Medicine: Principles and Practice, 2nd ed. Philadelphia: W.B. Saunders, 1989, pp. 734–745.

47. Stephen AM, Wiggins HS, Englyst HN, Cole TJ, Wayman BJ, Cummings JH. The effect of age, sex and level of intake of dietary fibre from wheat on large-bowel function in thirty healthy subjects. Br J Nutr 1986;56:349–361.

48. Silvaggio T, Mattison DR. Comparative approach to toxicokinetics. In: Paul M, ed. Occupational and Environmental Reproductive Hazards: A Guide for Clinicians. Baltimore: Williams and Wilkins, 1992, pp. 25–36.

49. Mattison DR, Malek A, Cistola C. Physiological adaptations to pregnancy: impact on pharmacokinetics. In: J. Aranda, S. Yaffe, eds. Pediatric Pharmacology: Therapeutic Principles in Practice, 2nd ed. 1992, pp. 81–96.

50. Keating FR, Jones JD, Elveback LR, Randall RV. The relation of age and sex to distribution of values in healthy adults of serum calcium inorganic phosphorus, magnesium, alkaline phosphatase, total protein, albumin, and blood urea. J Lab Clin Med 1969; 73:825–834.

51. Young CM, Blandin J, Tensuan R, Fryer HH. Body composition studies of older women, thirty to seventy years of age. Ann NY Acad Sci 1963;110:589–607. Cited in: Reference Man, ICRP 1975;23:42.

52. Hytten FE. Nutrition. In: Hytten FE, Chamberlain G, eds. Clinical Physiology in Obstetrics. Oxford: Blackwell, 1980, pp. 163–187.

53. Hytten FE. Weight gain in pregnancy. In: Hytten FE, Chamberlain G, eds. Clinical Physiology in Obstetrics. Oxford: Blackwell, 1980, pp. 3–42.

54. Sipes IG, Gandolfi AJ. Biotransformation of toxicants. In: Klaassen CD, Amdur MO, Doull J, eds. Casarett and Doull's Toxicology. New York: MacMillan, 1986, pp. 64–98.

55. Ljunggren H. Sex differences in body composition. In: Brozek J, ed. Human Body Composition: Approaches and Applications. Oxford: Pergamon Press, 1963, pp. 129–135.

56. Cunningham JJ. Body composition and resting metabolic rate: The myth of feminine metabolism. Am J Clin Nutr 1982;36:721–726.

57. Lewis PJ. Drug metabolism. In: Hytten FE, Chamberlain G, eds. Clinical Physiology in Obstetrics. Oxford: Blackwell, 1980, pp. 271–282.

58. Lewis PJ. Clinical Pharmacology in Obstetrics. Boston: Wright PSG, 1983.

59. Klaassen DC. Distribution, excretion and absorption of toxicants. In: Klaassen DC, Amdur MO, Doull J, eds. Casarett and Doull's Toxicology. New York: MacMillan, 1986, pp. 33–36.

60. Davison JM. The urinary system. In: Hytten FE, Chamberlain G, eds. Clinical Physiology in Obstetrics. Oxford: Blackwell, 1980, pp. 289–327.

61. Kirkwood C, Moore A, Hayes P, DeVane CL. Pelonero A. Influence of menstrual cycle and gender on alprazolam pharmacokinetics. Clin Pharmacol Ther 1991;50: 404–409.

62. Lew KH, Ludwing EA, Milad MA, et al. Gender-based effects on methynprednisolone pharmacokinetics and pharmacodynamics. Clin Pharmacol Ther 1993;54: 402–414.

63. Walle T, Walle K, Cowart TD, Conradi EC. Pathway selective sex differences in the metabolic clearance of propranolol inhuman subjects. Clin Pharmacol Ther 1989;46: 257–263.

64. Walle T, Walle K, Mathur RS, Palesch YY, Conradi EC. Propranolol metabolism in normal subjects: association with sex steroid hormones. Clin Pharmacol Ther 1994;56:127–132.

65. Walle UK, Fagan TC, Topmiller MJ, Conradi EC, Walle T. The influence of gender and sex steroid hormones on the plasma binding of propranolol enantiomers. Br J Clin Pharmacol 1994;37(1):21–25.

66. Carrillo JA, Benitez J. CYP1A2 activity, gender and smoking, as variables influencing the toxicity of caffeine. Br J Clin Pharmacol 1996;41(6):605–608.

67. Wang MQ, Nicholson ME, Jones CS, Fitzhugh EC, Westerfield CR. Acute alcohol intoxication, body composition and pharmacokinetics. Pharmacol Biochem Behav 1992;43:641–643.

68. Jones AW, Andersson L. Influence of age, gender and blood-alcohol concentration on the disappearance rate of alcohol from blood in drinking drivers. J Forensic Sci 1996;41(6):922–926.

69. Ammon E, Schafer C, Hofmann U, Klotz U. Disposition and first-pass metabolism of ethanol in humans: Is it gastric or hepatic and does it depend on gender? Clin Pharmacol Ther 1996;59:503–513.

70. Chen CJ, Chen CW, Wu MM, Kuo TL. Cancer potential in liver, lung, bladder and kidney due to ingested inorganic arsenic in drinking water. Br J Cancer 1992;66(5):888–892.

71. Tollestrup K, Daling JR, Allard J. Mortality in a cohort of orchard workers exposed to lead arsenate pesticide spray. Arch Environ Health 1995;50(3):221–229.

72. Gonsebatt ME, Vega L, Montero R, et al. Lymphocyte replicating ability in individuals exposed to arsenic via drinking water. Mutat Res 1994;313(2–3):293–299.

73. Lerda D. Sister chromatid exchange among individuals chronically exposed to arsenic in drinking water. Mutat Res 1994;312:111–120.

74. Bolognesi C, Parrini M, Bonassi S, Ianello G, Salanitto A. Cytogenetic analysis of a human population occupationally exposed to pesticides. Mutat Res 1993;285(2):239–249.

75. Oyeyinka GO. Age and sex differences in immunocompetence. Gerontology 1984;30:188–195.

76. Bonassi S, Bolognesi C, Abbondandolo A, et al. Influence of sex on cytogenetic endpoints: Evidence from a large human sample and review of the literature. Cancer Epidemiol Biomarkers Prev 1995;4:671–679.

77. Bush ML, Asplund PT, Miles KA, Ben-Jebria A, Ultman JS. Longitudinal distribution of O_3 absorption in the lung: Gender differences and intersubject variability. J Appl Physiol 1996;81(4):1651–1657.

78. Drechsler-Parks DM, Bedi JF, Horvath SM. Pulmonary function responses of young and older adult to mixtures of O_3, NO_2 and Pan. Toxicol Ind Health 1989;5: 505–517.

79. Rijcken B, Weiss ST. Longitudinal analysis of airway responsiveness and pulmonary function decline. Am J Respir Crit Care Med 1996;154:s246–s249.

80. Mattison DR, Thorgeirsson SS. Smoking and industrial pollution and their effects on menopause and ovarian cancer. Lancet 1978;1:187–188.

81. Spitz MR, Hoque A, Trizna Z, et al. Mutagen sensitivity as a risk factor for second malignant tumors following malignancies of the upper aerodigestive tract. J Natl Cancer Inst 1994;86(22):1681–1684.

82. Guinee DG Jr, Travis WD, Trivers GE, et al. Gender comparisons in human lung cancer: Analysis of p53 mutations, anti-p53 serum antibodies and C-erbB-2 expression. Carcinogenesis 1995;16(5):993–1002.

83. Su, Sheng JJ, Lipinskas TW. Ding X Expression of CYP2A genes in rodent and human nasal mucosa. Drug Metab Dispos 1996;24:884–890.

84. Davis DL, Hoel D, Fox J, Lopez AD. International trends in cancer mortality in France, West Germany, Italy, Japan, England, Wales and the United States. Ann NY Acad Sci 1990;609:5–48.

85. Griesemer RA, Eustis SL. Gender differences in animal bioassays for carcinogenicity. J Occup Med 1994;36:855–859.

86. Hayes WJ Jr. Dosage and other factors influencing toxicity. In: Hayes Jr WJ, Laws Jr ER, eds. Handbook of Pesticide Toxicology, Vol. 1. New York: Academic Press, 1991, pp. 39–105.

3

GENDER AND DEPRESSION

Joyce T. Bromberger

Depression is a ubiquitous term we use to refer to transient feelings of low mood or sadness that are occasional responses to the stresses of daily life. However, major depressive disorder, or clinical depression, is characterized by a persistent low mood or loss of interest or pleasure in one's usual activities in conjunction with other symptoms, such as decreased energy, disturbances in sleep and appetite, and feelings of worthlessness or guilt. Such symptoms are persistent and cause significant distress and/or interference with one's functioning (see Table 3–1 below for the primary criteria used to diagnose a major depressive episode.) Major depression is frequently a recurrent disorder[1,2] and in 12%–20% of cases is a chronic one.[3,4] However, it is treatable in many cases. There is increasing evidence that "subclinical or subsyndromal" depression, which reflects a constellation of symptoms that may not meet the full criteria identified below but which persists, is associated with significant morbidity.[5] This chapter is primarily concerned with clinical depression. Research that has been conducted on depressive symptoms and may have implications for clinical depression is also discussed.

EPIDEMIOLOGY OF DEPRESSION

Depression is a common illness that is frequently debilitating. It has been estimated that depressed individuals on average negatively affect three other peo-

Table 3–1. Criteria for Major Depressive Episode (MDE)

A. Five (or more) of the following symptoms have been present during the same
    2-week period and represent a change from previous functioning; at least one of the
    symptoms is either (*1*) depressed mood or (*2*) loss of interest or pleasure.

    1. Depressed, sad mood
    2. Decreased interest/pleasure in activities
    3. Significant weight loss/gain or decreased/increased appetite
    4. Insomnia or hypersomnia
    5. Psychomotor agitation or retardation
    6. Fatigue
    7. Feelings of worthlessness or excessive guilt
    8. Decreased ability to think or concentrate, or indecisiveness
    9. Recurrent thoughts of death, suicidal ideation with or without a plan or suicide
       attempt

B. The symptoms do not meet criteria for a mixed episode (manic and depressive
    symptoms together).
C. The symptoms cause clinically significant distress or impairment in social, occupa-
    tional, or other important areas of functioning.
D. The symptoms are not due to the direct physiological effects of a substance (e.g., a
    drug of abuse, a medication) or a general medical condition (e.g., hypothyroidism)
E. The symptoms are not better accounted for by bereavement, i.e., after the loss of a
    loved one.

[Reprinted with permission from the Diagnostic and Statistical Manual of Mental Disorders, Fourth
Edition. Copyright 1994 American Psychiatric Association[5a]]

ple during their illness.[6] The treatment of depression and lost productivity
represent a significant socio-economic cost,[7] estimated at $16.5 billion per
year.[8]

On average, rates of depression are twice as high in women as they are in
men. Epidemiologic studies conducted in the 1980s and 90s showed that these
relative differences are consistent across cultures despite the variation within
and between countries.[9,10] Studies show that the lifetime prevalence of major
depression in women ranges from 8% to 20%, indicating that as many as 1 in 5
women may experience a depressive episode at some time during their lives
(Fig. 3–1).

The predominance of women with depression is also observed in period
prevalence rates and for every age-group beginning with adolescence. Before
adolescence, rates of depression either do not differ between boys and girls or
may be somewhat higher in boys.[11,11a] Younger women, most notably those aged
15–24 years, appear to be at greater risk than women over age 50 (Fig. 3–2).
Women are also more likely to experience low-level chronic (dysthymia) or
subsyndromal depression.

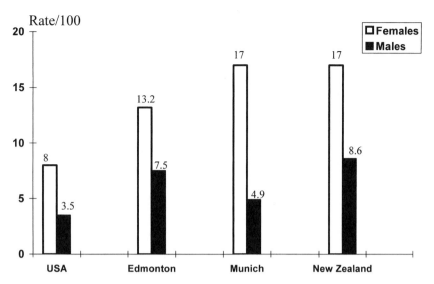

Figure 3–1. Lifetime rate/100 of major depression, age 26–64 [Reprinted with permission from Journal of Affective Disorders, Weissman et al., pages 77–84, 1993[9]]

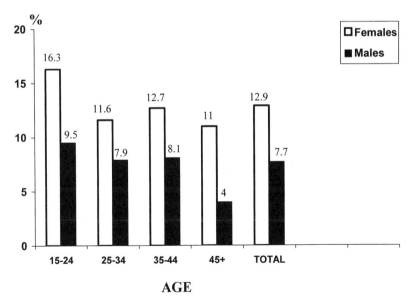

Figure 3–2. Rates of 12-month major depressive episode by sex and age [Reprinted from Kessler et al., 1993, page 81, with kind permission from Elsevier Science-NL, Sara Burgerhart-straat, 25, 1055 KV Amsterdam, The Netherlands[91]]

WHY DO MORE WOMEN THAN MEN BECOME DEPRESSED?

The clear and consistent gender differences in rates of depression across many cultures and the emergence of these conditions in early adolescence have generated extensive research investigating the factors and mechanisms that may account for these observations. Identifying mediators of depression is important in understanding causes of the specific vulnerability of women, and in expanding available and effective interventions. If a phenomenon is to be considered a mediator or mechanism, it needs to be a characteristic that is unique to or more common among women and that is associated with the outcome (depression). This chapter focuses on factors that meet both criteria. Many theories reflecting a wide range of factors have been proposed to explain the gender–depression relationship and an extensive literature has developed around them. These theories can be broadly categorized as artifactual, psychosocial, and biological/hormonal. There are few answers and no single theory offers a sufficient explanation of women's greater vulnerability to depression. Not surprisingly, the origins of gender differences in depression are probably best exemplified by the paradigm around which this book is organized: the interaction of biological factors with social-environmental, psychological, and genetic host vulnerability.

Artifactual Theories

In research, artifact refers to the consequence of the particular research methodology and does not represent a real finding. An artifact is a result of the ways in which we learn about the presence of an outcome, such as depression, rather than whether or not someone is actually depressed. It is an observation that does not reflect reality. Some researchers have argued that gender differences in the rates of depression reflect a response bias, such as men's unwillingness to admit to or seek help for depressive symptoms. Others suggest that men and women are equally susceptible to depression, but that depression in men often takes the form of acting out behaviors, such as drinking.[12] There is no evidence, however, of differences in reporting or expression of symptoms that is sufficient to explain the different rates of depression in women and men. For example, when Clancy and Gove[13] controlled for three types of response bias (perceived desirability, need for social approval, and tendency to deny), gender differences in symptoms of depression remained. It has also been found that men and women with similar levels of self-reported symptoms were equally likely to be diagnosed as depressed in a clinical interview.

Recent studies have focused on the influence of case definition, differential recall, and instability of diagnosis on the ratio of female-to-male prevalence rates. Some studies suggest that men are more likely than women to forget remote episodes[14,15] and thus underreport symptoms. Others[16,17] found no gender difference in the distribution of remote versus recent episodes of depression. Males and females equally underreported symptoms for more distant episodes.[17] Wilhelm and Parker[15] reported that when the threshold for caseness (i.e., number and severity of symptoms) was raised, the gender difference in depression rates decreased, whereas Fennig and colleagues[17] found no such change in the relative rates. There remains an ongoing interest in gender differences in depression rates as an artefact of ascertainment, case definition, and methodology more generally. However, the issue is less whether there is a real difference in the observed male–female ratio than it is the magnitude of the contribution of artefact to this difference.

Psychosocial Theories

Psychosocial explanations consider environmental, social, interpersonal, and psychological factors to be critical determinants in the development of depression. The factors typically identified are those that have been associated with the psychological and social aspects of the female gender role[18] and with depression. These include traits, such as being dependent and focused on the needs of others; roles, such as maternal and homemaker roles; and a history of victimization. The various psychosocial factors are not independent; they overlap and are reciprocal in many instances, as will be discussed below. However, for heuristic purposes, this section is organized around two key psychosocial domains: social–sex roles and personality traits. Although there is increasing evidence that exposure to childhood victimization, particularly sexual abuse, is implicated in the development of depression, a discussion of victimization is outside the scope of this text.

Social–Sex Roles. Social–sex role explanations attribute women's greater vulnerability to depression to characteristics of the specific roles women have in our society and the stresses and status attached to these. The sex-role theory of mental illness proposed over 20 years ago by Gove and Tudor[19] suggested that traditional female roles are inherently stressful and unsatisfying, whereas male involvement in both work and family roles is the source of men's better mental health. The mechanisms postulated for the psychological advantage of paid employment include the enhancement of self-esteem and confidence,[20] increased social support,[21] and modification or buffering of the negative and stressful aspects of being a housewife and/or mother.[22] Homemakers and mothers are said to have few resources for gratification and enhancing self-worth; these roles have low social status and can be restrictive, frustrating, and unrewarding. Low self-esteem,[23] social support,[24] and high stress[22,25] have all been shown to be associated with depression. For example, in a series of community and clinical studies of women, Brown and colleagues[22,23,26,27] showed that negative self-esteem predicted the onset of depression 1 year after initial assessment and that women with low marital support were more likely than those with high support to become depressed when they experienced a severe stressor.

However, evidence that the roles of homemaker and mother are directly associated with these depressogenic factors is not compelling. Additionally, results from the large body of research examining the relationship between employment status and depression are inconsistent, largely cross-sectional, and not convincing for a main effect of employment status. A significant limitation of the cross-sectional studies is the confound of the "healthy worker effect": healthier women are more likely to be in the work force. One of the few longitudinal studies examining the relationship between changes in employment status and changes in depressive symptom levels over 3 years found small increases in symptoms over time in all women except those who were not employed at study entry but were employed 3 years later (i.e., newly employed) (Fig. 3–3).[28]

In the last 5–10 years, it has become clearer that the impact of women's roles on their mental health is more strongly related to the quality of the specific experience than in role occupancy per se.[29] Studies tend to find that the impact of employment or other roles on women are related to the characteristics of the job or role and the associated balance of rewards and stresses.[30]

The theory that roles typically occupied by women generate more stress and fewer coping skills remains more of an assumption than an empirically substantiated finding. Studies comparing cumulative life event scores of men and

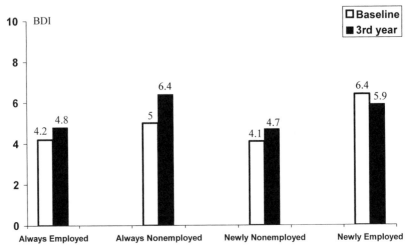

Figure 3–3. Mean Beck Depression Inventory scores, adjusted for education and marital status, of four employment groups [Reprinted with permission from American Journal of Public Health, Vol. 84, Bromberger and Matthews, page 204, Copyright American Public Health Association, Inc., 1994[28]]

women have not shown gender differences in exposure.[31–33] However, Wethington et al.[34] found that women reported more network events and deaths of loved ones and suggested that the psychological impact of such events as reflected in symptom levels was greater among women than among men. A recent study[35] of a community sample of 100 couples who experienced the same severe stressor assessed the impact of the event on the development of clinical depression. Among couples in which there were clear gender differences in their roles (i.e., women took more responsibility for activities and tasks typically considered part of a woman's role and had a relatively greater involvement in these), women were more likely to experience a depressive episode than men, following an event involving children, housing, or reproductive problems. The authors suggest that the differences in roles led to women being more likely to hold themselves responsible for such events, whereas men could distance themselves from them. It is noteworthy that 70% of the sample were working class (i.e., low socioeconomic status), which limits the extent to which the results can be generalized.

The discourse on the relative contribution of social-sex roles to the etiology of depression in women continues with no clear-cut conclusions. If such roles are salient, the various studies suggest that they are not inherently conducive or harmful to women's psychological well-being. It is likely that many facets of the roles themselves as well as what is brought to these roles in the form of personality traits and biology are important in understanding the origins of depression in women.

Personality Traits. The excess risk of depression among women has also been linked to developmental pathways involving gender differentiation in personality characteristics. Diverse theories (e.g., psychoanalytic and cognitive-behavioral) attribute gender differences in rates of depression to a variety of personality traits thought to be more common in women and linked to the female gender role. For example, sex-role theories of depression maintain that a vulnerability to depression develops as part of a socialization process that is different for females than males.[36] Females are expected and pressured to adopt personality characteristics and behaviors, such as being passive, dependent, nurturing, and understanding of others, considered appropriate for their gender but which may increase their risk of depression. According to the "gender intensification" theory,[37] this developmental process intensifies during early adolescence. As boys and girls begin to change biologically and physically at puberty, they become more aware of the significance of their gender and, in an effort to conform to expected gender roles, assume more of the traits and behaviors associated with being males or females in our society. Their behavior is reinforced by the increasing social pressures on and expectations of them to behave in ways stereotypically consistent with their gender. Several traits which will be discussed below have been found to be more common among pre-adolescent and adolescent girls than boys, suggesting that these early-appearing traits may interact with certain challenges of adolescence that lead to depression in adolescent girls.[36]

Spence and Helmreich[38] developed a measure that has been shown to discriminate between characteristics typically associated with female (emotional, passive) and male (assertive, dominant) gender roles. The female trait is commonly referred to as "expressive," which is associated with low instrumentality and high expressiveness, and the male trait as "instrumental," which refers to being task or action oriented. Consistent with this observation are findings that women tend to be more ruminative and self-focused, a specific type of passivity, when challenged or stressed.[39,40] For example, in a study in which individuals kept track of their naturally occurring moods and their responses to these moods for 30 consecutive days, when sad, women were more likely than men to go to their room alone and think about their feelings.[41] On the other hand, the perception that women tend to suppress angry feelings rather than express them directly[42] has limited empirical support.[43]

Many studies of various kinds, including those using cross-sectional, laboratory, and short-term naturalistic designs, have examined gender role–related personality traits as independent predictors of depression.[44,45] In a meta-analysis of 32 studies, Whitley[44] concluded that, irrespective of gender, instrumentality was inversely associated with both levels of depressive symptoms and general adjustment. Similar results were reported by Bromberger and Matthews[46] in a recent longitudinal study of middle-aged women. Traits were measured at study entry, along with a standard measure of depressive symptoms. Three years later, the less instrumental women showed a greater increase in depressive symptoms over baseline, after adjustment for potential confounders. Being highly expressive or nurturing was not associated with changes in symptoms,[46] which is consistent with Whitley's analysis. In stressful circumstances, instrumentality may be associated with active, problem-focused coping, which predicts psychological health in both men and women.[47,48] Thus the absence of instrumental characteristics would make a woman particularly susceptible to depressive symptoms when stressed.

A propensity toward focusing on one's feelings when stressed has been shown to be correlated with a depressive affect. Bromberger and Matthews's[46] study of middle-aged women found that women who were assessed as highly self-focused at study entry and who subsequently experienced a chronic stress were more symptomatic than all other women. Results of a prospective study of a younger sample of university students also indicated that those who were assessed as having a ruminative response style prior to the 1989 San Francisco Bay area earthquake had higher levels of depressed mood after the quake.[40] These results are consistent with behavioral-cognitive theories of depression proposing that the propensity to dwell on one's feelings or thoughts may render individuals vulnerable during times of negative events by increasing the accessibility of a negative schema or constructs and amplifying the accompanying negative emotions and cognitions.[49–51]

Other personality characteristics have been posited as being more common in women and contributing to the greater vulnerability of women to depression.[50,52] These include being dependent on relationships with others, especially men, for their emotional well-being, having self-defeating attributional tendencies, and perceiving little control over events and tasks. I have focused on a few selected traits likely to be linked to the development of depression in women.

Biological Hormonal Theories

A common explanation for gender differences in depression are biologic differences between men and women, specifically, reproductive-related biologic differences. A number of lines of research implicate reproductive hormones in the etiology of depression, but as will be seen, the data are inconsistent and subject to a range of methodological limitations.

Sex Steroids as Mediators of Depression. It has become increasingly clear that the physiological influence of ovarian steroids extends beyond their exertion on sexual and reproductive behavior. Estrogens are known to influence the structure and function of many organs and systems, including the brain. Studies have indicated that specific nuclear receptors for estrogen are found in certain areas of the brain, including the pituitary, hypothalamus, the limbic forebrain, and cerebral cortex, and that estrogens, progestins, and androgens affect a wide range of processes in the brain.[53] For example, these hormones affect neurofunctional processes, such as neurotransmission of chemical impulses between neurons in the central nervous system. Differential exposure to androgens and estrogens during perinatal development and in adulthood influences neurostructural differences in the brains of men and women. Ovarian steroids may contribute to depression in women at the level of their direct effect on neurotransmitter systems linked to depression or they may contribute indirectly at the level of psychophysiologic response to stress, as in the response of the hypothalamic–pituitary–adrenal (HPA) axis.

A major focus of research on the pathophysiology of depression has been on the roles of the neurotransmitter systems. A number of neurotransmitters have been implicated in the development and manifestation of depression, including monoamine, norepinephrine, and dopamine.[54] Recently, however, the serotonergic systems have received a lot of research attention. Preclinical studies have shown that these systems play an important role in regulating many physiologic functions that are often impaired in depressed patients, including sleep, appetite, and motor activity.[55] Studies of depressed patients have shown a decrease in serotonin (5-HT) turnover, a decreased uptake of serotonin into platelets, and fewer imipramine (IMI) binding sites on platelets.[54] Consistent with these findings is the efficacy of several recently developed selective serotonin re-uptake inhibitors, such as fluoxetine, sertraline, and paroxetine in the treatment of depression and amelioration of premenstrual symptoms.[56]

Effects of ovarian steroids, particularly estradiol, on processes involving neurotransmitter systems, including the dopaminergic, neuropeptide, GABA, and cholinergic systems, have been demonstrated in studies of rats.[53] A few small clinical studies of women suggest levels of estradiol are related to alterations in the concentrations and availability of neurotransmitter amines.[54]

Neurotransmitters play a role in a number of systems implicated in major depression and may be influenced by them as well. For example, serotoninergic structures may alter the negative feedback effects of cortisol on HPA axis function, which would result in hypercortisolemia, one of the most consistent biologic correlates of major depression.[55] Increased secretion of cortisol is also a part of the general adaptational response to stress. The stress response is a complex system that interacts with many regions of the brain in the regulation of emotion, cognitive function, behavior, and immune and reproductive functioning.[56] In the case of the reproductive system, there are data showing that aspects of its functioning, such as the production of luteinizing hormone (LH), follicle-stimulating hormone (FSH), and estradiol are inhibited by responses to stress by various components of the HPA axis. At the same time, gender differences in stress responses have been described in animal experiments suggesting that sex hormones may be involved in regulating the HPA axis; for example, female rats showed higher levels of plasma corticosterone than male rats.[57] The limited human data are inconsistent and difficult to interpret. In response to administration of ovine corticotropin-releasing hormone (oCRH), plasma levels of adrenocorticotropin hormone (ACTH) were higher in teenage boys than girls[58] and lower in young adult men than in women,[59] but in both studies the cortisol levels were similar in males and females. In a study of depressed men and women, Young and colleagues[60] reported that postmenopausal women had a higher rate of dexamethasone resistance (i.e., nonsuppression of cortisol) than did either men or premenopausal women.

Despite the inconsistent findings and the need for further research, the implication of these studies is that gonadal hormones interact in some complex way with the central nervous system. Stress has long been shown to be correlated with depression and recent studies provide evidence of it being causally related to onset.[27,61] Thus, if women are more biologically sensitive or responsive to stress than men, irrespective of rates of exposure, this would suggest one potential pathway by which sex hormones may mediate gender and depression.

There are many biological processes and innumerable and complicated interactions among them, many not yet clearly elucidated, that are potentially involved in the putative link between gonadal hormones and depressive illness. This discussion has focused on the activational effects of sex steroids. However, it is also possible that any organizational and structural influences gonadal hormones have on the brain may contribute to differences in cognitive styles, learning abilities, and regulation of emotions, as well as to neuronal connectivity at the cortical level.

DEPRESSION IN THE LIFE CYCLE OF WOMEN

The biological explanation of greater female vulnerability to depression involves the dysregulation or imbalance of the ovarian hormones. In particular, this dysregulation is thought to occur during periods of significant or rapid change in levels of gonadal hormones: during puberty, premenstrually, postpartum, and at menopause. During these life cycle events, there may be absolute changes in steroid hormone levels (e.g., decreases in estrogen and progesterone in the postpartum period) or alterations in the ratio of estrogen to progesterone (e.g., premenstrually). This theory has emerged from epidemiologic data and from a large number of anecdotal and clinical reports suggesting that some women become depressed during times of significant or rapid changes in the levels of ovarian hormones. The following sections will focus on four reproductive periods of women's lives as potential points of biological vulnerability to major depression. Another layer of complexity is added by the fact that each of the reproductive transitions is a time of psychological and social changes as well. For each type of reproductive transition, the available data on the epidemiology of depression and on hypothesized hormonal associations are presented.

Puberty

As noted earlier, significant differences in the rates of depression in boys and girls start to emerge around the time of puberty, between 11 and 14 years of age[11,62,63] (Fig. 3–4). Efforts to understand the source of the differences are complicated by the constellation of changes that occur at this time. Puberty marks a biological, psychological, and social transition from childhood to adolescence that is characterized by complex interactions within each domain and among them. For example, the external physical changes that occur in girls even before the onset of menarche may influence their feelings about themselves, their relationship to family, and the expectations of them by their family, friends, and social environment generally. Classic psychoanalytic theories have held the view that physiological changes linked to new sexual feelings create anxiety and "psychological instability," including depression.[64] There are numerous ways, including the previously discussed impact of personality charac-

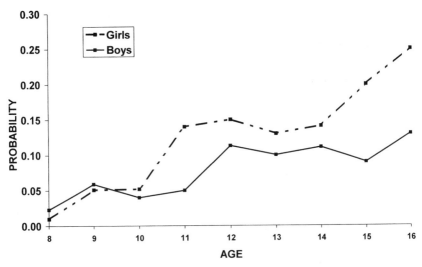

Figure 3–4. Effects of gender and age on depression. Odds ratio for gender = 1.63 (1.42 −1.89)** for age = 1.21 (1.17 −1.25)** [Reprinted from Development and Psychopathology, Vol. 1, No. 1, Angold and Rutter, page 13, with the permission of Cambridge University Press[11]]

teristics, in which the risk for depression might be elevated in females at this juncture.

The biological transition to puberty is a process involving increased gonadotropin pulse frequency and amplitude, including frequent pulses of luteinizing hormone (LH) that begin during sleep and promote maturation of secondary sex characteristics.[65] This activity sets in motion the mature, daily, pulsatile gonadotropin-releasing hormone (GnRH), production of LH and follicle-stimulating hormone (FSH), and fluctuations in estrogen and progesterone in females. The alterations in these endocrine parameters have generated considerable interest in the relationship of reproductive hormones to depression in adolescents and women.

A hormonal etiology for depression at puberty has been assessed indirectly by analyzing age or physical morphological stage, and in some cases, directly by evaluating hormonal measures. Marshall and Tanner's[66] categorization of the physical stages marking the transition from pre-adolescence to adulthood has been a relatively easy way to classify maturational status. Studies have used classifications based on reports of physical characteristics provided by adolescents or mothers, in some studies using Tanner pictures,[67] and physical examination.[68]

An epidemiologic study conducted in the Isle of Wight using a crude observational measure of pubertal status found it was more strongly associated with depressive symptoms than was age.[69] Results from a more recent prospective epidemiologic investigation of children aged 9–16 years, the Great Smoky Mountains Study, also showed that the increased risk of depression in girls occurred in mid-puberty (Tanner III) and was independent of age[11a]. In addition, a British study that examined the effects of age, gender, and pubertal status on rates of depression in a clinical sample of approximately 3,000 boys and girls, ages 8 to 16 years showed a clear effect for age and gender; rates of various constructs of depression (e.g., symptoms, syndrome, ICD-9) for boys and girls began to diverge around 11 years of age and became significantly different by 14 years (Fig. 3–4).[11] Subsequent analyses for boys and girls separately showed only an effect for age and none for pubertal status. Although these data suggest that change in maturation, a presumptive surrogate for hormone levels, was not related to depression, in some cases a determination of pubertal status was based on a "superficial observation" of the child and not on a physical examination. Additionally, hormone levels were not measured. Given that anovulatory cycles may predominate for up to 2 years after menarche with concomitant variability in ovarian estrogen levels,[65] even a physical examination may not be highly correlated with actual hormone concentrations at any one point in time.

Because endocrine and psychosocial changes usually co-occur, it is difficult to distinguish the role of hormones per se. Most child and adolescent epidemiologic studies have either not assessed hormonal or pubertal status or not used adequate measures to do so. The studies that have examined the associations of depression with levels of gonadal hormones and gonadotropins in prepubertal and pubertal boys and girls report mixed results that reflect a variety of complex relations among hormones and negative affect. For example, studies have found that low concentrations of DHEAS (an adrenal androgen) were related to elevated depression;[70] and that levels of FSH high for chronological age were positively related to negative affect.[71] Brooks-Gunn and Warren[68] found a positive curvilinear correlation between depressive symptoms and estrogen for girls in the middle stages of puberty, but not early or late stages, suggesting an association with rapidly rising estrogen. However, stressful life events accounted for more variance than did hormone levels.

Although studies point to an effect of hormonal changes at puberty on depressive affect, they have many methodological problems, including small sample sizes and the use of single serum specimens (in some cases over 6–12 months) for hormonal assays. The latter is a problem because gonadal steroid and gonadotropin levels in premenarcheal girls are even more variable than those measured during the normal adult female menstrual cycle.

If gonadal hormones are related to the divergence in gender rates of depression at adolescence, the relationship may be mediated by the neuropeptide oxytocin. Recently, Frank and Young[71a] suggested that oxytocin, a complex and multipurpose peptide that undergoes a fivefold increase at puberty (in both males and females), may be more important than the sex steroids in explaining the marked rise in rates of depression among adolescent girls compared to their male counterparts. Based on animal data indicating that oxytocin is related to affiliative behavior, i.e., attachment and bonding (e.g., maternal-infant) in females but not males[71b,71c], Young and Frank argue that the "biological stage is set" for an intensified need for pair-bonding and interpersonal relationships in females. If this need is actually or perceived to be unmet or frustrated, depression may result. Indeed, Frank's recent study of adolescent depression found that girls with major depression were significantly more likely to have experienced a severe interpersonal event in the 6 months prior to depression onset than were depressed adolescent boys or nondepressed boys or girls.[71d]It is too early to know whether this hypothesis will be supported by subsequent research, but it does provide an example of the way in which biological and psychosocial phenomena may interact to put women at risk for depression.

Menstrual Cycle

The phase of the menstrual cycle just prior to the start of menses has been associated with mood changes, such as increased depression or anxiety. Severe premenstrual symptoms that impair functioning are referred to as PMS (premenstrual syndrome), a term that has become part of our common vocabulary. Reports of phase-specific mood changes (either transient and mild, or severe, as in PMS) coinciding with specific patterns of sex hormone levels suggest that sex hormones are associated with mood swings, and by extrapolation, may relate to clinical depression.

Menstrual cycle–associated dysphoric mood or PMS may contribute to gender differences in rates of depressive illness by being included in the observed prevalence rates of major depression, by increasing biologic vulnerability to depressive illness in women, or by confounding studies of past depressive history. However, the extent to which mood changes occur normally during the menstrual cycle and the prevalence of a significant disorder (i.e., PMS) have yet to be determined.

The normal adult menstrual cycle is characterized by shifts in levels of gonadal steroids and gonadotropins. In the luteal phase, after the surge in the gonadotropins, progesterone levels peak above those of estradiol and both start a rapid decline about 7 days before the onset of menses (menstrual cycle blood). During this premenstrual period, women are thought to experience more frequently a variety of irritable, anxious, and depressive mood changes along with physical symptoms, such as breast tenderness, headaches, and bloating. All of these symptoms appear to subside once menses begin.[72,73] However, there is a wide variation in the prevalence of such symptoms (30% to 75%) and they may vary across cultures.[74] Studies that have examined the relationship between measured hormone levels in menstruating women have not found a correlation between hormones and depressed mood.[75]

We do not know whether the symptoms of depression and anxiety associated with the premenstruum constitute a discrete psychiatric disorder, commonly known as PMS; an exacerbation of an ongoing depressive disorder; its residual symptoms; or a subtype of clinical depression.[76,77] Studies of clinical samples have reported much higher rates of prior major depression in PMS subjects than in controls.[76,78] On the other hand, after reviewing the literature on premenstrual syndromes and analyzing a large data set, the DSM-IV work group concluded that there is a subset of women with severe premenstrual mood syndromes that should be considered for further study as having a specific psychiatric disorder (designated as premenstrual dysphoric disorder [PMDD] in Diagnostic and Statistical Manual of Mental Disorders, 4th edition). The criteria and utility of this diagnosis have yet to be determined.[79,80]

The prevalence of such syndromes or disorders has been difficult to estimate because of the lack of agreement on their definition and because of differences in the composition of study populations.[81,82] For example, over 150 physical and emotional symptoms have been associated with PMS, suggesting a very heterogenous phenomenon. Earlier investigations of the prevalence of mood changes used retrospective questionnaires, did not include endocrinologic data on cycle phase, and recruited samples of women with menstrual problems. Using retrospective reports has been shown to be a highly problematic way of obtaining data for both mild and severe symptoms, as such reports are not confirmed by prospective daily ratings over several months in as many as 50% of women who previously reported significant premenstrual symptoms.[83] More reliable estimates based on DSM-III-R and prospective ratings report prevalence rates of premenstrual disorder in the range of 3%–5% in several community samples.[81]

The contributions of gonadotropins and gonadal hormones to the pathophysiology of PMS have been assessed directly in small clinical studies using prospective diaries to document symptoms. In general, these studies provide negligible support for a detectable effect of changing levels of any of these hormones on mood.[84] Alterations in estradiol, progesterone, LH, FSH, and testosterone have been assessed by several groups of researchers. Some researchers found no differences in the patterns of changes in any hormones among women diagnosed with PMS versus a control group[85,86]; another found a positive association between increases in estradiol and progesterone levels and symptoms in the luteal phase.[87] A recent study suggests that androgens may play a role in PMS; Eriksson and colleagues[88] found that serum concentrations of free testosterone were significantly higher in 11 PMS subjects than in controls throughout the menstrual cycle, but levels of progesterone, total testosterone, and dehydroepiandrosterone sulphate (DHEAS) did not differ between groups. At this point in time, there does not appear to be substantial evidence that differences in levels of one or more sex hormones explain why some women experience significant and disabling symptoms, including depression, premenstrually.

Postpartum

The postpartum period (i.e, within the first few months after childbirth) may be a time of increased risk for major depression. The estimates of the prevalence of depression during this period range from 10% to 15%[89,90] and are similar to those reported in a recent epidemiologic study of the prevalence of psychiatric disorders in over 8,000 individuals.[91] Whether postpartum depression is more common than depression at other times remains debatable. What has been documented is that 50% to 80% of postpartum women experience a brief period of dysphoria, typically called the "baby blues," which is characterized by a few days of crying episodes, tension, irritability, and sensitivity after childbirth.[92] The prevalence of the "blues," the psychological and social changes involving the increased demands of a new baby and often decreased feelings of self-efficacy, and the large and rapid decreases in estrogen and progesterone levels after delivery have focused attention on the postpartum period as a time of vulnerability to depression.

Clinical depression that occurs in the few months after delivery is associated with the same psychosocial factors as depression that occurs at other times, including marital conflict, low instrumental and emotional support, and negative life stress (although the stressors at this particular time are often specifically related to childcare).[93] To a mother, an infant usually brings increased emotional and physical demands, decreased sleep, fewer opportunities for social interaction, and depending on the mother's life circumstances, an increased need to juggle various responsibilities for work, home, and other children.

The sudden drop after delivery of very high progesterone and estradiol levels has generated a lot of interest in the link between these changes and the onset of depression postpartum. In rats, progesterone has been shown to have a sedative effect. At one time it was thought that the withdrawal of progesterone in late pregnancy and the early puerperium was responsible for some cases of depression postpartum. However, several studies in humans assessing plasma levels of total and free progesterone show no relationship between progesterone and mood.[94–96] Similarly, estrogen levels have shown only a weak association with the blues[94] and none with clinical depression.[95] On the other hand, a group of British researchers recently reported that in a double-blind, placebo-controlled study of 61 women with major depression that began within 3 months of childbirth, women who were treated with two 100-µg 17 β-estradiol patches changed twice a week improved more quickly and to a significantly greater extent than did women who were given placebo patches.[97] This may be the only clinical trial using estradiol to treat depression that had its onset postpartum, and the dosage of estradiol used was about four times that typically used in hormone replacement therapy.

Despite the magnitude of the hormonal changes after childbirth and the coincident onset of depression, the available data provide little evidence that such changes are directly related to this disorder. There is also no data to suggest how hormonal patterns postpartum might contribute to the initiation of an episode of depression. However, it may be that for some vulnerable subsets of women (e.g., those with a history of depression, cumulative stressors, low marital and other support), the hormonal environment after delivery acts as a precipitant to depression.

Menopause

The cessation of menses and reproductive function occurs around the age of 51 on average. Historically, menopause has been linked to numerous untoward symptoms, including insomnia, irritability, nervousness, and especially, depression. At one time, it was thought that involutional melancholia (menopausal depression) was a distinct clinical depressive entity and a definition for it was included in the second edition of the *Diagnostic and Statistical Manual* (the classification and definition of psychiatric disorders). In the late 1970s, Weissman[98] demonstrated from a review of studies that there was no empirical evidence of a unique menopausal depressive disorder and the classification was omitted from subsequent editions of the manual.

Recent epidemiologic investigations of prevalence rates of psychiatric disorders do not show that women in their 40's and 50's have elevated rates of depression,[91,99] as would be expected if the biologic or social aspects of menopause were associated with depression (Fig. 3–2). However, the overall rates in the broad age stratum (40–54 years) may conceal variations related to specific phases in the menopausal transition or to subsets of vulnerable women.

In studies of menopause, depression has been measured primarily using checklists of symptoms and in some recent studies, self-report measures of depression, such as the Center for Epidemiologic Studies of Depression Scale (CES-D).[100] Most studies have been cross-sectional[101–103] and fewer have been longitudinal investigations.[104–107] Some studies suggest an increase in levels of symptomatology during the perimenopause[108] but overall, the research has yielded unconvincing evidence of significant associations between depressive symptoms and either the perimenopause or postmenopause. However, self-report questionnaires that assess only the previous 2 weeks provide a crude and limited picture of women's emotional experiences during the long and complex menopausal transition. Furthermore, such approaches do not yield good data on clinical disorder. To date, only one epidemiologic study has assessed categories of "mental disability" including depressive syndrome, rather than symptoms, and it found that a current episode of psychiatric illness was associated with a history of mental illness whereas self-reported menopausal status was not.[109]

Despite the numerous studies attempting to assess the relationship between menopause and depression, the data are limited by the cross-sectional methodology or by the measures and technology used. There is an absence of well-designed prospective studies assessing clinical depression, bleeding patterns, and hormones with state-of-the-art measures. Women continue to report depression and anxiety associated with changes in their menstrual cycle. The dialogue and debate concerning the emotional impact of menopause and the midlife period generally are ongoing.

The menopausal transition is a time of decline in ovarian hormone levels leading to the cessation of menses. It is also a time of a shift in roles, responsibilities, relationships, and phase-specific events, such as the illness and death of parents, the maturation of children, and the departure of children from home. It is difficult to disentangle the contribution of these multiple factors to the development of depression during this period, not only because it is hard to separate the influence of biology from that of the loss of the mothering role, for instance, but because they co-occur over an extended period of time.

Psychosocial perspectives view midlife as a stage in the life cycle that is accompanied by specific challenges that may promote depression. According to these theories, women are vulnerable to depression in midlife because of the changes in their roles, the stressors that accompany life events, and the psychological impact of biological changes. A few studies suggest that stresses women experience at this time of life influence mood more than menopausal status.[105,110]

For most women, before they stop menstruating, the pattern of their menstrual cycles, including duration, frequency, and amount of bleeding, begins to change and becomes less predictable. It has been estimated that on average, this transitional phase, or perimenopause, takes 3 to 4 years.[111] Although the ovaries continue to produce testosterone, the concentrations of ovarian estrogen and progesterone become negligible and those of LH and FSH increase.[112] However, the process by which this occurs is uncertain and the changes themselves are not well characterized nor well understood. For example, it is not clear that sex steroids decrease steadily; they may wax and wane in unpredictable ways that include periods of hyperestrogenic as well as hypoestrogenic production.[113]

The impact of sex steroids on transient depressed mood and major depression during peri- and postmenopause has long been a subject of controversy. Several lines of research using different paradigms have reported varying results. These include studies of the relationships between levels of estradiol, progesterone, and androgens and mood in peri- and postmenopausal women; the effects of hormone replacement therapy (HRT) on mood or the usefulness of HRT for treatment of depression or depressive symptoms in postmenopausal women; and the circulating levels of sex-steroid hormones in surgically meno-pausal women who were and were not taking some type of hormone replace-ment regimen. Because the daily variability in sex-steroid hormone levels in-creases during the perimenopause, their measurement is even more complex than when women are menstruating regularly.

Most studies of menopausal women have failed to find an association be-tween hormone levels and depressed mood. However, early studies examining the impact of estrogen replacement therapy on mood were methodologically flawed. Many did not use double-blind designs; they used measures of depres-sive symptoms with unknown reliability and validity, and they were conducted in samples that included both naturally and surgically menopausal women. A re-cent double-blind study,[114] comparing two different doses of estrogen with placebo in asymptomatic women who had undergone a hysterectomy, found that at the end of 3 months, the depression scores of women receiving estrogen decreased significantly whereas those of women taking placebo did not signifi-cantly change.

In prospective clinical studies with surgically and naturally postmenopausal women in their 40's and 50's without a psychiatric disorder, Sherwin found evi-dence of an association between circulating sex-steroid hormone levels and mood.[115,116] In the case of the surgically postmenopausal women, those who had received estrogen or a combined estrogen–testosterone drug intramuscularly once a month for the previous 2 years had more positive moods than a group who had not received treatment.[115] A study of naturally menopausal women ran-domly assigned to one of four cyclical hormone regimens that included estro-gen at one of two doses (.625 or 1.25 mg) followed by either 5 mg of progestin (medroxyprogesterone acetate) or placebo showed that women who were taking progestin reported more negative mood than those on placebo.[116] These find-ings, in addition to those of other studies,[117] indicate that progestins may attenu-ate any positive effects of estrogen. Although this suggests an association be-tween mood and sex steroids, postmenopausal women produce very little progesterone and estradiol. Therefore, it is not clear how clinical trial results are related to fluctuations in endogenous hormones. Additionally, the outcomes measured were general affect rather than depressive symptoms, as assessed by a standard instrument, and none of the women was clinically depressed.

GONADAL HORMONES IN THE GENESIS AND TREATMENT OF MAJOR DEPRESSION

Data on the role of gonadal hormones in depressed patients are limited. A case–control study of regularly menstruating women, comparing serum levels of sex steroids in untreated patients with controls, showed no difference in mean progesterone or estradiol concentrations but did reveal significant differences in testosterone.[118] After treatment, testosterone levels remained high, but were no longer significantly different from those of controls. There were no significant differences between untreated patients and controls in concentrations of estradiol, progesterone, LH, and FSH. Although the serum estradiol levels were similar in untreated patients and controls (65.9 vs. 69.4), there was a significant negative correlation between estradiol levels and the severity of symptoms among patients, as measured by the Hamilton Depression Scale, a frequently used standard measure of depression severity. This suggests that if there is a relationship between estradiol and depression, it may be detectable only at the highest levels of depression severity.

Studies of clinically depressed patients have not shown improvement with estrogen replacement treatment.[119,120] One frequently cited exception reported that women with severe treatment-resistant depression improved after treatment with estrogen, but very high doses of estrogen were used.[121] None of the studies assessed serum levels of estradiol which vary even with fixed dosing and can cause supra-physiologic levels. In an effort to address some of the limitations of previous research, a new randomized, double-blind study has recently been undertaken to test the efficacy of estrogen treatment for mildly to moderately depressed postmenopausal women. (B.G. Pollock and M. Wylie, personal communication).

SUMMARY

From their early teens, women are at twice the risk for major depression as men. It does not appear that during postpartum and menopause they are, on average, at significantly greater risk than at other times. However, the averages may not reveal the entire story. Indeed, women who are particularly self-focused and passive may represent a subset of vulnerable women. They may be more negatively affected by life stressors during times of reproductive fluctuations than at other times of their lives or more vulnerable than their counterparts who are not so stressed. On the other hand, it also seems clear that the female gender role attributes of emotional understanding and concern about the well-being of others are not associated with depressed mood in younger or older women. There is some evidence that occupying a particular role or roles themselves is not deleterious but that an imbalance of stresses and rewards in the role(s) in which the former outweigh the later may induce negative affect.

The evidence that sex steroids play an etiologic or contributory role in major depression is inconsistent and difficult to interpret. Each of various gonadal hormones (including estradiol, progestins, and testosterone) have been implicated in some type of depressive phenomenon by at least one study. Given the absence of a consistent relationship between measured or inferred estradiol or androgen hormone levels, it is likely that the responsiveness of and interaction among various systems is likely involved in depression. The growing evidence that estradiol influences multiple areas of the brain and is involved in the actions of multiple neurotransmitter systems suggests that it contributes to either the development or maintenance of clinical depression. Continued research is needed to elucidate the biological activity of sex hormones outside the reproductive system. Equally important are efforts to assess the psychological, social, and environmental factors that no doubt interact with each other and with biological and genetic factors.

REFERENCES

1. Zis AP, Goodwin FK. Major affective disorder as a recurrent illness. A critical review. Arch Gen Psychiatry 1979;36:835–839.

2. Klerman GL. Treatment of recurrent unipolar major depressive disorder. Commentary on the Pittsburgh study. Arch Gen Psychiatry 1990;47:1158–1162.

3. Keller MB, Klerman GL, Lavori PW, et al. Long term outcome of major depression: Clinical and public health significance. JAMA 1984;252:788–792.

4. Scott J. Chronic depression. Br J Psychiatry 1988;153:287–289.

5. Wells KB, Stewart A, Hays RD, et al. The functioning and well-being of depressed patients: Results from the Medical Outcomes Study. JAMA 1989;262:914–919.

5a. Diagnostic and Statistical Manual of Mental Disorders, Fourth Edition. Washington, DC: American Psychiatric Association, 1994.

6. Sartorius N. Research on affective disorders within the frame-work of the WHO program. In Schou M, Stromgren E, eds. Aarhus Symposia: Origin, Prevention, and Treatment of Affective Disorders. London: Academic Press, 1979, pp. 207–213.

7. Judd LL, Paulus MP, Wells KB, Rapaport MH. Socioeconomic burden of subsyndromal depressive symptoms and major depression in a sample of the general population. Am J Psychiatry 1996;153:1411–1417.

8. Munoz R. Depression prevention research: Conceptual and practical considerations. In: Munoz R, ed. Depression prevention: Research directions. Washington, DC: Hemisphere, 1987, pp. 2–10.

9. Weissman MM, Bland R, Joyce PR, et al. Sex differences in rates of depression: Cross-national perspectives. J Affect Disord 1993;29:77–84.

10. Culbertson FM. Depression and gender. An International review. Am Psychol 1997;52:25–31.

11. Angold A, Rutter M. Effects of age and pubertal status on depression in a large clinical sample. Dev Psychopathol 1992;4:5–28.

11a. Angold A, Costello EJ, Worthman CM. Puberty and depression: the roles of age, pubertal status and pubertal timing. Psychol Med 1998;28:51–61.

12. Nolen-Hoeksema S. Sex differences in unipolar depression: Evidence and theory. Psychol Bull 1987;101:259–282.

13. Clancy K, Gove W. Sex differences in mental illness: An analysis of response bias in self-reports. Am J Sociol 1974;80:205–216.

14. Angst J, Dobler-Mikola A. Do the diagnostic criteria determine the sex ratio in depression. J Affect Disord 1984;7:189–198.

15. Wihelm K, Parker G. Sex differences in lifetime depression rates: Fact or artefact? Psychol Med 1995;24:97–111.

16. Coryell W, Endicott J, Keller M. Major depression in a nonclinical sample: Demographic and clinical risk factors for first onset. Arch Gen Psychiatry 1992;49: 117–125.

17. Fennig S, Schwartz JE, Bromet EJ. Are diagnostic criteria, time of episode and occupational impairment important determinants of the female: male ratio for major depression? J Affect Disord 1994;30:147–154.

18. McGrath E, Keita GP, Strickland BR, Russo NF, eds. Women and Depression. Risk Factors and Treatment Issues. Washington, DC: American Psychological Association, 1990.

19. Gove WR, Tudor JF. Adult sex roles and mental illness. Am J Sociol 1973;78 :812–835.

20. Baruch GK, Barnett R. Role quality, multiple role involvement, and psychological well-being in midlife women. J Pers Soc Psychol 1986;51:578–585.

21. Hibbard JH, Pope CR. Employment status, employment characteristics, and women's health. Women Health 1985;10:59–77.

22. Brown GW, Harris T. Social Origins of Depression: A Study of Psychiatric Disorder in Women. London: Tavistock Publications, 1978.

23. Brown GW, Bifulco A, Veiel HOF, Andrews B. Self-esteem and depression. II. Social correlates of self-esteem. Soc Psychiatry Psychiatr Epidemiol 1990;25:225–234.

24. Cohen S, Wills TA. Stress, social support, and the buffering hypothesis. Psychol Bull 1985;89:310–357.

25. Gruen RJ. Stress and depression: Toward the development of integrative models. In: Goldberger L, Breznitz S, eds. Handbook of Stress: Theoretical and Clinical Aspects. New York: Free Press, 1993, pp. 550–569.

26. Brown GW, Andrews B, Harris T, et al. Social support, self-esteem and depression. Psychol Med 1986;16:813–831.

27. Brown GW, Bifulco A, Harris TO. Life events, vulnerability and onset of depression: Some refinements. Br J Psychiatry 1986:150:30–42.

28. Bromberger JT, Matthews KA. Employment status and depressive symptoms in middle-aged women: A longitudinal investigation. Am J Public Health 1994;84: 202–206.

29. Barnett RC, Baruch GK. Social roles, gender, and psychological distress. In: Barnett RC, Biener L, Baruch GK, eds. Gender and Stress. New York: Free Press, 1987, pp. 122–141.

30. Stephens MAP, Franks MM, Townsend AL. Stress and rewards in women's multiple roles: The case of women in the middle. Psychol Aging 1994;9:45–52.

31. Bebbington P, Hurry J, Tennant C, Sturt E Wing JK. Epidemiology of mental disorders in Camberwell. Psychol Med 1981;11:561–579.

32. Dohrenwend BS. Social status and stressful life events. J Pers Soc Psychol 1973;9:203–214.

33. Kessler RC, McLeod JD. Sex differences in vulnerability to undesirable life events. Am Sociol Rev 1984;49:620–631.

34. Wethington E, McLeod JD, Kessler RC. The importance of life events for explaining sex differences in psychological distress. In: Barnett RC, Biener L, Baruch GK, eds. Gender and Stress. New York: Free Press, 1987, pp. 144–156.

35. Nazroo JY, Edwards AC, Brown GW. Gender differences in the onset of depression following a shared life event: A study of couples. Psychol Med 1997;27:9–19.

36. Nolen-Hoeksema S, Girgus JS. The emergence of gender differences in depression during adolescence. Psychol Aging 1994;115:424–443.

37. Hill JP, Lynch ME. The intensification of gender-related role expectations during early adolescence. In: Brooks-Gunn J, Petersen AC, eds. Girls at Puberty. NY: Plenum Press, 1983, pp. 201–228.

38. Spence JT, Helmreich R. Masculinity and Femininity: Their Psychological Dimensions, Correlates and Antecedents. Austin, TX: University of Texas Press, 1979.

39. Ingram RE, Cruet D, Johnson BR, Wisnicki KS. Self-focused attention, gender role, and vulnerability to negative affect. J Pers Soc Psychol 1988;55:967–978.

40. Nolen-Hoeksema S, Morrow J. A prospective study of depression and post-traumatic stress symptoms after a natural disaster: The 1989 Loma Prieta earthquake. J Pers Soc Psychol 1991;61:115–121.

41. Nolen-Hoeksema S, Morrow J, Fredrickson BL. Response styles and the duration of episodes of depressed mood. J Abnorm Psychol 1993;102:20–28.

42. Alexander GG, French TM, eds. Studies in Psychosomatic Medicine: An Approach to the Cause and Treatment of Vegetative Disturbances. New York: Ronald, 1948.

43. Haynes S, Levine S, Scotch N, et al. The relationship of psychosocial factors to coronary heart disease in the Framingham Study: 1. Methods and risk factors. J Epidemiol 1978;107:362–383.

44. Whitley BE Jr. Sex-role orientation and psychological well-being: Two meta-analyses. Sex Roles 1984;12:207–225.

45. Nolen-Hoeksema S, Parker LE, Larson J. Ruminative coping with depressed mood following loss. J Pers Soc Psychol 1994;67:92–104.

46. Bromberger JT, Matthews KA. A "feminine" model of vulnerability to depressive symptoms: A longitudinal investigation of middle-aged women. J Pers Soc Psychol 1996;70:591–598.

47. Aspinwall LG, Taylor SE. Modeling cognitive adaptation: A longitudinal investigation of the impact of individual differences and coping on college adjustment and performance. J Pers Soc Psychol 1992;6:989–1003.

48. Holohan CJ, Moos RH. Life stressors, personal and social resources, and depression: A 4-year structural model. J Abnorm Psychol 1991;100:131–138.

49. Beck AT, Rush AJ, Shaw BF, Emery G. Cognitive Therapy of Depression. New York: Guilford Press, 1979.

50. Nolen-Hoeksema S. Sex Differences in Depression. Stanford, CA: Stanford University Press, 1990.

51. Teasdale JD. Cognitive vulnerability to persistent depression. Cognit Emotion 1988;2:247–274.

52. Sprock J, Yoder CY. Women and depression: An update on the report of the APA Task Force. Sex Roles 1997;36:269–303.

53. McEwen BS. Ovarian steroids have diverse effects on brain structure. In: Berg G, Hammar M, eds. The Modern Management of the Menopause. A Perspective for the 21st Century. New York: Parthenon, 1994, pp. 269–278.

54. Halbreich U, Lumley LA. The multiple interactional biological process that might lead to depression and gender differences in its appearance. J Affect Disord 1993; 29:159–173.

55. Gold PW, Frederick K, Goodwin MD, Chrousos GP. Clinical and biochemical manifestations of depression. Relation to the neurobiology of stress. N Engl J Med 1988; 319:413–419.

56. Chrousos GP, Gold PW. The concepts of stress and stress system disorders. Overview of physical and behavioral homeostasis. JAMA 1992;267:1244–1252.

57. Vamvakopoulos NC, Chrousos GP. Evidence of direct estrogenic regulation of human corticotropin releasing hormone gene expression. Potential implications for the sexual dimorphism of the stress response and immune/inflammatory reaction. J Clin Invest 1993;92:1896–1902.

58. Dorn LD, Burgess ES, Susman EJ, et al. Response to oCRH in depressed and nondepressed adolescents: Does gender make a difference? J Am Acad Child Psychiatry 1996;35:764–773.

59. Gallucci WT, Baum A, Laue L, et al. Sex differences in sensitivity of the hypothalamic pituitary adrenal axis. Health Psychol 1993;12:420–425.

60. Young EA, Katun J, Haskett RF, et al. Dissociation between pituitary and adrenal suppression to dexamethasone in depression. Arch Gen Psychiatry 1993;50: 395–403.

61. Frank E, Anderson B, Reynolds CF III, et al. Life events and the research diagnostic criteria endogenouse subtype. A confirmation of the distinction using the Bedford College methods. Arch Gen Psychiatry 1994;51:519–524.

62. Bebbington PE. Editorial: Sex and depression. Psychol Med 1998; 28:1–8.

63. McGee R, Feehan M, Williams S, et al. DMS-III disorders in a large sample of adolescents. J Am Acad Child Psychiatry 1990;29:611–619.

64. Freud A. Adolescence as a developmental disturbance. In: Kaplan G, Lebovici S, eds. Adolescence: Psychosocial Perspectives. New York: Basic Books, 1969, pp. 5–10.

65. Ferin M, Jewelewicz R, Warren M. The Menstrual Cycle. Physiology, Reproductive Disorders, and Infertility. New York: Oxford University Press, 1993, pp. 78–91.

66. Marshall WA, Tanner JM. Variations in pattern of pubertal changes in girls. Arch Dis Child 1969;44:291–303.

67. Peterson AC, Sarigiani PA, Kennedy RE. Adolescent depression: Why more girls? J Youth Adolesc 1991;20:247–271.

68. Brooks-Gunn J, Warren MP. Biological and social contributions to negative affect in young adolescent girls. Child Dev 1989;60:40–55.

69. Rutter M, Tizard J, Whitmore K. The Selection of Children with Psychiatric Disorder. Education, Health and Behavior. London: Longman, 1970.

70. Nottelmann ED, Inoff-Germain G, Susman EJ, Chrousos GP. Hormones and behavior at puberty. In: Bancroft J, Reinisch JM, eds. Adolescence and Puberty. New York: Oxford University Press, 1990, pp. 88–123.

71. Susman EJ, Nottelmann ED, Inoff-Germain GE, et al. The relation of relative hormone levels and physical development and socio-emotional behavior in young adolescents. J Youth Adolesc 1985;14:245–264.

71a. Frank E, Young E. Pubertal changes and adolescent challenges: Why rates of depression rise precipitously for girls between ages 10 and 15. In: Frank E, ed. Sex, Society and Madness: Gender and Psychopathology. Washington: American Psychiatric Press. (In press).

71b. Insel TR, Hulihan TJ. A gender-specific mechanism for pair bonding: oxytocin and partner preference formation in monogamous voles. Behav Neurosci 1995;109(4): 782–789.

71c. Carter CS, Williams JR, Witt DM, Insel TR. Oxytocin and social bonding. Ann New York Acad Sci 1992;652:204–211.

71d. Frank E. Assessment of life stress in depressed adolescents. Paper presented at the Annual Meeting of the Society for Research in Child Development, Washington, DC, April 1997.

72. Dennerstein L, Burrows GD. Affect and menstrual cycle. J Affect Disord 1979;1:77–92.

73. Merikangas KR, Foeldenyi M, Angst J. The Zurich Study. XIX. Patterns of menstrual disturbances in the community: Results of the Zurich Cohort Study. Eur Arch Psychiatry Clin Neurosci 1993;243:23–32.

74. Dan AJ, Monagle L. Sociocultural influences on women's experiences of perimenstrual symptoms. In: Gold JH, Severino SK, eds. Premenstrual Dyspohorias. Myths and Realities. Washington, DC: American Psychiatric Press, 1994, pp. 201–230.

75. Laessle RG, Tuschl RJ, Schweiger U, Pirke KM. Mood changes and physical complaints during the normal menstrual cycle in healthy young women. Psychoneuroendocrinology 1990;15:131–138.

76. Endicott J. The menstrual cycle and mood disorders. J Affect Disord 1993;29: 193–200.

77. Warner P, Bancroft J, Dixson A, Hampson M. The relationship between perimenstrual depressive mood and depressive illness. J Affect Disord 1991;23:9–23.

78. Pearlstein TB, Frank E, Rivera-Tovar A, et al. Prevalence of axis I and axis II disorders in women with late luteal phase dysphoric disorder. J Affect Disord 1990;20: 129–134.

79. Hurt SW, Schnurr PP, Severino SK, et al. Late luteal phase dysphoric disorder in 670 women evaluated for premenstrual complaints. Am J Psychiatry 1992;149:525–530.

80. Severino SK, Gold JH. Summation. In: JH Gold, SK Severino, eds. Premenstrual Dyspohorias. Myths and Realities. Washington, DC: American Psychiatric Press, 1994, pp. 231–248.

81. Rivera-Tovar AD, Frank E. Late luteal phase dysphoric disorder in young women. Am J Psychiatry 1990;147:1634–1636.

82. Rivera-Tovar AD, Pilkonis P, Frank E. Symptom patterns in late luteal-phase dysphoric disorder. J Psychopathol Behav Assess 1992;14:189–199.

83. Rubinow DR, Roy-Byrne P. Premenstrual syndromes: Overview from a methodologic perspective. Am J Psychiatry 1984:163–172.

84. Parry BL. Biological correlates of premenstrual complaints. In: Gold JH, Severino SK, eds. Premenstrual Dyspohorias. Myths and Realities. Washington, DC: American Psychiatric Press, 1994, pp. 47–66.

85. Rubinow DR, Hoban G, Grover GN, et al. Changes in plasma hormones across the menstrual cycle in patients with menstrually related mood disorders and in control subjects. Am J Obstet Gynecol 1988;158:5–11.

86. Watts JFF, Butt WR, Edwards LR, et al. Hormonal studies in women with premenstrual tension. Br J Obstet Gynecol 1985;92:247–255.

87. Hammarback S, Damber JE, Backstom T, et al. Relationship between symptom severity and hormone changes in women with premenstrual syndrome. J Clin Endocrinol Metab 1989;68:125–130.

88. Eriksson E, Sundblad C, Lisjo P, et al. Serum levels of androgens are higher in women with premenstrual irritability and dysphoria than in controls. Psychoneuroendocrinology 1992;17:195–204.

89. O'Hara MW, Schlechte JA, Lewis DA, Varner MW. Controlled prospective study of postpartum mood disorders: Psychological, environmental, and hormonal variables. J Abnorm Psychol 1991;100:63–73.

90. Kumar R, Robson KM. A prospective study of emotional disorders in childbearing women. Br J Psychiatry 1984;144:35–47.

91. Kessler RC, McGonagle KA, Swartz M, et al. Sex and depression in the National Commorbidity Survey I: Lifetime prevalence, chronicity and recurrence. J Affect Disord 1993;29:85–96.

92. Hopkins J, Marcus M, Campbell SB. Postpartum depression: A critical review. Psychol Bull 1984;95:498–515.

93. Campbell SB, Cohn JF, Flanagan C, et al. Course and correlates of postpartum depression during the transition to parenthood. Dev Pscyhopathol 1992;4:29–47.

94. O'Hara MW, Neunaber DJ, Zekoski EM. A prospective study of postpartum depression: Prevalence, course, and predictive factors. J Abnorm Psychol 1984;93:158–171.

95. Harris B. Biological and hormonal aspects of postpartum depressed mood. Working towards strategies for prophylaxis and treatment. Br J Psychiatry 1994;164:288–292.

96. Harris B, Lovett L, Smith J, et al. Cardiff puerperal mood and hormone study. III. Postnatal depression at 5 to 6 weeks postpartum, and its hormonal correlates across the peripartum period. Br J Psychiatry 1996;168:739–744.

97. Gregoire AJP, Kumar R, Everitt B, et al. Transdermal oestrogen for treatment of severe postnatal depression. Lancet 1996;347:930–933.

98. Weissman MM. The myth of involutional melancholia. JAMA 1979;242:742–744.

99. Weissman MM, Bruce ML, Leaf PJ, et al. Affective disorders in psychiatric disorders in America: The epidemiologic catchment area study. In: Robins LN, Regier DA, eds. Psychiatric Disorders in America: The Epidemiologic Catchment Area Study. New York: Free Press, 1992, pp. 53–80.

100. Radloff LS. The CES-D scale: A self-report depression scale for research in the general population. Appl Psychol Measur 1977;1:385–401.

101. Greene JG, Cooke DJ. Life stress and symptoms at the climacterium. Br J Psychiatry 1980;136:486–491.

102. Neugarten BL, Kraines RJ. "Menopause" symptoms in women of various ages. Psychosom Med 1965;27:266–273.

103. Porter M, Penny GC, Russell D, et al. A population based survey of women's experience of the menopause. Br J Obstet Gynaecol 1996;103:1025–1028.

104. Hunter M. The South-East England longitudinal study of the climacteric and postmenopause. Maturitas 1992;14:117–126.

105. Kaufert PA, Gilbert P, Tate R. The Manitoba Project: A re-examination of the link between menopause and depression. Maturitas 1992;14:143–155.

106. Matthews KA, Wing RR, Kuller LH, et al. Influence of the perimenopause on cardiovascular risk factors and symptoms of middle-aged health women. Arch Intern Med 1994;154:2349–2355.

107. McKinlay JB, McKinlay SM, Brambilla D. The relative contributions of endocrine changes and social circumstances to depression in mid-aged women. J Health Soc Behav 1987;28:345–363.

108. Matthews KA, Bromberger J, Egeland G. Behavioral antecedents and consequences of the menopause. In: Korenman SG, ed. The Menopause. Norwell, MA: Serono Symposia, 1990, pp. 1–15.

109. Hallstrom T, Samuelsson S. Mental health in the climacteric: The longitudinal study of women in Gothenburg. Acta Obstet Gynecol Scand [Suppl] 1985;130:13–18.

110. Bromberger JT, Matthews KA. A longitudinal study of the effects of pessimism, trait anxiety, and life stress on depressive symptoms in middle-aged women. Psychol Aging 1996;11:207–213.

111. McKinlay SM, Brambilla DJ, Posner JG. The normal menopause transition. Maturitas 1992;14:103–115.

112. Sherman BM, West JH, Korenman SG. Menopausal transition: Analysis of LH, FSH, estradiol, and progesterone concentrations during menstrual cycles of older women. J Clin Endocrinol Metab 1976;42:629–636.

113. Santoro N, Brown JR, Skurnick J, et al. Perimenopausal reproductive hormone excretion differs markedly from that of women with premature ovarian failure (POF). Presented at the 75th Annual Meeting of the Endocrine Society. Las Vegas, NV, June 1993, #1060A.

114. Ditkoff EC, Crary WG, Cristo M, Lobo RA. Estrogen improves psychological function in asymptomatic postmenopausal women. Obstet Gynecol 1991;78:991–995.

115. Sherwin BB. Affective changes with estrogen and androgen replacement therapy in surgically menopausal women. J Affect Disord 1988;14:177–187.

116. Sherwin BB. The impact of different doses of estrogen and progestin on mood and sexual behavior in postmenopausal women. J Clin Endocrinol Metab 1991;72:336–343.

117. Backstrom T. Effects of natural and synthetic gestagens on mood and brain excitability. In: Berg G, Hammar M, eds. The Modern Management of the Menopause. A Perspective for the 21st Century. New York: Parthenon, 1994, pp. 295–300.

118. Baischer W, Koinig G, Hartmann B, et al. Hypothalamic-pituitary-gonadal axis in depressed premenopausal women: Elevated blood testosterone concentrations compared to normal controls. Psychoneuroendocrinology 1995;20:553–559.

119. Schneider MA, Brotherton PL, Hailes J. The effect of exogenous oestrogens on depression in menopausal women. Med J Aust 1977;2:162–163.

120. Oppenheim G, Zohar J, Shapiro B, Belmaker RH. The role of estrogen in treating resistant depression. In: Zohar V, Belmaker RH, eds. Treating Resistant Depression. New York: PMA Publishing Corp, 1987, pp. 357–365.

121. Klaiber EL, Broverman DM, Vogel W, Kobayashi T. Estrogen therapy for severe persistent depressions in women. Arch Gen Psychiatry 1979;36:550–554.

4

COGNITION AND FRAILTY IN OLDER WOMEN: SOCIOECONOMIC AND PHYSIOLOGIC INFLUENCES

Anne B. Newman

This chapter deals with the influence of biology and socioeconomics on functional status and disability in women. Women live longer than men and experience more of the morbidity associated with longevity. However, some socioeconomic and biologic features seem to moderate the progression to dementia and frailty among the elderly. The influence of such factors as education, social support, and sex steroid hormones on diseases of aging is evaluated below. Methodological issues such as how to measure functional status and disability among women, including cognitive function, are also discussed.

LIFE EXPECTANCY AND ACTIVE LIFE EXPECTANCY

Improvement in infant and maternal health earlier in this century contributed to the increased life expectancy of women. Mortality rates have also declined among older women. From 1960 to 1990, mortality rates declined by 43% in women aged 65–74, 32% in those aged 75–84, and 24% in those aged 85 or more.[1] The number of adults aged 65 and older is increasing twice as fast as the total population. Over half of girls born today should reach their 85th birthday, and women reaching age 65 today can expect to live on average an additional 18 years. The most rapidly growing group is the "oldest old,"[2] those over age 85. In this group, women outnumber men by a ratio of 2.6 to 1.[3,4] Throughout life, beginning even at conception, the risk of mortality for women is less than for men.

Despite a substantial survival advantage over men, older women are at increased risk of dependency. This is related to both biologic and psychosocial factors. For example, the increased life expectancy of women and the tendency of women to be younger than their husbands lead to a higher risk of widowhood. Thus, older women are more likely to live alone in old age without the support of a caregiver. While half of the men aged 85 and older live with their wives, only 10% of women this age live with their husbands.[2] Consequently, one-quarter of women aged 85 and older live in nursing homes compared with 10% of men this age[5] (Fig. 4–1). Clearly, the burden of disability with aging should be of personal concern to all women.

While total life expectancy is a useful measure of the health status of a population, it does not reflect functional status and quality of life. As our population has aged and the prevalence of chronic disease has increased, the focus of health care and disease prevention in older adults has shifted from the reduction of mortality to the reduction of morbidity and improvement in quality of life.[6] Morbidity can be defined in many ways, including number of hospital days, doctor visits, diagnoses, and days of reduced activity. These methods are associated with, but do not describe the impact of, chronic disease on daily life. The functional impact of chronic disease in older adults is often quantified by the disability associated with multiple chronic conditions and illnesses. The period of life before disability occurs has been termed "active life expectancy." Ultimately, the success of preventive health interventions for older adults must be demonstrated by a reduction in morbidity or an increase in active life expectancy, resulting from a reduction in years of disability. An increase in active life expectancy has been targeted as one of the most important goals for the year 2000 by the U.S. Department of Health and Human Services.[7]

Because the total number of older people is increasing, it has become apparent that the number of dependent, disabled, older people will increase unless the burden of chronic conditions in old age can be reduced. Gains in total life expectancy have been accompanied by increases in active life expectancy and disabled life expectancy.[8,9] Data from the established populations of the Epidemiologic Study of the Elderly (EPESE) have been used to calculate both of these periods using life-table methods (Table 4–1). The absolute number of years of remaining life that is expected to be disabled is 1.4 to 1.7 years in older men and 2.7 to 3.8 years in older women. This absolute number of years of disability is fairly stable across 10-year age-groups from 65 to 85 years of age in both men and women, but because remaining life expectancy is shorter in the oldest groups, the proportion of remaining life that is disabled increases from about 15% in women at age 65 to about 45% in women at age 85. For men, the proportion of remaining life expectancy that is disabled is less at all ages, ranging from about 10% at age 65 to about 30%–40% at age 85. For African-Americans, active life expectancy is less before age 75 than for whites, but is higher after age 75. The biologic basis of these differences is not well understood. It is possible that the longer life expectancy in women is due to a higher reserve ca-

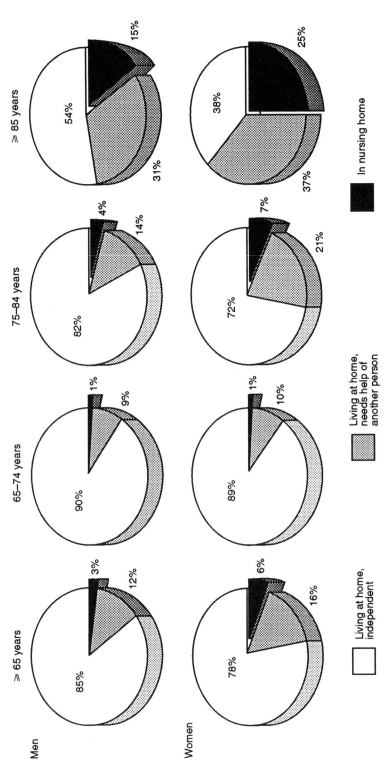

Figure 4–1. Percentage of the population that lives at home independently, at home but with the help of another person, or in a nursing home [Reprinted with permission from "The Aging of America," Vol. 263, No. 17, page 2337, Copyright 1990, American Medical Association[5]]

Table 4–1. Total Life Expectancy, Active Life Expectancy, and Disabled Life Expectancy at 65, 75, and 85 Years of Age, According to Sex and Race (in Years)

SUBGROUP	AT AGE 65			AT AGE 75			AT AGE 85		
	TOTAL	ACTIVE	DISABLED	TOTAL	ACTIVE	DISABLED	TOTAL	ACTIVE	DISABLED
Men									
Black	11.4	10.0	1.4	7.6	6.0	1.6	4.6	3.0	1.7
White	12.6	11.2	1.4	7.1	5.7	1.5	3.6	2.1	1.5
Women									
Black	18.7	15.9	2.8	13.4	10.4	3.0	9.0	5.8	3.2
White	18.6	16.0	2.7	11.8	9.0	2.8	6.9	3.9	3.0

[Reprinted from New England Journal of Medicine, Vol 329(2), Guralnik, et al., page 113, July 1993[9]]

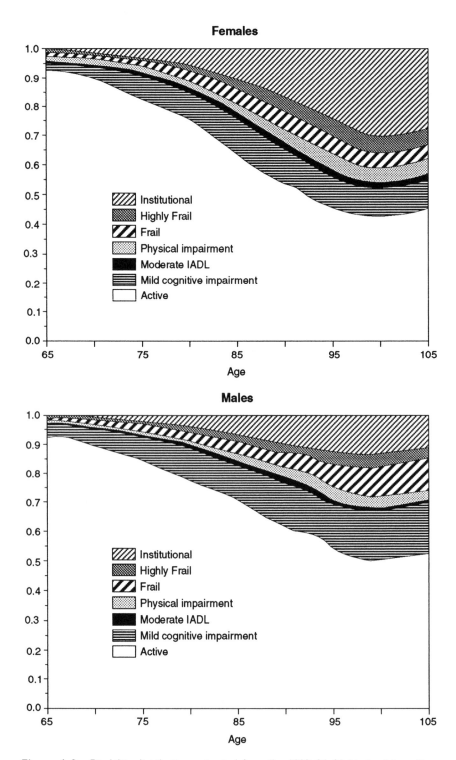

Figure 4–2. Disability distribution estimated from the 1982–84–89 National Long Term Care Survey [Reprinted from Journal of Gerontology, Vol. 48, Manton, et al., page 24, September 1993[12]]

pacity, including a tolerance of more disability. For older African-American women, those who are higher educated have the highest survival rates of all groups after age 75.[9] This group represents a unique survival cohort for the study of successful aging.

Although the number of older adults with disability represents a substantial public health burden, it should be noted that at all ages, most remaining life expectancy is free of disability. Furthermore, the proportion of remaining life that is disabled does not continue to increase after age 85 (Fig. 4–2). This is due to an eventual balance between the competing risks of mortality and increasing disablement.

There has been an ongoing debate about the potential for compressing the period of disability or morbidity at the end of life.[10,11] It appears that at least for much of this century, the increase in life expectancy has been associated with an increased duration of chronic disease. There is limited evidence that the prevalence of disability is decreasing; however, it is being closely evaluated. Some new evidence suggests that disability may be declining. Using disability rates and institutionalization incidences from the National Long-term Care Survey, Manton et al. recently reported a decline in disability since 1984.[12]

DISABILITY: DEFINITION AND METHODS

Disability in older adults is usually due to the combined presence of multiple comorbid conditions and to the decreased physiologic reserve that occurs with aging.[13] For example, disability from the most common disease of older women, osteoarthritis, is greatly compounded by another common condition, heart disease, and both together compound disability with increasing age.[14]

Disability is usually defined in terms of difficulty reported in performing essential tasks that are necessary for living in the community. These include self-care tasks, or *activities of daily living* (ADLs); household and community activities such as housekeeping, cooking, and financial management, or *instrumental activities of daily living* (IADLs); and sometimes, mobility tasks. As a measure of morbidity, disability has been shown to be related to number of bed or hospital days, comorbidity, institutionalization, and mortality. It is also related to care needs, thus making it a useful measure for health services research.[15]

Disability in ADLs and IADLs reflects the impact of both physical and cognitive impairments of an individual on complex task performance. The methods by which disability or function have been ascertained in most epidemiologic studies is by self-report. Most commonly, a self-report of any difficulty with task performance is defined as disability. Other methods include assessing the frequency of an individual's needing assistance and the self-report of ability. At least 43 different published indices of disability have been identified.[16]

These variations can create major differences in the reported prevalence of disability. For example, a report of any difficulty reflects less severe impairment than a report of needing the help of another person. In addition to these problems of self-reporting disability, cognitively impaired individuals underreport disability, relative to an observer or proxy. Proxy response is also problematic in that proxies tend to overreport disability, relative to the patient's report[17] or observed performance.[18,19]

Particularly important for the understanding of disability in women is the gender bias found in many IADL questionnaires. Many of the activities included are household tasks, the majority of which are done by women (cleaning, shopping, meal preparation). There may also be bias by ethnicity due to different social expectations about performance, although it is likely that much of this difference may be attributed to actual higher rates of disease related to ethnicity.

In more recent epidemiologic studies, self-report data have been supplemented by direct assessment of performance.[20] Measurements usually include gait speed, grip strength, and timed performance of more complex tasks. Such measures are more reproducible, and they are less influenced by language, culture, or gender. They are also likely to be more sensitive to change in function. Measurements of gait speed, balance, and chair stands in the EPESE study have been shown to be associated with subsequent institutionalization and incident disability,[21,22] thus indicating that change in performance may serve as a useful intermediate outcome measure in studies of disability.

Assessment indicating poorer performance has also been associated with self-reported disability in the Cardiovascular Health Study[23] and the Women's Health and Aging Study.[24] The combination of poor performance and self-reported disability was associated with recurrent falling in women in the Study of Osteoporotic Fractures (SOF).[25] Performance measures are likely to be more sensitive to change in function and early decline than self-report. However, most measures were developed to distinguish disabled from non-disabled adults and thus tend to be limited in the ability to distinguish among individuals functioning in the normal range.[26] More work needs to be done to develop tests that are sufficiently challenging to distinguish individuals at higher levels of function.

DISABILITY AND COGNITIVE FUNCTION

Cognitive impairment is a major cause of disability and a major contributing factor to the need for institutional care.[27] The proportion of disability in a community due to cognitive impairment is more difficult to assess directly than physical impairment, as early impairment is often not recognized and such individuals are unlikely to attribute disability to cognitive impairment. In addition, dementia is underreported in medical records. The prevalence of dementia in older adults living in the community is best detected by cognitive screening tests. It has been found to be substantial, increasing from 5% to 30% from age 65 to 85.[28,29] Screening tests for dementia are now included in most epidemiologic studies of older adults. These tests were developed to distinguish demented from nondemented individuals and do not discriminate well in the normal range. Another major problem with the interpretation of cognitive tests is that performance on these tests is strongly influenced by education. However, the test scores are not in and of themselves diagnostic for dementia. Diagnosis requires documentation of decline from a prior level of function; educational attainment is often used as a proxy for prior function.

The diagnosis of dementia also requires documented decline in cognitive performance to a degree that interferes with daily life. Tests for dementia should be combined with assessment of disability. Intelligence tests may be better able to detect early changes in performance within the normal range, which are analogous to subclinical disability.

To assess higher-functioning adults, including those with post-high-school education and those functioning in the normal range, tests assessing normal intelligence in healthy adults have been adopted in many studies. For example, the Digit Symbol Substitution Test, which is included in the Wechsler Intelligence Scale, has been shown to be a predictor of mortality in the Western Collaborative Group Study[30] and the Cardiovascular Health Study.[31] It is hypothesized that this test measures processing speed in the central nervous system. Such tests may measure cognitive reserve or detect early cognitive loss.

DISABILITY AND COMORBIDITY

Most older adults have more than one chronic condition,[32] thus in the study of any one disease or condition of older adults, the presence and severity of other comorbid conditions must be evaluated (Fig. 4–3). In a national U.S. survey, half of those over age 60 had two or more chronic conditions and a quarter had three or more. These conditions are also associated with a high prevalence of medication use. As stated above, disability may summarize the simultaneous effects of multiple diseases and conditions. In addition, disability may also account for the severity of conditions.

Comorbidity can be assessed by simple counts of diagnosed medical conditions or by direct assessment of organ function. Charlson et al. described a method of combining diagnoses by organ system and severity that has been widely used in clinical studies.[33] Assessment of comorbidity is crucial for making valid comparisons between patient groups.[34] Although disability increases with the number of comorbid conditions, it is not the same as comorbidity, as some diseases have greater functional consequences than others.[35] For example,

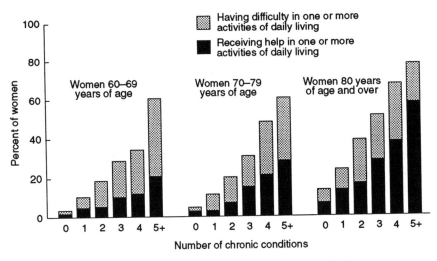

Figure 4–3. Prevalence of women 60 years of age and over having difficulty in one or more activities of daily living by number of chronic conditions and age-group [Reprinted with permission from Advance Data from Vital and Health Statistics, No. 170, Guralnik, et al., page 7, May 1989, Copyright 1989, Massachusetts Medical Society. All rights reserved[32]]

arthritis, when severe, is more likely to cause functional impairment than heart disease. Hypertension, on the other hand, has no direct functional impact. Therefore, the number of conditions does not explain disability.

Few studies have evaluated the specific type of disability attributable to specific diseases and conditions. Recent data from the Cardiovascular Health Study (CHS)[35] show that most disability is attributable to arthritis and other musculoskeletal disease, particularly among women. In women age 65 and older, 55% who had difficulty with one or more ADLs or IADLs attributed this to arthritis (Table 4–2). In the study of osteoporotic fractures, conditions associated with at least a 50% increase in the prevalence of disability included diabetes, stroke, Parkinsonism, cataracts, osteoarthritis, and osteoporosis. Back pain and fracture history were independently associated with disability (Table 4–3). More work needs to be done in further evaluating the types of arthritis and musculoskeletal conditions leading to disability and the interactions of comorbid conditions contributing to disability.

DISABILITY AND FRAILTY

Disability is not equivalent to frailty. Frailty can be defined as a state of vulnerability to adverse health outcomes, including morbidity and mortality. Frailty is due to a lack of physiologic reserve of the organism or critical organ systems to respond to environmental stress.[36] Therefore, disability is more likely to occur in frail individuals, who are at risk because of decreased physiologic reserve.

Table 4–2. Diseases Reported to Cause Difficulty with Physical Tasks

	MEN			WOMEN		
	PERCENT OF PERSONS $N = 765^a$		PERCENT OF TASKS $N = 1655^b$	PERCENT OF PERSONS $N = 1520^a$		PERCENT OF TASKS $N = 4053^b$
Arthritis or other musculoskeletal diseases	38.6	(290)*	32.9	55.1	(830)	46.5
Cancer	0.5	(4)	0.3	0.9	(13)	0.6
Diabetes	1.1	(8)	1.4	1.1	(17)	0.8
Heart disease	15.7	(118)	11.7	12.9	(194)	10.6
Hypertension	0.4	(3)	0.2	1.7	(25)	0.9
Injury	10.1	(76)	7.5	13.2	(198)**	9.7
Lung disease	7.3	(55)	7.4	5.4	(81)	4.2
Mental disorders	0.1	(1)	0.1	0.6	(9)**	0.4
Old age	12.9	(97)**	8.0	11.3	(170)***	6.8
Stroke*	5.3	(40)	8.7	1.8	(27)	2.1
Other	28.6	(215)	21.8	28.1	(424)	17.5

Numbers in parentheses are number of participants.

^{a}Total number of participants reporting difficulty.

^{b}Total number of tasks in which there was difficulty.

*Significant gender differences, Chi-Square test, $P < 0.01$.

**Chi-Square test for trend with gender, $P < 0.01$, percent increases with age.

***Chi-Square test for association within race, within gender, $P < 0.01$, non-white greater than white.

[Reprinted from Journal of the American Geriatrics Society, Vol. 42, No. 10, Ettinger, et al., Page 1040, October 1994[35]]

Table 4–3. Multi-variate Model of Impaired Function[a]

VARIABLES	ODDS RATIO (95% CI)[b]	P-VALUE
Diabetes	1.20 (0.93–1.54)	0.17
Stroke	1.47 (1.04–2.08)	0.03
Parkinsonism	2.28 (1.11–4.67)	0.02
Cataracts	1.23 (1.03–1.45)	0.02
Osteoarthritis	2.29 (1.85–2.82)	0.0001
Back pain	1.66 (1.35–2.04)	0.0001
Osteoporosis	1.62 (1.34–1.96)	0.0001
Hip fracture since age 50	2.40 (1.57–3.65)	0.0001

[a]Impaired function defined as difficulty performing three or more physical and instrumental ADLs.
[b]Odds ratios were calculated with the use of multiple logistic regression ($n = 9052$).

[Reprinted from Journal of American Geriatrics Society, Vol. 42(5), Ensrud, et al., page 486, 1994[42]]

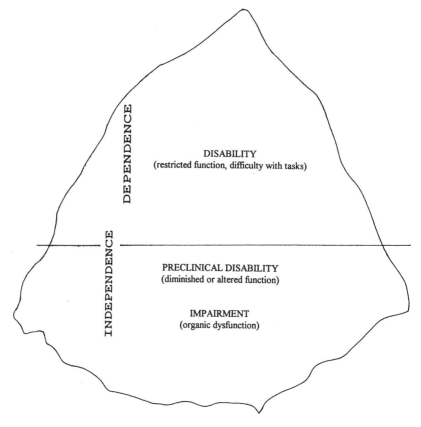

Figure 4–4. The iceberg of disability. Note that clinical recognition of disability generally occurs when independence is affected. The states below the waterline are hypothesized to include both impairment and preclinical disability. [Reprinted from the Journal of Aging and Health, Vol. 3, No. 2, Fried, et al., page 289, May 1991[37]]

Closer scrutiny of those at risk reveals that with more careful measurement, early changes in function or adaptations to impairment can be detected before frank disability is reported.[37] These changes have been referred to as "subclinical disability" (Fig. 4–4). The use of performance-based measures of function has demonstrated that prior to the development of frank disability, relatively poorer performance can be detected.[21,22] Much of the literature regarding frailty in older adults has subsumed both the at-risk and the disabled under the term frailty. Others consider only the most disabled to be frail.[38] The use of performance measures of function, such as strength measures, cognitive assessment, and task performance, has been coupled with the use of technologies to measure specific impairments of important, corresponding organ systems to better define those at risk. For example, poorer muscle strength as well as low bone mass predict hip fracture and disability in older women. MRI of the brain has been added to data on cognitive performance to predict cognitive decline. As more detailed data on performance and organ impairment are analyzed, we will be more able to distinguish those with subclinical disability as frail.

Thus frailty, when defined as at risk, is multidimensional and somewhat difficult to assess at a systemic level. A model of the path to disability and handicap that has been proposed by the World Health Organization is often used as a conceptual framework for the study of risk factors for disability.[39] In this model (Fig. 4–5), impairment is defined as an abnormality in the function or structure of a psychological, physiological, or anatomical system (organ level), while disability is defined as an abnormality in the person (organism level). Most

DISEASE ·······> IMPAIRMENT ·······> DISABILITY ·······> HANDICAP

Impairment
In the context of health experience, an impairment is any loss or abnormality of psychologic, physiologic, or anatomic structure or function

Disability
In the context of health experience, a disability is any restriction or lack (resulting from an impairment) of ability to perform an activity in the manner or with the range considered normal for a human being

Handicap
In the context of health experience, a handicap is a disadvantage for a given individual, resulting from an impairment or a disability, that limits or prevents the fulfilment of a role that is normal (depending on age, sex, and social and cultural factors) for that individual

Figure 4–5. World Health Organization model of impairment, disability, and handicap [Reprinted with permission from World Health Organization, page 27–30, 1980[39]]

studies of the mediators of the transition from robust to frail health use these definitions to classify levels of complexity in the study of frailty.

RISK FACTORS FOR PHYSICAL DISABILITY AND FRAILTY

Important factors in the path from health to disability and frailty in old age have been identified in evaluating health outcomes for specific chronic diseases. For example, much of the interest in estrogen and its effect on aging comes from its important role in the pathogenesis of both osteoporosis and coronary artery disease.

Other potential mediators of disability and frailty have been identified from the study of aging. Important changes in the endocrine and immune systems that are seen in aging animals and humans are currently under evaluation in population studies. Several of these mediators are related to physical disability and frailty as well as to cognitive disability and dementia. Clinical diseases including stroke, heart disease, and osteoporosis all contribute to disability.[35,40–42] Because the risk factors for and mediators of many of these specific conditions have been discussed in other chapters, only factors that pertain to disability in general will be reviewed here.

PSYCHOSOCIAL FACTORS

Several psychological, social, and economic factors have been shown to be related to health outcomes; the role of social support to health outcomes in older adults has been reviewed recently.[43] For older women, the factors that have emerged as most significant with respect to disability and cognitive function include education, and caregiving related to social support and depression.

Education is generally protective against multiple adverse health outcomes, although its relation to physical function has shown conflicting results. In the McArthur Study of Successful Aging, those individuals with higher education had higher physical function at baseline but were more likely to show decline after 3 years of follow-up.[26] Among older African-Americans and Caucasians, education has a greater effect on active life expectancy than race (Table 4–4). In all age, race, and gender groups, those with higher education had better functional status and fewer years of disability. The longest remaining and active life expectancy was seen among African-American women over age 75, who had significantly more years of both active and total life expectancy than white women, particularly those who had 12 or more years of education. These African-American women were likely to live another 17.1 years, with 13.5 years of active life expectancy. The relationship of education to active life expectancy has important implications for the prevention of disability. Women with higher education have been shown to have better, lifelong health practices.[44] Increases in the level of education achieved by women during this cen-

Table 4–4. Total Life Expectancy, Active Life Expectancy, and Disabled Life Expectancy in Women at 65, 75, and 85 Years of Age, According to Educational Status (in years)

SUBGROUP[a]	AT AGE 65			AT AGE 75			AT AGE 85		
	TOTAL	ACTIVE	DISABLED	TOTAL	ACTIVE	DISABLED	TOTAL	ACTIVE	DISABLED
Lower education									
Black	18.2	15.6	2.7	13.0	10.1	2.9	8.7	5.6	3.1
White	17.8	15.2	2.6	11.1	8.4	2.7	6.4	3.5	2.9
Higher education									
Black	22.8	19.5	3.3	17.1	13.5	3.6	12.2	8.4	3.8
White	21.1	18.0	3.0	13.9	10.7	3.2	8.6	5.2	3.4

[a] A lower education level was defined as less than 12 years of school completed, and a higher education level as 12 years or more.

[Reprinted from New England Journal of Medicine, Vol. 329(2), Guralnik, et al., page 113, July 1993[a]]

tury may translate into future reductions in the period of disability an improvement in active life expectancy.

A second important social factor that is particularly common in women is
that women are frequently caregivers for a disabled spouse or parent. While
having social support and contacts has been shown to be an independent predictor of independent functioning,[45] the importance of providing support as a caregiver has only more recently been studied.[46] Caregiving provides an important
social role as well as a major stress on the caregivers; those caring for patients
with dementia are particularly at risk for poorer health.[47–49]

Depressive symptoms are also related to function,[23] although the direction
of the association is not clear. Depressive symptoms are more common in disabled people but appear to be attenuated by increased social support.[50] Older
women have higher rates of depressive symptomatology than men, perhaps because they have increased rates of disability.[51] Alternatively, those with depression are more likely to report impairment. In a study of performance in older
men and women, however, depression score or history of a nervous or emotional disorder was independently associated with lower scores for gait speed,
chair stand, and grip strength in women. Psychological factors contributed more
to performance than measures of prevalent disease, which suggests that motiva-
tion has a large effect on performance.[52]

BEHAVIORAL AND COHORT FACTORS

Behavioral factors such as smoking, physical activity, and obesity have been
studied in relation to specific diseases and mortality as well as to disability.
Much of these data reflect the experience of the specific age-cohort studied.
Studies of older women today may differ from future studies because of differences in life experience in successive cohorts. Older women in the 1990s, who
were born between 1900 and 1920, compared with future cohorts of women
born after 1930 experienced higher rates of maternal mortality and childhood
infectious diseases, including measles, polio, small pox, and a major influenza
epidemic in 1917. Nutritional deficiencies were more common during their
childhood, and antibiotics were not available until the 1930s. There are also
huge differences in education level in successive birth cohorts (Table 4–4). Improvements in public health may improve health outcomes in future cohorts of
older women.

One of the most dramatic changes in behavior affecting public health over
the course of this century is the increase in cigarette smoking in women, which
has already led to a rise in lung cancer in women. Rates of exposure to cigarette
smoke in the older-women cohorts are relatively low, ranging from 10% to
15%.[40–42] Future studies may show increases in lung cancer and osteoporosis as
well as increased effects on disability, as the prevalence of smoking has in-

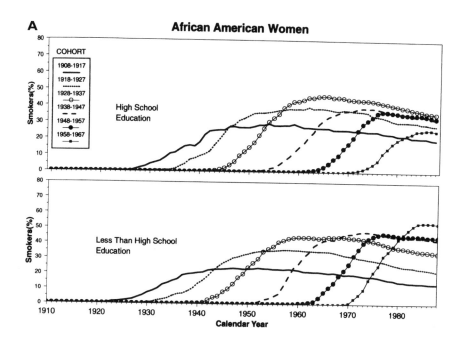

A

African American Women

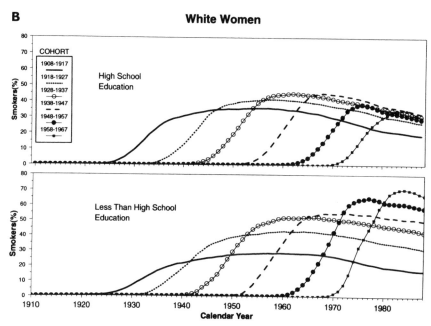

B

White Women

Figure 4–6. Smoking prevalence among birth cohorts of African-American women **(A)** [Reprinted with permission from American Journal of Public Health, Vol. 86, No. 2, Escobedo and Peddicord, page 234, February 1996, Copyright 1996, American Public Health Association[57]] and white woman **(B)** by educational attainment, 1978–1980, 1987, 1988 National Health Interview Surveys[57] [Reprinted from American Journal of Public Health, Vol. 86, No. 2, Escobedo and Peddicord, page 233, February 1996[57]]

101

creased with successive cohorts, especially among those women with less than a high school education (Fig 4–6a,b).[53]

In studies of disability in older women, smoking is significantly associated with disability, although its effect is diminished when adjusted for smoking-related comorbid conditions.[42] Continued smoking predicts a subsequent decline in function as measured by self-report[38] and performance[43] as well as increased cardiovascular morbidity and mortality.[54]

Obesity also contributes to disability in women.[40,42,55] In the Study of Osteoporotic Fractures, measurement of function was assessed by self-reported difficulty in 6 ADLs and IADLs. For each 5 kg/m^2 of body mass index (BMI) the risk of subsequent self-reported disability was increased by 65%—independent of age, comorbidity, and other factors. Obesity also predicts a decline in physical performance.[26] The association between disability and obesity may be mediated by its association with osteoarthritis.[53,56]

Physical activity in relation to disability is difficult to assess cross-sectionally as disability would be expected to limit the physical activity. Nevertheless, it is plausible that physical activity could increase functional reserve and thus be protective against disability. Once disability occurs, further inactivity may accelerate the process, causing further loss of bone and muscle mass and loss of strength and endurance.[36] Higher-functioning older adults report higher participation in moderate and strenuous exercise and are more likely to maintain performance.[45]

Several intervention trials of various types of exercise have demonstrated that performance can be improved. Muscle strength and mass are increased with resistance exercise,[58] balance is improved with training,[59,60] and arthritic pain is relieved and distance walked is improved with either strength training or endurance training.[61] These studies have demonstrated that physical function, even at advanced ages, is plastic. Evidence is also mounting that improvements in function can be maintained and can prevent adverse health outcomes such as falls and hip fracture.[59] In addition, there is adequate evidence that exercise improves risk factors such as lipids and bone density for many chronic conditions associated with disability in old age.[62,63]

SARCOPENIA

Aging is associated with a loss of muscle and bone mass and a relative increase in the proportion of fat mass. The loss in bone mass (osteoporosis) has been shown to be related to multiple disease- and age-associated factors; this is discussed in Chapter 8. Muscle strength is directly related to muscle mass. The difference in strength between men and women can be accounted for in part by the lower muscle mass in women.[64,65] The loss of muscle mass with age is called "sarcopenia".[66]

Numerous factors have been hypothesized to influence the decline in muscle mass during old age. These include hormonal factors such as estrogen and adrenal androgens, body weight, physical activity, smoking, poor health, and genetic factors.[67] Few studies have been done to assess these factors or to evaluate the relationship of muscle mass and strength with function and disability. It seems likely that decline in physical function among older adults may be related in part to loss of muscle mass and strength.[68]

Future research will identify the factors associated with sarcopenia and loss of strength and function, the goal being to identify factors amenable to intervention. Interventions already under study include exercise, as well as nutritional and trophic factor supplementation.[69-71]

HORMONES

Age-related changes in endocrine function are likely to contribute to frailty through decline in muscle mass, strength, and neuromuscular function that characterize aged individuals. In women the loss of ovarian estrogen after menopause has been studied most extensively, particularly regarding the effects of estrogen replacement on cardiovascular disease and osteoporosis and on cognitive function and genitourinary function.[44] Although estrogen replacement therapy is associated with lower cardiovascular disease mortality and higher bone mass, it has not been associated with less disability.[42]

Estrogen levels in women vary significantly with obesity and body fat distribution. Obesity is also negatively associated with sex steroid–binding globulin, which binds estrogens and androgens and is a marker of androgenicity. Body fat distribution and the different hormonal patterns associated with abdominal obesity may have specific effects on the health of older women. Postmenopausal estrogen levels are largely determined by the peripheral aromatization of plasma adrenal androstenedione to estrone. Abdominal obesity appears to be associated with a relatively more androgenic profile and thus may be less protective than peripheral adiposity against loss of lean mass.[72]

Other hormonal factors appear to be important in the maintenance of strength and muscle mass. Dehyroepiandrosterone (DHEA) is an adrenal precursor to both androgens and estrogens. Serum levels of DHEA and DHEA sulfate are lower in older adults and lower in men, but not women, with cardiovascular disease.[73,74] Higher levels correspond with preserved function in older men and women.[75] DHEA has been shown to increase muscle mass in patients with chronic diseases such as AIDS and lupus. Thus, this drug holds promise as a potential method to limit the loss of lean mass that occurs with aging. Androgenic effects are associated with its use in women, including potential adverse effects on lipid profile.[76] DHEA also has a role in the regulation of insulin sensitivity and insulin-like growth factor-1. Treatment of women with lower doses of DHEA, perhaps in combination with estrogen, may prove to be an effective strategy to prevent frailty in women.[77]

Growth hormone is another important trophic factor that decreases with age, leading to a decline in function in older adults. Decreased basal and pulsatile secretion of growth hormone and insulin-like growth factor may contribute to decreased muscle and bone mass in both men and women.[78] Trials of growth hormone replacement have been conducted in men only and have shown significant increases in muscle (2.5 kg) and bone mass (5.1%), although no improvement in strength or exercise tolerance has occurred.[79] These changes do not increase function, but they may prevent levels of muscle mass from reaching critical thresholds and delay the onset of disability. More research is needed to determine long-term effects on function.[77]

DEMENTIA AND COGNITIVE FUNCTION

Dementia is a syndrome with numerous potential etiologies, including alcohol use, head trauma, and vitamin deficiencies.[80] Over 90% of cases, however, are attributed to Alzheimer's disease and vascular disease. Variations in classification of dementia subtypes have led to some variation in the prevalence, although there is general agreement that about 5% of the population is affected at age 65, and the rate increases to over a third of those individuals over 80.[29] Several risk factors for dementia have been evaluated; the most important of these for women are level of education and estrogen exposure. Risk factors for vascular disease also contribute indirectly to cognitive impairment by causing small strokes and perhaps brain atrophy. Recently, new information about genetic markers of dementia have been explored, including the phenotype of apolipoprotein E.

Higher education has been shown consistently to prevent dementia and cognitive decline.[81,82] The relationship of education to dementia is confounded by the fact that the screening and diagnostic tests for cognitive disfunction are strongly influenced by level of education. Higher education is in part a marker for higher socioeconomic status, thus it may be a surrogate for better health practices or lower exposure to illness or injury. Education may develop brain capacity early in the life span, thus increasing cognitive reserve that could delay the appearance of impairment. It may also be that individuals with higher brain capacity receive more education because of ability, thus making education a marker of a high reserve capacity. A recent long-term follow-up of a group of nuns showed that those with more complex language skills in writing samples were less likely to be diagnosed as demented over 50 years later. This suggests that the development of dementia is related to lower reserve capacity and cognitive ability in youth.[83]

Estrogen replacement therapy has been evaluated as a treatment for dementia as well as a protective factor in maintaining cognitive function in women during late life. Estrogen has been shown to increase cholinergic function,[84] which is deficient in Alzheimer's disease, and may effect other neurotransmitters as well. In addition, estrogen may exert a beneficial effect on cognitive function by improving blood flow or decreasing the risk of stroke. A case-controlled study of Alzheimer's disease showed a reduced odds ratio (0.69, 95% CI 0.46–1.03) of dementia in estrogen users. Risk was also associated with increased dose, longer use, and factors related to endogenous estrogen levels.[85] In contrast, a large study of cognitive function in women from the Rancho Bernardo cohort showed no association between estrogen use and cognitive function.[86] Because estrogen replacement therapy has many other potential benefits for older women and because dementia has such a devastating impact on independence and quality of life during old age, a clinical trial of estrogen to prevent dementia has been added to the Women's Health Initiative. The Women's Health Initiative is a 10-year, randomized clinical trial of the effects of estrogen replacement therapy on cardiovascular disease and stroke.

Cardiovascular disease, including stroke and hypertension, has also been associated with cognitive loss of function in late life. Up to half of the cases of dementia in a representative sample of 85-year-olds in Gothenburg, Sweden, met criteria for vascular dementia.[28] In a U.S. survey, vascular dementia was much less commonly diagnosed, although dementia was more common.[29] Although cardiovascular disease is more common among men, vascular dementia and Alzheimer's dementia have similar prevalence and severity in men and women. Higher systolic blood pressure has been associated with cognitive performance almost 30 years later in men in the Honolulu Heart Study.[86a] Unfortunately, many early cohort studies were conducted with men only, so long-term follow-up data for women are more rare. Nevertheless, it is likely that the relationship of vascular disease to cognitive decline is similar in men and women.[87]

Finally, genetic factors for the development of dementia and cognitive impairment have been identified, especifically those associated with Alzheimer's disease. Alzheimer's disease is clinically defined by the presence of established criteria, including loss of memory and at least two other cognitive functions, such as language impairment and visual–spacial difficulties, with no other cause, such as stroke or trauma, to explain the deficits.[80] Pathologic criteria include the presence of widespread senile plaques and neurofibrillary tangles throughout the cerebral cortex. There are 6 known mutations on chromosome 21 that are associated with early-onset Alzheimer's; these are related to an abnormal amyloid precursor protein, a component of the senile plaque. Abnormal chromosome 19 is associated with late-onset Alzheimer's disease.[88] Variable genes on chromosome 19 lead to the production of the 4 different alleles of apolipoprotein E (APO-E4). APO-E4 is a risk factor for Alzheimer's disease and apparently causes the deposition of beta-amyloid. This gene is associated not only with clinical dementia but also with the deposition of beta-amyloid in the brain of older adults who are not demented.[89] Although women appear to be affected at the same rate as men, the number of women affected is greater because of their longer survival.

CONCLUSIONS

Much has been learned about health and disability in older women by the study of specific chronic diseases and the syndrome of frailty. Although women are more likely to live with disability than men, many factors related to disability, such as psychosocial and behavioral factors, are amenable to modification and prevention. Care must be taken with further research in evaluating the experiences, environmental factors, and behavior of younger cohorts on outcomes, particularly with regard to the increased rates of smoking among younger cohorts. Continued efforts are needed to promote heathy lifestyles and behavior for young women.

One of the lessons of the study of disability in old age is that multiple conditions need to be considered simultaneously to understand active life expectancy. Most women will have more than one chronic condition and each has specific biologic mediators. The focus on active life expectancy as an outcome allows multiple diseases and conditions to be evaluated simultaneously. The risk factors for geriatric syndromes, including physical disability and dementia, overlap. A goal of future research on interventions should be to modify shared risk factors and assess multiple outcomes.[44,90] The Women's Health Initiative Clinical Trial of Estrogen Replacement is an important example of this. Outcomes to be evaluated include cardiovascular disease, osteoporosis, breast cancer, dementia, and function and quality of life.

The study of individual conditions can result in arbitrary distinctions between aging and disease. Since many conditions are present, perhaps subclinically, in older adults, a better approach is to quantitate the degree of pathology and identify risk factors for progression. For example, the Study of Osteoporotic Fractures has taken this approach to the study of decline in bone mass by identifying factors associated with bone loss in addition to assessing factors related to falls and fractures. The study of osteoarthritis would benefit from a similar approach but has been hindered by the insensitivity of knee X-rays in detecting changes in joint pathology. There are several other conditions contributing to disability in women that would also benefit from further study, including hearing and visual impairment.

The research on hormones and trophic factors in aging is promising, but it must be subject to randomized trials. Outcomes should include both physical and cognitive function. Given the marked difference in survival and active life expectancy between men and women, sex steroid hormones would appear to hold promise for explaining some of the gender differences.

The importance of education's role in protecting against disability and cognitive loss also needs to be clarified. There are probably significant genetic and environmental factors related to education that explain its strong effect on active life expectancy. Finally, as women are more likely to be providing care to others, social support must be looked at in terms of both support received and support given.

In summary, the study of disability and dementia in older women requires a cross-cutting approach. Young women have bright prospects for a long, healthy, active life, but we can do better.

REFERENCES

1. National Center for Health Statistics. Moss AF, Parson VL. Current estimates from the National Health Interview Survey, United States, 1985. Vital and Health Statistics, Ser. 10, No. 160; DHHS Publ. No. 8601558. Washingtion, DC: Public Health Service, 1986; pp. 13, 82–83, 106, 118.

2. Campion EW. The oldest old. New Engl J Med 1994;330(25):1819–1820.

3. Bureau of the Census. Current Population Reports. Special Studies. Sixty-Five plus in America. Washington, DC: Government Printing Office, 1993 (P23-178RV).

4. Day JC. Bureau of the Census. Current Population Reports. Population Projections of the United States by Age, Sex, Race, and Hispanic Origin: 1993 to 2050 (middle series). Washington, DC: Government Printing Office, 1993, P 25–1104.

5. Schneider EL, Guralnik JM. The aging of America: Impact on health care costs. JAMA 1990;263(17):2335–2340.

6. Fried LP, Bush TL. Morbidity as a focus of preventive health care in the elderly. Epidemiol Rev 1988;10:48–64.

7. Healthy People 2000: National Health Promotion and Disease Prevention Objectives. Washington, DC: Department of Health and Human Services, 1990.

8. Branch LG, Guralnik JM, Foley DJ, et al. Active life expectancy for 10,000 caucasian men and women in three communities. J Gerontol 1991;46(4):M145–M150.

9. Guralnik JM, Land KC, Blazer D, Fillenbaum GG, Branch LG. Educational status and active life expectancy among older blacks and whites. New Engl J Med 1993:329(2):110–116.

10. Fries JF. Aging, natural death, and the compression of morbidity. N Engl J Med 1980;303:130–135.

11. Black PH, Levy EM. Aging, natural death, and the compression of morbidity: Another view. N Engl J Med 1983;309:854–855.

12. Manton KG, Corder LS, Stallard E. Estimates of change in chronic disability and institutional incidence and prevalence rates in the U.S. elderly population from the 1982, 1984, and 1989 National Long Term Care Survey. J Gerontol 1993;48(4): 5153–5166.

13. Verbrugge LM, Lepkowski JM, Imanaka Y. Comorbidity and its impact on disability. Milbank Mem Fund Q 1989;67(suppl 2):13–57.

14. Ettinger WH, Davis MA, Neuhaus JM, Mallon KM. Long-term physical functioning in persons with knee osteoarthritis from NHANESI: Effects of comorbid medical conditions. J Clin Epidemiol 1994;47:809–815.

15. Branch LG, Meyers AR. Assessing physical function in the elderly. Clin Geriatr Med 1987;3(1):29–51.

16. Feinstein AR, Josephy BR, Wells CK. Scientific and clinical problems in indexes of functional disability. Ann Intern Med 1986;105:413–420.

17. Magaziner J, Simonsick EM, Kashner TM, Hebel JR. Patient–proxy response comparability on measures of patient health and functional status. J Clin Epidemiol 1988;41(11):1065–1074.

18. Pinholt EM, Kroenke K, Hanley JR, et al. Functional assessment of the elderly. Arch Int Med 1987;147:484–488.

19. Elam, JT, Beaver T, El Derwi D, Applegate WB, Graney MJ, Miller ST. Comparison of sources of functional report with observed functional ability of frail older persons. Gerontologist 1989;28:(suppl 308). [Abstract].

20. Guralnik JM, Branch LG, Cummings SR, Curb JD. Physical performance measures in aging research. J Gerontol 1989;44(5):M141–M146.

21. Guralnik JM, Simonsick EM, Ferrucci L, et al. A short physical performance battery assessing lower extremity function: Association with self-reported disability and prediction of mortality and nursing home admission. J Gerontol 1994;49(2):M85–M94.

22. Guralnik JM, Ferrucci L, Simonsick EM, Salive ME, Wallace RB. Lower-extremity function in persons over the age of 70 years as a predictor of subsequent disability. N Engl J Med 1995;332:556–561.

23. Fried LP, Ettinger WH, Hermanson B, Newman AB, Gardin J for the CHS Collaborative Research Group. Physical disability in older adults: A physiological approach. J Clin Epidemiol 1994;47:747–760.

24. Ferrucci L, Guralnik JM, Bandeen-Roche KJ, Lafferty ME, Pahor M, Fried LP. Physical performance measures. In: Guralnik JM, Fried LP, Simonsick EM, Kasper JD, Lafferty ME, eds. The Women's Health and Aging Study: Health and Social Characteristics of Older Women with Disability. National Institute on Aging, 1995, pp. 35–41.

25. Nevitt MC, Cummings SR, Kidd S, Black D. Risk factors for recurrent nonsyncopal falls. JAMA 1989;261(18):2663–2668.

26. Seeman TE, Charpentier PA, Berkman LF, et al. Predicting changes in physical performance in a high-functioning elderly cohort: MacArthur studies of successful aging. J Gerintol 1994;49(3):M97–M108.

27. Shapiro E, Tate R. Who is really at risk of institutionalization? Gerontologist 1988;28:237.

28. Skoog I, Nilsson L, Palmertz B, Andreasson LA, Svanborg A. A population-based study of dementia in 85-year-olds. New Engl J Med 1993;328(3):153–158.

29. Evans DA, Funkenstein HH, Albert MS, et al. Prevalence of Alzheimer's disease in a community population of older persons. JAMA 1989;262(18):2551–2556.

30. Swan GE, Carmelli D, LaRue A. Performance on the Digit Symbol Substitution Test and a 5-year mortality in the Western Collaborative Group Study. Am J Epidemiol 1995;141(1):32–40.

31. Fried LP, Kronmal RA, Newman AB, et al. Risk factors for five-year mortality in older adults: The Cardiovascular Health Study. JAMA. 1998;279:585–592.

32. Guralnik JM, LaCroix AZ, Everett DF, Kovar MG. Aging in the Eighties: The Prevalence of Co-morbidity and its Association with Disability. Advanced Data from Vital and Health Statistics, No. 170. Baltimore: National Center for Health Statistics, 1989.

33. Charlson ME, Pompei P, Ales KL, MacKenzie CR. A new method of classifying prognostic comorbidity in longitudinal studies: Development and validation. J Chron Dis 1987;40(5):373–383.

34. Greenfield S, Apolone G, McNeil BJ, Cleary PD. The importance of co-existent disease in the occurrence of postoperative complications and one-year recovery in patients undergoing total hip replacement. Comorbidity and outcomes after hip replacement. Med Care 1993;31:141–154.

35. Ettinger WH, Fried LP, Harris T, Shemanski L, Schulz R, Robbins J. Self-reported causes of physical disability in older people: The Cardiovascular Health Study. J Am Geriatr Soc 1994;42(1):1035–1044.

36. Fried LP. Frailty, 3rd ed. In: Hazzard WR, Bierman EL, Blass JP, Ettinger WH, Halter JB, eds. Principles of Geriatric Medicine and Gerontology. New York: McGraw-Hill, 1994, pp. 1149–1156.

37. Fried LP, Herdman SJ, Kuhn KE, Rubin G, Turano K. Preclinical disability: Hypothesis about the bottom of the iceberg. J Aging Health 1991;3(2):285–300.

38. Manton KG, Stallard E, Liu K. Forecasts of active life expectancy: Policy and fiscal implications. J Gerontol 1993 Special Issue, Sept.;48:11–26.

39. World Health Organization. International Classification of Impairments, Disabilities, and Handicaps. Geneva; World Health Organization, 1980.

40. LaCroix AZ, Guralnik JM, Berkman LF, Wallace RB, Satterfield S. Maintaining mobility in late life. Am J Epidemiol 1993;137(8):858–869.

41. Pinsky JL, Branch LG, Jette AM, et al. Framingham Disability Study: Relationships of disability to cardiovascular risk factors among persons free of diagnosed cardiovascular disease. Am J Public Health 1985;122:644–656.

42. Ensrud KE, Nevitt MC, Yunis C, et al. Correlates of impaired function in older women. JAMA Geriatr Soc 1994;42(5):481–489.

43. Schulz R and Rau MT. Social Support through the life course. In: Cohen S, Syme SL, eds. Social Support and Health. New York: Academic Press, 1985, pp. 136–149.

44. Grady D, Rubin SM, Petitti DB, et al. Hormone therapy to prevent disease and prolong life in postmenopausal women. Ann Intern Med 1992;117(12):1016–1037.

45. Seeman TE, Berkman LF, Charpentier PA, Blazer DG, Albert MS, Tinetti ME. Behavioral and psychosocial predictors of physical performance: MacArthur Studies of Successful Aging. J Gerontol 1995;50A(4):M177–M183.

46. Schulz R, Williamson GM. Psychosocial behavioral dimensions of physical frailty. J Gerontol 1993;48:39–43.

47. Williamson GM, Schulz R. Relationship orientation, quality of prior relationship and distress among caregivers of Alzheimer's patients. Psychol Aging 1990;5:502–510.

48. Schulz R, Visintainer P, Williamson GM. Psychiatric and physical morbidity effects of caregiving. J Gerontol 1990;45:P181–191.

49. Schulz R, Newsom J, Mittlemark M, Burton L, Hirsch C, Jackson S. Health effects of caregiving: The Caregiver Health Effects Study. Ann Behav Med. 1997;19:110–116.

50. Newsom JT, Schulz R. Social support as a mediator in the relation between functional status and quality of life in older adults. Psychol Aging 1996;11(1):34–44.

51. Blazer D, Hughes DC, George LK. The epidemiology of depression in an elderly community population. Gerontol Soc Am 1987;27(3):281–287.

52. Hirsch CH, Fried LP, Harris T, Fitzpatrick A, Enright P, Schulz R. Correlates of performance-based measures of muscle function in the elderly: the Cardiovascular Health Study. J Gerontol Med Sci 1997; Vol 52A(4):M192–M200.

53. Felson DT. Epidemiology of hip and knee osteoarthritis. Epidemiol Rev 1988; 10:1–28.

54. Kuller LH, Shemanski L, Psaty BM, et al. Subclinical disease as an independent risk factor for cardiovascualr disease. Circulation 1995;92(4):720–726.

55. Pinsky JL, Leaverton PE, Stokes J. Predictors of good function: The Framingham Study. J Chron Dis 1987;40(Suppl 1):159S–167S.

56. Felson DT. The epidemiology of knee osteoarthritis: Results from the Framingham Osteoarthritis Study. Semin Arthritis Rheum 1990;20(3):42–50.

57. Escobedo LG, Peddicord JP. Smoking prevalence in US birth cohorts: The influence of gender and education. Am J Pub Health 1996;86(2):233–234.

58. Fiatarone MA, O'Neil EF, Ryan ND, et al. Exercise training and nutritional supplementation for physical frailty in very elderly people. N Engl J Med 1994;330:1769–1975.

59. Wolf SL, Barhart HX, Kutner NG, et al. Reducing frailty and falls in older persons: An investigation of Tai Chi and computerized balance training. J Am Geriatr Soc 1996;44(5):489–497.

60. Wolfson L, Whipple R, Derby C, et al. Balance and strength training in older adults: Intervention gains and Tai Chi maintenance. J Am Geriatr Soc 1996;44(5):498–506.

61. Ettinger WH, Burns R, Messier SP, et al. A randomized trail comparing aerobic exercise and resistance exercise with a health education program in older adults with knee osteoarthritis. JAMA 1997;277(1):25–31.

62. King AC, Haskell WL, Young DR, et al. Long-term effects of varying intensities and formats of physical activity on participation rates, fitness and lipoproteins in men and women aged 50 to 65 years. Circulation 1995;91:2596–2604.

63. Shaw JM, Snow-Harter C. Osteoporosis and physical activity. Phys Activity Fitness Res Dig 1995;2:1–6.

64. Reed RL, Pearlmutter L, Yochum K, Meredith KE, Mooradian AD. The relationship between muscle mass and strength in the elderly. J Am Geriatr Soc 1991; 39:555–561.

65. Hurley BF. Age, gender and muscular strength. J Gerontol Series A 1995; 50A (special issue):41–44.

66. Evans WJ. What is sarcopenia? J Gerontol Series A 1995; 50A (special issue):5–8.

67. Harris T. Muscle mass and strength: Relation to function in population studies. J Nutr 1997;127:1004S–1006S.

68. Dutta C. Significance of sarcopenia in the elderly. J Nutr 1997;127:992S–993S.

69. Evans WJ. Effects of exercise on body composition and functional capacity in the elderly. J Gerontol Series A 1995;50A:147–150.

70. Schwartz RS. Trophic factor supplementation: Effect on the age-associated changes in body composition. J Gerontol Series A 1995; 50A:151–156.

71. Weindruch R. Interventions based on the possibility that oxidative stress contributes to sarcopenia. J Gerontol Series A 1995;50A:157–161.

72. Kaye SA, Folsom AR, Soler JT, Prineas RJ, Potter JD. Associations of body mass and fat distribution with sex hormone concentrations in postmenopausal women. Int J Epidemiol 1991;20(1):151–156.

73. Herbert J. The age of dehydroepiandrosterone. Lancet 1995;345:1193–1194.

74. Barrett-Connor E, Khaw K, Yen SCC. A prospective study of DNEAS, mortality and cardiovascular disease. N Engl J Med 1986;315:1519–1524.

75. Berkman LF, Seeman TE, Albert M, et al. High, usual and impaired functioning in community-dwelling older men and women: Findings from the MacArthur Foundation Research Network on successful aging. J Clin Epidemiol 1993;46(10):1129–1140.

76. Morales AJ, Nolan JJ, Nelson JC, Yen SSC. Effects of replacement dose of dehydroepiandrosterone in men and women of advancing age. J Clin Endocrinol Metab 1994;78(6):1360–1367.

77. Casson PR, Buster JE. DHEA administration to humans: Panacea or palaver? Semin Reprod Endocrinol 1995;13(4):247–256.

78. Ho KY, Evans WS, Blizzard RM, et al. Effects of sex and age on 24-hour profile of growth hormone secretion in men and women: Importance of endogenous estradiol concentrations. J Clin Endocrinol Metab 1987;64:51–58.

79. Baum HB, Biller BM, Finkelstein JS, et al. Effects of physiologic growth hormone therapy on bone density and body composition in patients with adult-onset growth hormone deficiency. Ann Intern Med 1996;125:883–890.

80. Geldmacher DS, Whitehouse PJ. Evaluation of dementia. N Engl J Med 1996;335(5):330–336.

81. Farmer ME, Kittner SJ, Rae DS, Bartko JJ, Regier DA. Education and change in cognitive function: The Epidemiologic Catchment Area Study. Ann Epidemiol 1995; 5(1):1–7.

82. Albert MS, Jones K, Savage CR, et al. Predictors of cognitive change in older persons: MacArthur Studies of Successful Aging. Psych Aging 1995;10(4):578–589.

83. Snowdon DA, Demper SJ, Mortimer JA, Greiner LH, Wekstein DR, Markesbery WR. Linguistic ability in early life and cognitive function and Alzheimer's disease in late life: Findings from the nun study. JAMA 1996;272(7)528–532.

84. Luine V. Estradiol increases choline acetyltransferase activity in specific basal forebrain nuclei and projection areas of female rats. Exp Neurol 1985;89:484–490.

85. Paganini-Hill A, Henderson VW. Estrogen deficiency and risk of Alzheimer's disease in women. Am J Epidemiol 1994;140(3):256–261.

86. Barrett-Connor E, Kritz-Silverstein D. Estrogen replacement therapy and cognitive function in older women. JAMA 1993;269(20):2637–2640.

86a. Launer LJ, Masaki K, Petrovich H, et al. The association between midlife blood pressure levels and late-life cognitive function: The Honolulu-Asia Aging Study. JAMA 1995;274:1846–1851.

87. Breteler MMB, Claus JJ, Diederick EG, Hofman A. Cardiovascular disease and distribution of cognitive function in elderly people: The Rotterdam Study. BMJ 1994; 308:1064–1068.

88. Shua-Haim JR, Gross JS. Alzheimer's syndrome, not Alzheimer's disease. J Am Geriatr Soc 1996;44:96–97.

89. Polvikoski T, Sulkava R, Haltia M, et al. Apolipoprotein E, dementia, and cortical deposition of β-amyloid protein. New Engl J Med 1995;333(19):1242–1247.

90. Tinetti ME, Inouye SK, Gill TM, Doucette JT. Shared risk factors for falls, incontinence, and functional dependence. JAMA 1995;273(17):1348–1353.

5

VIOLENCE AGAINST WOMEN

Elaine J. Alpert

Violence, an enormous problem in U.S. society, affects men and women very differently. Overall, women are less likely than men to become victims of violent crime, but they are ten times more likely than men to be assaulted, raped, robbed, or murdered by a current or former intimate partner. Nearly 95% of all assaults against men are perpetrated by strangers (50%) or acquaintances (44%); only 5% of known assailants of males are current or former intimate partners (2%), or other relatives (3%). In contrast, women are nearly equally likely to report being assaulted by strangers (31%); acquaintances (35%); and either intimate partners (28%) or other relatives (5%).[1-3]

Violence against women is endemic in society and affects the lives and health of millions of women, as well as their families and communities. Published surveys indicate that females ages 12 and over sustain nearly 5 million violent assaults per year, of which 1 million are perpetrated by intimate partners,[2] and that as many as 4 million women per year are physically assaulted by current or former intimate partners.[4,5]

The effects of violence against women are numerous and far-reaching, with deleterious consequences across the life span for the victimized individual, her children and other dependents, extended family, friends, community, and society at-large. However, the complexities and limitations inherent in interpreting violence and other abuse solely as a gender issue become apparent when one acknowledges the prevalence of intimate partner violence in lesbian and gay male relationships, the existence of a small proportion of cases of victimization by women of male partners, and the occurrence of child abuse and neglect at the hands of female as well as male caregivers.

This chapter provides an overview of selected issues related to violence against adolescent and adult women, with particular attention to intimate partner violence, sexual assault, and homicide. Evolutionary, biological, psychological, social, and cultural factors that may contribute to the occurrence of violence against women are discussed.

NOMENCLATURE AND DEFINITIONS

A scholarly understanding of the scope of violence against women requires examination of the influence and interactions of gender, culture, socioeconomic status, and role expectations. It is equally important to examine the context of abuse relative to the people (i.e., victims, perpetrators, bystanders, children and other family members) and institutions (i.e., health care, legal and criminal justice, work sites, schools, community, religions) involved. Such a broad conceptualization invites both research and clinical debate regarding definitions, causes, and methods of violence intervention and prevention.

Universal agreement has not been, nor can be, attained by scholars or activists in assigning a precise definition to the term "violence against women." Perspectives on this problem are informed by one's training and orientation. For example, researchers in criminal justice define violence by reportable or otherwise measurable criminal outcomes (i.e., felony assault, homicide, rape). Mental health perspectives are more expansive than those of criminal justice, viewing violent acts and behavior in terms of their impact on the abused individual (i.e., injury, illness, chronic pain, anxiety, depression, post-traumatic stress disorder, substance abuse). For example, the American Psychological Association Task Force on Male Violence Against Women defines violence against women as "physical, visual, verbal, or sexual acts that are experienced by a woman or a girl as a threat, invasion, or assault and that have the effect of hurting her or degrading her and/or taking away her ability to control contact (intimate or otherwise) with another individual." The effects of psychological abuse are felt to be more difficult to recover from than physical injuries, and may therefore have a more deleterious and long-lasting impact on victims of violence. Information about the psychological and physical effects of violence against women is typically collected by researchers subscribing to a mental health orientation, and would be found less commonly in criminal-justice surveillance data sets.[6]

Yet a third lens for viewing violence against women is that of feminist theory, which includes the constructs of gender and power. Feminist theory opposes the notion that norms of ideology and behavior should be shaped by the interests of the dominant class, i.e., males. Thus, androcentric values and attitudes, assumed by men to be normative, influence and even dominate social interactions. Indeed, at the extreme, "the social institutions of marriage and family . . . may promote, maintain, and even support [violence against women]."[7]

Central to feminist philosophy is the idea that women's lives and experiences should be examined in context, from their own frames of reference.

Taking into account the basic tenets of each perspective, then, the broad term "violence against women" can be seen as encompassing a range of purposeful individual and institutional behaviors and responses that, alone or in combination, intimidate and control women, either individually or as a group. The analysis of violence against women involves a variety of related terms, such as family, domestic, relationship, intimate partner, or dating violence; spouse abuse; woman battering; elder abuse; incest; rape; and sexual assault. These terms underscore the broad range of contexts within which females experience violence, and the difficulty of capturing all situations under any one heading. Although beyond the scope of this chapter, state and culturally sanctioned human rights abuses, as well as both open and surreptitious exploitation of girls and women, are important to incorporate in a broad conceptualization of violence against women. Such abuses include genital mutilation, systematic abortion of female fetuses, female infanticide, rape in the context of war crimes, forced marriage, sexual slavery (e.g., the "comfort women" of World War II), the sale of girls and young women into prostitution, and both child and adult pornography.

Family violence is a major subset of the larger problem of violence against women and has been defined as "intentional intimidation, physical and/or sexual abuse or battering of children, adults or elders by a family member, intimate partner, or caretaker."[8] The expanded nature of "family" in society to include unmarried partners, same-gender partners, extended kinships, step- or otherwise nonbiological families, and other types of relationships should also be considered in the context of family violence.

SOURCES OF DATA

Accurate data collection is clearly crucial to confirm, disprove, or refine hypotheses of the determinants of violence. It is equally important to inform the design, implementation, and evaluation of interventions, and to guide more effective allocation of resources for prevention and treatment. However, the magnitude of the problem of violence against women has been a subject of active discussion and debate, in part because of complexities inherent in arriving at "gold-standard" definitions,[9] inconsistent data collection, and underreporting of violent acts. Unfortunately, there have been few reliable population studies even in more established fields such as child abuse and neglect. Discussion of violence is further confused by divergent conclusions drawn from different data sources and by hypotheses that cannot be optimally tested by examining available data sets.

Surveillance data, such as the National Crime Victimization Survey (NCVS)[1,2] and the Uniform Crime Reports (UCR), focus on criminal victimization of women and are collected via self-report during structured telephone interviews (NCVS) or through information offered voluntarily to the FBI as monthly incident reports by police departments (UCR). The deliberate focus of both surveys on criminal acts and outcomes can help to address trends over time because they are validated, regularly reported, and consistently accrued.[10] However, each data set has limitations, particularly the potential for underreporting. For example, NCVS respondents may minimize the frequency and severity of their victimization, may not consider their abuse to represent criminal behavior because of its occurrence in the home, or may not be alone at the time of the telephone interview and thus may not feel safe to disclose their abuse. UCR data do not provide details regarding victim–offender relationships, and they include only the proportion of violent offenses known to the police (neglecting the substantial proportion of nonfatal assaults that go unreported).[11]

The National Institute of Justice (NIJ) and the Family and Intimate Violence Prevention Team of the National Center for Injury Prevention and Control recently conducted a random-digit national phone survey in which 8,000 men and 8,000 women were queried about their experiences with violence by intimate partners, acquaintances, and strangers.[12] Once analyzed, the results of this survey will be compared with existing data derived from the revised NCVS[2] to determine whether the NCVS is sufficient to assess the extent of violence against women, or whether a separate survey is needed to generate more accurate surveillance data.

A variety of public and private organizations including schools, police departments, hospital emergency departments, medical examiner's offices, and rape crisis centers can serve as excellent sources of data regarding rates and types of victimization, and often they provide detailed data that describe a particular area's characteristics and needs. However, statistics from such sources may be unreliably collected, incomplete, out of date, or not easily generalizable to other areas or cultures or to the population at-large. For example, until recently, instruction about intimate partner violence and elder mistreatment were not standard components of medical education, and thus the majority of currently practicing physicians have received little or no formal education about the medical or behavioral manifestations of these types of abuse.[13] Thus, medical records rarely contain explicit information such as "diagnoses" or detailed descriptions of patterns of domestic or elder abuse, although trained researchers can sometimes extract useful data from a careful review of medical records.

Two additional national population-based studies that assess the extent of domestic violence in the U.S. have been published.[4,5] Straus, Gelles, and Steinmetz surveyed one adult member of each of 2,143 two-parent families to determine the frequency and causes of spousal abuse. From this data set, Straus and colleagues concluded that nearly 2 million married women per year are kicked, bitten, punched, hit with an object, beaten up, threatened with a gun or knife, or attacked with a gun or knife by a spouse. The 1985 Family Violence Survey reported similar findings.

Perhaps the most important qualitative information that can be sought in the field of violence against women is from survivors of abuse themselves.[14–18] Other valuable insights can be gleaned by examining ethnographic and related in-depth studies of the experiences of health care providers caring for victims and perpetrators of abuse.[19,20] Listening to the stories of survivors and providers helps advocates, clinicians, and researchers better direct services, resources, and inquiry, and contributes a vital dimension to both understanding and preventing violence.

EPIDEMIOLOGY

Intimate Partner Violence

Domestic violence, or intimate partner violence, can be defined as "intentional violent or controlling behavior by a person who is currently, or was previously, in an intimate relationship with the victim,"[21] or alternatively, as a "pattern of assaultive and coercive behaviors used in the context of dating or intimate relationships."[22] The spectrum of intimate partner violence includes not only physical injury but also sexual assault, social isolation, intimidating verbal abuse, threats, humiliation, economic deprivation, and the restriction of access to transportation and other resources.[23] Tactics such as these are often used by the perpetrator to maintain control over the victim by engendering fear and uncertainty.

Wilt and Olson[24] reviewed the available literature regarding annual incidence and lifetime prevalence of domestic violence and determined that at least 9% of U.S. women have been victims of severe domestic violence at some point in their lives, and at least 30% have experienced some form of abuse at the hands of an intimate partner. Indeed, the vast majority of those who are abused in intimate or dating relationships are women, accounting for greater than 95% of adolescent and adult victims.[2]

Rates of violence against women by intimate partners are consistent across racial, ethnic, and geographic boundaries, but young, poor, and unmarried women appear to be at especially high risk of being victims of violence by current or former partners.[2,25] Furthermore, women separated from their husbands are three times as likely as divorced women, and about 25 times as likely as married women, to have suffered a recent rape, sexual assault, aggravated assault, simple assault, or robbery perpetrated by a current or former spouse.[2]

Thirty percent of all injuries suffered by adult women who report for emergency care are attributable to battering,[26] and the lifetime prevalence of victimization (child or adult) for females who present for any reason to emergency facilities has been reported to be as high as 54%.[27] Although precise incidence and prevalence estimates are difficult to establish, relationship violence appears to be as common in gay and lesbian relationships as in heterosexual liaisons.[28,29]

Rape and Sexual Assault

Rape and sexual assault are common and devastating crimes, with long-lasting adverse consequences for victims. Although sexual assault of adults and children is a problem of enormous medical, public health, and criminal justice importance, reliable incidence data are difficult to accrue because of issues of definition, data collection methodology, and reluctance on the part of many victims to report. Although it is believed that fewer than half of all sexual crimes are ever reported, it is estimated that at least 20% of adult women, 15% of college women, and 12% of adolescent females have endured some form of sexual abuse or assault.[30] Five hundred thousand rapes and sexual assaults per year are estimated to occur to females age 12 and up. Girls and women are the victims in approximately 95% of all reported sexual assaults; males constitute the remaining 5%.[2] More than half of reported sexual assault crimes against women are completed rapes (34%) or attempted rapes (28%).[2] In contrast to the stereotyped image of the rapist as a cunning stranger hiding in the bushes, waiting to ambush an innocent passerby, most sexual assault is perpetrated by a current or former intimate partner (26%), other relative (3%), or acquaintance or friend (53%). Indeed, less than one in five (18%) of all sexual assaults or rapes are committed by strangers.[2] Sexual assault can also occur within married relationships, usually within the context of ongoing domestic violence.

Victims of sexual assault can suffer physical as well as psychological consequences, including injury, unintended pregnancy, sexually transmitted diseases, sexual dysfunction, guilt, insomnia, anxiety, depression, post-traumatic stress disorder, and alcohol and other substance abuse.[31]

Homicide

The United States has the highest homicide rate (9 per 100,000 population) of any industrialized nation in the world. Victims of homicide are likely to be male (78%) and relatively young (65% under age 35).[32] For males 15 through 24 years of age, the annual U.S. homicide rate (21.9 deaths per 100,000 population) is 4.4 times higher than that of Scotland, the country with the next highest rate.[33] The statistics are particularly dismal for young black males in the United States, whose annual death rate due to homicide (85.6 per 100,000) is more than seven times that of young white males. In fact, homicide, the 12th leading cause of death nationwide, is the leading cause of death for U.S. black males between the ages of 15 and 24.[34,35]

Although women are less at risk for homicide than men, when murdered, they are much more likely to be killed by current or former intimate partners than are men. In 1994, current or former husbands or boyfriends killed 28% of female murder victims, whereas only 3% of male homicide victims were killed by current or former intimate partners.[2]

Child Abuse and Children Who Witness Violence

Domestic violence affects not only the women who suffer directly from abuse but also the estimated 3.3 million children each year who are exposed to domestic violence in their own homes.[36] Long-term behavioral effects have been described in children who have witnessed violence and can be as harmful to the healthy development of children as having been victimized themselves.[37–39] Children who witness violence may show signs and symptoms of post-traumatic stress disorder, particularly if the children are young, if the violence is repeated, and if it occurs near to them.[40] A study at Children's Hospital in Boston showed that 40% to 59% of mothers of abused children were themselves currently or previously physically abused,[41] highlighting life cycle and family systems issues involved in the intergenerational scope and perpetuation of violence.

THEORIES OF CAUSATION

What causes violence in general and violence against women in particular? Identifying the cause(s) of any health or social welfare problem is instrumental in developing optimal treatment and is crucial for designing effective strategies for prevention.[12] There is general agreement among researchers, statisticians, health care providers, and other experts from scientific and advocacy communities that violence against women is a complex and multifaceted problem that is heterogeneous in both its origins and effects. Most research to date on this topic has been limited to the examination of single biological, pathophysiological, or sociological causes, although at least one recent study has tested more complex interrelationships using a multivariate statistical approach.[42] Such an approach to analysis is important, as it is clear that violent behavior arises from complex interactions among individual biological, psychosocial, and cultural influences.[43]

Evolution

How much influence evolutionary and biological factors have over present-day human behavior is a matter of much debate. In an evolutionary sense, it has been postulated that sexual behavior is directed at maximizing the chances that one's genes will be passed on, thus ensuring the perpetuation of the species. In this context, males were "best served by mating with as many fertile females as possible to increase their chance of impregnating one of them; females, who have the tasks of pregnancy and nurturing the young, are often better served by pair bonding."[43] Thus, differences in sexual behavior between males and females may at least in part have helped foster successful reproduction in human ancestors. Evolutionary theory can also contribute to explaining the origins of violence against women, in that sexual jealousy, domination, and possessiveness—behaviors that frequently characterize perpetrators of intimate partner violence—may in fact represent a distortion of the evolutionary drive to assure paternity and thus success of the species.

Evolutionary explanations of physical and sexual aggression are clearly not sufficient to illuminate the cause(s) of violence against women. Rape is a crime of violence, not an act of reproduction. Many rapes involve oral or anal, and not vaginal, penetration. Indeed, some rapes and other sexual assaults involve the use of objects designed to hurt or control the victim without any attempt at penile intercourse. A small proportion of rape victims are male.

Biology

Most research on biological or physiological correlates of violence against women have focused on animal research regarding the action of steroid hormones (particularly testosterone); neurotransmitters (particularly norepinephrine, gamma aminobutyric acid, serotonin, and dopamine); and structural, posttraumatic, or functional disorders of brain function.[6,43] In human males, there appears to be an association between aggressive behavior and elevated serum testosterone levels, but neither a causal nor incremental relationship has been established. Other studies have demonstrated correlations between low levels of serotonin and aggressive behavior.[44,45] Traumatic brain injury has been reported to precede violent behavior in certain individuals, however, it is unclear how many of these injuries result directly from child abuse, or how many of these individuals may have witnessed violence as children.[43] Once again, association remains far from causation.

Physical size may contribute to, but does not appear to cause, violent behavior. Men are generally physically larger and stronger than women and are thus more likely to inflict injury during a physical assault. Many women may choose not to initiate behavior designed to dominate men by physical force or threat of force because of their smaller physical size.

Personality and Psychopathology

Most research about the personality profiles of batterers or sexual offenders has been conducted on men who are incarcerated or who are court mandated to batterer intervention programs. Thus, these studies are not felt to be representative of the population at-large, or even of batterers or sexual offenders in general, as most perpetrators are not in jail, in treatment, or even identified. Furthermore, most studies of perpetrators rely on self-report or on interviews with victims and are thus subject to underreporting by both victim and perpetrator because of both recall and reporting bias. Indeed, victims and batterers appear to minimize the frequency and severity of abusive incidents, when parallel corroboration with police reports and victims' medical records are obtained.[46–49] Some researchers have found a high prevalence of borderline personality disorder and antisocial personality disorder in batterers.[50,51] Others maintain that batterers are a heterogeneous group, with no single pathologic personality disorder that adequately describes them. There is general agreement, however, that batterers tend to be self-focused and to view the use of power (accompanied by intimidation and physical violence in many cases) over their partners as a legitimate and even necessary tool to maintain dominance in the relationship.[52,53]

RISK FACTORS FOR VICTIMIZATION

The risk of victimization among women is, to a large extent, a function of perpetrator—not victim—behavior and attributes. Despite extensive research directed at discerning causative or permissive factors for victimization, there appears to be no specific biological basis, personality type, or cluster of attitudinal characteristics that underlie or predict victimization from intimate partner abuse or sexual assault.[54] However, adolescent and adult victims of sexual assault are reported to have a higher prevalence of prior child sexual abuse than non-victims.[55] Research has shown that young age, low socioeconomic status, unmarried status, prior physical or sexual abuse, and possibly witnessing the abuse of caregivers are risk factors (although not causes) for both physical and sexual victimization.[25,55] However, by far the most significant risk factor for a person becoming a victim of intimate violence is simply being female.

Sociological and Cultural Explanatory Models of Victimization

Stark and Flitcraft[56] have summarized research on the social and cultural causes of violence against intimate partners and have defined three explanatory models: the gender–politics model, the interpersonal violence model, and the family violence model. Each has merit in explaining some aspects of intimate violence, but none is sufficient to delineate the causes of violence against women.

Gender–politics model. This model derives from feminist theory and asserts that family violence and violence against women are inextricably linked. Family violence can be explained as one outcome of an historically entrenched pattern (rejected by feminist theorists as inappropriate and repugnant) of male control over women that extends throughout the life cycle of the family and is reinforced by societal institutions, laws, and existing cultural norms. Walker[57] states that the "feminist political gender analysis has reframed violence against women as one of misuse of power by men who have been socialized into believing they have the right to control the women in their lives, even through violent means." Smith[58] asserts that violence against women develops and continues as an extension of patriarchal traditions that allow, and in fact, encourage, men to assert control over their wives and children. Efforts by women to assert their own personal, psychological, or financial independence are perceived as threats to men's sense of authority as heads of the household. Additionally, women as well as men have been socialized to accept male authority in relationships.[59] The gender–politics model explains the customs and laws that historically have legitimized and condoned violence against women (even those in non-cohabitating dating relationships). However, this model alone is not sufficient to explain violence against women. Panzer and Eilenberg write, "While providing an important perspective on the consequences for women of social norms that condone the use and misuse of power, the gender–politics model falls short of offering a complete explanation. After all, what prevents the majority of men from beating their female partners?"[59] This model also does not explain the occurrence of abuse in gay and lesbian relationships.

Interpersonal violence model. This model contends that dysfunctional behavior, psychiatric problems, or inadequate coping skills lead to violent conflict in relationships. According to this model, "violence arises among adults who lack the skill to cope non-violently with stress or conflict."[50] This theory adequately explains why some couples resolve conflicts nonviolently, whereas physical abuse is the outcome for others. However, this model has important shortcomings that limit its utility. Identifiable conflict between partners does not precede every episode of violence—for example, a man who perceives that his mate is having an affair (when in fact she may be out shopping) may become angry, accusing, and violent upon the unsuspecting woman's return home. The interpersonal violence model also does not explain why more women than men are abused in their own homes. Although women may strike back in self-defense when assaulted by intimates, the context of domestic violence is largely gendered. That is, partner violence is generally characterized by the threat or use of force by a male partner to intimidate and control a female victim and those persons (usually children or other close relatives) or things (personal property or keepsakes) that are important to her.

Family violence model. This model suggests that family violence is considered to be normative because of the nature of the closeness and intensity of family structures, and it is perpetuated by socially accepted norms of privacy in family relationships, even in cases of severe violence and abuse. The family violence model explains why violence is condoned as a means by which to address conflicts in the home, for example, using spanking as a form of discipline ("spare the rod, spoil the child"), or using violence against women to maintain hierarchy, order, and authority in the household. This model also explains why many men who resort to violence in order to enforce control over their wives and children do not replicate this behavior in non-family relationships, such as in the work or community setting. This model is supported by principles of social learning theory that maintain that violent behavior is learned behavior, often acquired by witnessing such acts during early childhood. Patterns of violent behavior become ingrained within families as acceptable, automatic, and even necessary responses to real or perceived conflict, and are transmitted intergenerationally. This model, however, is also insufficient in explaining the origins of violence against women in particular, or of family violence. Although being abused or neglected as a child does increase a male child's risk of delinquency, adult criminal behavior, and adult violent behavior,[60] most abused children do not resort to violence later in life, and most abusive men were not themselves abused as children.[61]

ALCOHOL AND OTHER SUBSTANCES OF ABUSE AND VIOLENCE AGAINST WOMEN

The relationship between intoxication with alcohol and other substances of abuse, and violence against women, has been investigated extensively.[62–64] Brookoff et al.[65] evaluated victim and perpetrator characteristics in domestic assaults for which police were summoned and determined that 92% of the assailants and 42% of the victims had used alcohol or other drugs on the day of the assault and that 45% of the assailants used drugs or alcohol to the point of intoxication on a daily basis for at least 1 month prior to the assault. Overall, alcohol is thought to be a contributing factor in the majority of domestic assaults.[66]

Alcoholism and drug abuse are more prevalent among abused women than non-abused women. Indeed, it is estimated that fully half of all alcoholic women have been victimized as children or as adults.[67] Furthermore, although alcohol abuse may precede, and possibly contribute to, the onset of abuse in some women, alcohol abuse is often a consequence, rather than a cause, of child physical or sexual abuse or of violence against adult women.[68,69]

Alcohol use, in the context of acute intoxication as well as with chronic use, compromises the battered woman's ability to identify danger and access help, and it may contribute to keeping her trapped in an abusive relationship. Health care providers and others who could serve as resources for battered women may view the alcoholic or drug-abusing battered woman as unworthy, unimportant, "asking for it," or even deserving of abuse. A woman's alcohol or drug problem is often viewed as provocation of violence, and the use of violence against such women is somehow seen as excusable, justifiable, or even necessary. Alcoholic battered women are thus doubly isolated—because of their abuse and because of their alcoholism.

Thus, although alcohol use correlates strongly with, and indeed has been shown to be a risk factor for, marital aggression, a causal link between alcohol use and violence against women has clearly not been established, and the nature of the association most likely represents a complex interplay of physiological, psychological, social, and cultural factors.

VIOLENCE AGAINST WOMEN AND ITS RELATION TO VIOLENCE IN THE ENTERTAINMENT MEDIA

Violence on television, in movies, in video games, and in music videos has harmful effects on viewers of all ages. Research has shown that portrayals of violence, particularly sexual violence, depicted as "entertainment," have contributed significantly to both aggression-related attitudes and to aggressive behavior in children, teens, and adults.[70] The 1972 Surgeon General's Scientific Advisory Committee on Television and Social Behavior reviewed published literature and new research commissioned for its charge and reported a significant correlation between viewing television and the development of aggressive behavioral traits. Furthermore, a direct and causal link between exposure to violent imagery on television and subsequent violent behavior was demonstrated.[71] A report by the National Institute of Mental Health in 1982 on television and behavior,[72] which reviewed research findings published since the 1972 Surgeon General's report, concluded that "violence on television does lead to aggressive behavior by children and teenagers." In 1985, the American Psychological Association published a position statement that recognized that televised violence had a causal effect on aggressive behavior.[73] Several other studies and reports support the same conclusion. Viewing media violence, especially if the protagonist or hero partakes in violent behavior, if the violence is portrayed as humorous or consequence-free, and if the violence is repetitive, can alter for viewers the apparent social norms associated with violence, teach children and adolescents in particular "social scripts" about violence, and create or support attitudes that condone violence and desensitize viewers to its effects. Sexualized violence against women that is presented as entertainment has especially deleterious consequences. Too frequently, violence against women is portrayed quite graphically in television and movies, and often it has implicit or even explicit sexual overtones. Males who view sexually violent material (much of it R-rated and thus easily available to adolescents), can become sexually aroused and may report callous attitudes toward rape.[70] Additional research indicates a correlation between such arousal patterns and attitudes, and real-life aggressive behavior toward women.[74] Donnerstein et al. assert quite cogently, "It is not unreasonable to assume that a young adolescent's first exposure to sex will come in the form of a mildly erotic, but violent scene from a rented video or a late-night cable movie. To a young adolescent who is searching for information about relationships, sexual violence in popular films may be a potent source of influence on initial attitudes toward sexuality."[70] Clearly, the problem of media portrayals of violence against women, particularly sexual violence, is quite serious and serves to reinforce misogynistic stereotypes that have been quite damaging to women's self-esteem, empowerment, and safety.

THE PREVENTION OF VIOLENCE AGAINST WOMEN

Violence against women has become an urgent and visible societal issue largely because of the determined grass-roots advocacy of the feminist movement beginning in the 1960s. The health care response to violence against women followed the lead of the women's rights movement and has evolved considerably over the past two decades, in parallel with advances in public health, criminal justice, social policy, and emerging societal opinion in opposition to the abuse of women and children. This response has moved most recently toward efforts directed at the primary prevention of violence and abuse, which entails structural and cultural changes that would promote violence-free life and greater respect between individuals.

Initial efforts in the 1960s and 1970s were largely (and appropriately) tertiary prevention oriented, directed towards rescuing women in the throes of desperate crises. Battered women's shelters and safe home networks emerged at this time, as did abuse prevention statutes in many states. The image of the battered woman in the health care setting was of a bruised and bloodied trauma victim being treated in an emergency facility. The focus was on the injury rather than its cause, and there was little awareness of the cyclical and progressive nature of abuse, the intergenerational transmission of violence, and of the central therapeutic concepts of safety, confidentiality, support, and empowerment.

The 1980s and early 1990s brought concepts of secondary prevention to the forefront. Routine screening for abuse in both primary care and emergency health care settings has become the standard of care, although the standard has not yet been universally met because many providers have not been trained in how to screen and assess at-risk patients and to intervene on their behalf. In law enforcement, ongoing training of police and court personnel and the growth of the victim's rights movement (in concert with federal and state statutes supporting victim–witness advocates in the court system) has focused attention on early, multidisciplinary intervention for battered women and their children. A new awareness of widespread and deleterious effects on children when they witness violence between caregivers has recently emerged. New knowledge about the relationship between domestic violence and homelessness[75,76] has helped to focus services for homeless women and children more appropriately on safety and economic empowerment and has allowed for the passage in many states of legislation protecting battered homeless women from having public assistance terminated.

Much ground has been gained in the move to protect and empower vulnerable populations against victimization, but there is still a very long way to go. Without abandoning the safety net and early intervention programs of the last two decades, the new horizon for an integrated societal response to violence against women must now be directed toward primary prevention. Strategies to reduce or prevent violence against women must involve more than individual- or case-based approaches; broad structural and cultural changes must be made in the way both perpetrators and victims are treated. Every member of society deserves to live a violence-free life, the basic prerequisites of which include rights to education, safe housing, employment, basic health care, self-determination, and respect. It is the responsibility of every member of society to advocate for, and model, non-violence. Health care providers can incorporate discussions about healthy dating and intimate relationships into routine health visits with teens and young adults so that their future children have a better chance of growing up in a violence-free environment. Community policing, including violence and drug abuse prevention programs in schools, can potentially have a profoundly positive effect on young boys and girls and foster stability and lower crime rates in neighborhoods. Efforts toward reducing gratuitous, consequence-free violence in the entertainment media can help model more positive behavior and reverse the recent trend toward the portrayal of women as objects of pleasure and of violence as consequence-free or even enjoyable. Teachers, clergy, community leaders, and neighbors can serve as trusted sources of support for children and adults who are at risk or in danger, and can help model proactive, non-violent, and respectful behavior.

The rewards for the primary prevention of violence will be seen in the next generation, but not without the concerted energy and cooperation of every person and group in society.

REFERENCES

1. Bachman R. Violence Against Women: A National Crime Victimization Survey Report. U.S. Department of Justice, Office of Justice Programs, Bureau of Justice Statistics, NCJ-145325. Washington, DC: Government Printing Office, January 1994.

2. Bachman R, Saltzman LE. Violence Against Women: Estimates from the Redesigned Survey. U.S. Department of Justice, Office of Justice Programs, Bureau of Jus-

tice Statistics, NCJ-154348. Washington, DC: Government Printing Office, August 1995.

3. Bureau of Justice Statistics Selected Findings. Violence Between Intimates. U.S. Department of Justice, Office of Justice Programs. NCJ-149259, 1994.

4. Straus MA, Gelles RJ, Steinmetz SK. Behind Closed Doors: Violence in the American Family. New York: Anchor Press/Doubleday, 1980.

5. Straus MA, Gelles RJ. How violent are American families? Estimates from the National Family Violence Resurvey and other studies. In: Straus MA, Gelles RJ, eds. Physical Violence in American Families: Risk Factors and Adaptations to Violence in 8,145 Families. New Brunswick, NJ: Transaction, 1990, pp. 95–112.

6. National Research Council. Crowell NA, Burgess AW, eds. Understanding Violence Against Women. Washington, DC: National Academy Press, 1996.

7. Bograd M. Feminist perspectives on wife abuse: An introduction. In: Yllo K, Bograd M, eds. Feminist Perspectives on Wife Abuse. Newbury Park, CA: Sage Publications, 1988, pp. 11–26.

8. Alpert EJ, Cohen S, Sege RD. Family violence: An overview. Acad Med 1997;72(suppl):S3–S6.

9. Flitcraft A. Learning from the paradoxes of domestic violence. JAMA 1997;277:1400–1401.

10. Isaac N, Prothrow-Stith D. Violence. In: Allen KM, Phillips JM, eds. Women's Health Across the Lifespan. New York: Lippincott, 1997, pp. 439–453.

11. Barancik JI, Chatterjee BF, Greene YZ, Mekenzie EM, Fife B. Northeastern Ohio Trauma Study: I. Magnitude of the problem. Am J Public Health 1983;73:746–751.

12. Saltzman LE, Johnson D. CDC's Family and Intimate Violence Prevention Team: Basing programs on science. J Am Med Wom Assoc 1996;51:83–86.

13. Alpert EJ. Report of the Committee on Violence. Waltham, MA: Massachusetts Medical Society, 1995.

14. Smith PH, Tessaro I, Earp JL. Women's experiences with battering: A conceptualization from qualitative research. Womens Health Issues 1995;5:173–182.

15. Herman J. Trauma and Recovery. New York: Basic Books, 1992.

16. Warshaw C, Poirier S. Case and commentary: Hidden stories of women. Second Opin 1991;17:48–61.

17. Anonymous. Lone Bear's story. Med Encounter 1996;12:2–6.

18. Campbell JC, Pliska MJ, Taylor W, Sheridan D. Battered women's experiences in the emergency department. J Emerg Nurs 1994;20:280–288.

19. Cohen S, DeVos E, Newberger E. Barriers to physician identification and treatment of family violence: Lessons from five communities. Acad Med 1997;72(Suppl):S19–S25.

20. Sugg NK, Inui T. Primary care physicians' response to domestic violence: Opening Pandora's box. JAMA 1992;267:3157–3160.

21. Massachusetts Medical Society Committee on Violence, Alpert EJ (chair). Partner Violence: How to Recognize and Treat Victims of Abuse, 2nd ed. Waltham, MA: Massachusetts Medical Society, 1996.

22. Ganley A. Understanding domestic violence. In: Ganley A, Warshaw C, Salber P, eds. Improving the Health Care Response to Domestic Violence: A Resource Manual for Health Care Providers. San Francisco: Family Violence Prevention Fund, 1995, pp. 15–45.

23. Flitcraft AH, Hadley SM, Hendricks-Matthews MB, McLeer SC, Warshaw C. Diagnostic and Treatment Guidelines on Domestic Violence. Chicago: American Medical Association, 1992.

24. Wilt S, Olson S. Prevalence of domestic violence in the United States. J Am Med Wom Assoc 1996;51:77–82.

25. McCauley J, Kern DE, Kolodner K, et al. The 'battering syndrome': prevalence and clinical characteristics of domestic violence in primary care internal medicine practices. Ann Intern Med 1995;737–746.

26. McLeer SV, Anwar R. A study of battered women presenting in an emergency department. Am J Public Health 1989;79:65–66.

27. Abbott J, Johnson R, Koziol-McLain J, Lowenstein SR. Domestic violence against women: Incidence and prevalence in an emergency department population. JAMA 1995;273:1763–1767.

28. Brand PA, Kidd AH. Frequency of physical aggression in heterosexual and female homosexual dyads. Psychol Rep 1986;59:1307–1313.

29. Lobel K. Naming the Violence: Speaking Out About Lesbian Battering. Seattle: Seal Press, 1986.

30. Koss MP. Hidden rape: Sexual aggression and victimization in a national sample of students in higher education. In: Burgess AW, ed. Rape and Sexual Assault. New York: Garland Publishing, 1988, pp. 2:3–25.

31. Schwartz IL. Sexual violence against women: Prevalence, consequences, societal factors, and prevention. Am J Prev Med 1991;7:363–373.

32. Perkins C, Klaus P. Criminal Victimization 1994. Bureau of Justice Statistics Bulletin, U.S. Department of Justice, Office of Justice Programs, NCJ-158022, 1996.

33. Fingerhut LA, Kleinman JC. International and interstate comparisons of homicide among young males. JAMA 1990;263:3292–3294.

34. Centers for Disease Control and Prevention. Homicide among young black males—United States, 1978–1987. MMWR CDC Surveill Summ 1990;39:869–872.

35. National Center for Injury Prevention and Control. 1994: 10 Leading Causes of Death. Atlanta: Centers for Disease Control and Prevention, 1997.

36. Carlson BE. Children's observations of interparental violence. In: Roberts AR, ed. Battered Women and Their Families. New York: Springer-Verlag, 1984, pp. 147–167.

37. Zuckerman B, Augustyn M, Groves BM, Parker S. Silent victims revisited: The special case of domestic violence. Pediatrics 1995;84:511–513.

38. Hughes HH. Psychological and behavioral correlates of family violence in child witness and victims. Am J Orthopsychiatry 1988;58:77–90.

39. Silvern L, Kaersvang L. The traumatized children of violent marriages. Child Welfare 1989;68:421–436.

40. Garabino J, Kostelny K, Dubrow N. What children can tell us about living in danger. Am Psychol 1991;46:376–383.

41. McKibben L, DeVos E, Newberger EH. Victimization of mothers of abused children: A controlled study. Pediatrics 1989;84:531–535.

42. McKenry PC, Julian TW, Gavazzi SM. Toward a biopsychosocial model of domestic violence. J Marriage Fam 1995;57:307–320.

43. Reiss AJ, Roth JA. Understanding and Preventing Violence. Panel on the Understanding and Control of Violent Behavior, Committee on Law and Justice, National Research Council. Washington, DC: National Academy Press, 1993.

44. Brown GL, Goodwin FK, Ballenger JC, Goyer PF, Major LF. Aggression in humans correlates with cerebrospinal fluid amine metabolites. Psychiatry Res 1979;1:131–139.

45. Coccaro EF, Siever LJ, Klar HM, Maurer G. Serotonergic studies in patients with affective and personality disorders. Arch Gen Psychiatry 1989;46:587–598.

46. Edelson J, Brygger MP. Gender differences in reporting violence. Paper presented at the Third Annual Family Violence Research Conference, 1987, Durham, NH.

47. Jouriles EN, O'Leary D. Interspousal reliability of reports of marital violence. J Consult Clin Psychol 1985;53(3):419–421.

48. Sonkin D, Martin D, Walker L. The Male Batterer: A Treatment Approach. New York: Springer-Verlag, 1985.

49. Szinovacz M. Using couple data as a methodological tool: The case of marital violence. J Marriage Fam 1983;45:633–644.

50. Hamberger LK, Hastings JE. Personality correlates of men who abuse their partners: A cross-validational study. J Fam Violence 1986;1:323–346.

51. Hart SD, Dutton DG, Newlove T. The prevalence of personality disorder among wife assaulters. J Pers Disorders 1993;7:328–340.

52. Gondolf EW. Who are those guys? Toward a behavioral typology of batterers. Violence Vict 1988;3:187–203.

53. Sanders DG. A typology of men who batter. Am J Orthopsychiatry 1992;62:264–275.

54. Hotaling GT, Sugarman DV. An analysis of risk markers in husband to wife violence: The current state of knowledge. Violence Vict 1986;1:101–124.

55. Browne A, Finkelhor D. The impact of child sexual abuse: A review of the research. Psychol Bull 1986;99:66–77.

56. Stark E, Flitcraft AH. Spouse Abuse, 13th ed. In: Last JM, Wallace RB, eds. Public Health & Preventative Medicine. Appleton & Lange, 1992.

57. Walker L. Psychology and violence against women. Am Psychol 1989;44:695–702.

58. Smith MD. Patriarchal ideology and wife beating: A test of a feminist hypothesis. Violence Vict 1990;5:257–273.

59. Panzer P, Eilenberg J. Gender and violence. In: Violence Against Women in the United States: A Comprehensive Background Paper. New York: The Commonwealth Fund Commission on Women's Health, 1995, pp. 25–32.

60. Widom CS. The cycle of violence. Science 1989;244:160–166.

61. Stark E, Flitcraft A. Women and children at risk: A feminist perspective on child abuse. Int J Health Serv 1988;18:97–118.

62. Leonard KE. Drinking patterns and intoxication in marital violence: Review, critique, and future directions of research. In: Martin SE, ed. Alcohol and Interpersonal Violence: Fostering Multidisciplinary Perspectives. Washington, DC: U.S. Department of Health and Human Services, Public Health Service, NIH Publication No. 93-3496, 1993.

63. Hotaling GT, Sugarman DB. An analysis of risk markers in husband to wife violence: The current state of knowledge. Violence Vict 1986;1:101–124.

64. Kantor GK, Straus MA. The "drunken bum" theory of wife beating. Soc Probl 1987;34:213–231.

65. Brookoff D, O'Brien KK, Cook CS, Thompson TD, Williams C. Characteristics of participants in domestic violence: Assessment at the scene of domestic assault. JAMA 1997;277:1369–1373.

66. U.S. Department of Health and Human Services. Eighth Special Report to the U.S. Congress on Alcohol and Health. Washington, DC: U.S. Government Printing Office, 1993.

67. Stark E, Flitcraft AH. Spouse abuse. In: Rosenberg M, Fenley MA, eds. Violence in America: A Public Health Approach. New York: Oxford University Press, 1991, pp. 123–154.

68. Hilberman E, Munson K. Sixty battered women. Victimology: An International Journal 1977;2(8):460–470.

69. Report of the National Council on Alcoholism and Drug Dependence, Inc. New York, 1995.

70. Donnerstein E, Slaby RG, Eron LD. The mass media and youth aggression. In: Eron LD, Gentry JH, Schlegel P, eds. Reason to Hope: A Psychosocial Perspective on Violence and Youth. Washington, DC: American Psychological Association, 1994, pp. 219–250.

71. Surgeon General's Scientific Advisory Committee on Television and Social Behavior. Television and Growing Up: The Impact of Televised Violence. Washington, DC: U.S. Government Printing Office, 1972.

72. National Institute of Mental Health. Television and Behavior: Ten Years of Scientific Progress and Implications for the Eighties, Summary Report (Vol. 1). Washington, DC: U.S. Government Printing Office, 1982.

73. APA Commission on Violence and Youth. Violence and Youth: Psychology's Response. Washington, DC: Public Interest Directorate, American Psychological Association, 1993.

74. Malamuth NM. Predictors of naturalistic sexual aggression. J Pers Soc Psychol 1986;50:953–962.

75. Richie BE, Johnsen C. Abuse histories among newly incarcerated women in a New York City jail. J Am Wom Assoc 1996;51:111–117.

76. Bassuk EL, Weinreb LF, Buckner JC, Browne A, Salomon A, Bassuk SS. The characteristics and needs of sheltered homeless and low-income housed mothers. JAMA 1996;276:640–646.

II

SEX STEROID HORMONES

6

HORMONES IN WOMEN

Kathleen D. Ryan

There are many endocrine glands whose normal functioning is required for good health in women and men. However, the hormones secreted by the endocrine system to regulate reproduction in women, and the hormones and endocrine glands that make fertility, pregnancy, and lactation possible, are unique to women and at times contribute in a unique way to the physiology of health and (eventually) to the pathophysiology of or susceptibility to disease in women. This chapter will describe the basic mechanisms underlying the hormonal milieu in normal, healthy women to provide a foundation for considering the issues of women's health.

ENDOCRINE REGULATION OF THE MENSTRUAL CYCLE

The organ systems whose functions are critical to a discussion of the human reproductive cycle are the hypothalamo–pituitary axis, the ovary, and the uterus. The hypothalamus is neural tissue located at the base of the brain, and it has a direct vascular connection (portal vasculature) to the anterior pituitary gland which rests beneath it. This vascular connection is a "portal system," that is, a collection of veins that begin and end in capillary beds (the capillary beds of the hypothalamus and of the pituitary). There is no direct neural connection between the brain and the anterior pituitary gland. Specific neurons in the hypothalamus secrete a peptide, gonadotropic hormone-releasing hormone (GnRH), into the portal vasculature. At the pituitary, GnRH binds to specific receptors on the gonadotropes, cells that produce luteinizing hormone (LH) and follicle-stimulating hormone (FSH), together termed the gonadotropic hormones. These gonadotropins drive ovarian secretion of the peptide inhibin and the steroid hormones estradiol and progesterone. The sex steroids support the female phenotype (appearance) and regulate changes in the cell structure of the uterine lining or endometrium. This chapter will review the physiological mechanisms regulating ovarian function and show how this cyclic function changes throughout the reproductive life span of human females. More detailed information may be found in references 1–5.

EVENTS OF THE OVARIAN CYCLE

Basic Ovarian Activity, Independent of Cyclicity

At birth, humans possess nearly 500,000 follicles in two ovaries that provide the substrate for the ovarian cycle. Most of these are primordial follicles defined by their simple structure and resting state; primordial follicles consist of an ovum (or egg) surrounded by a single layer of flattened epithelial cells (Fig. 6–1A). In such follicles, the ovum has 46 chromosomes and is about 70% of eventual maximum size. From the viewpoint of menstrual cycle regulation, the seminal characteristics of primordial follicles are that (a) follicles can remain in the primordial state for as long as 50 or more years, (b) factors that initiate movement of primordial follicles into the proliferating pool are unknown, and (c) once a follicle leaves the primordial state, it will ovulate or become atretic. That is, once a follicle begins to develop beyond the primordial state, it is committed to a program with no other resting states and will progress to ovulation or become atretic. Follicles that have left the resting state are referred to as the "proliferating pool." Follicles enter the proliferating pool from the time of formation of the ovary in utero and the process continues until functional follicles are depleted from the ovaries around 50 years of age in humans.

The process through which a primordial follicle leaves the resting state and starts to grow is termed "recruitment," which is thought to occur continuously; the analogy used is that of a dripping faucet—a slow, but continuous activation of one follicle at a time. This model explains why there are often groups of follicles that are very close in stage of development, but only very rarely are even two follicles at identical stages of development. Once recruited, follicles enter into the *menstrual cycle–independent phase* of the follicle life cycle. During this interval (approximately 6–8 weeks duration), the ovum increases in size, the cells surrounding the ovum become cuboidal (square in shape), begin to proliferate, and become enclosed in a basement membrane. These cells become the granulosa cell compartment of the follicle. Outside the basement membrane another layer of cells organizes into the theca cell compartment of the follicle. The replicating granulosa and theca cells cause a substantial increase in overall size of the follicles and these two compartments become the endocrine effectors

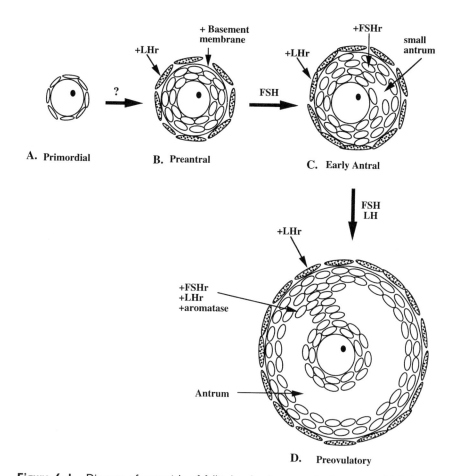

A. Primordial B. Preantral C. Early Antral

D. Preovulatory

Figure 6–1. Diagram of essentials of follicular development. **A:** Structure of follicles in resting stage: primordial follicle. Ovum with nucleus, surrounded by single layer of flattened epithelial cells. Follicles can remain in this stage indefinitely. **B:** First phase of active growth of follicles after recruitment from resting stage. Differentiation of theca (stippled cells) with LH receptor, establishment of basement membrane enclosing replicating granulosa cells. Granulosa cell layer of preantral follicles can vary from 2 cell layers (newly recruited follicles) to 9–15 cell layers (large preantral follicles). This stage can take 5–8 weeks. **C:** Follicle at beginning of rapid growth phase: early antral follicle. Under stimulus of increased FSH, rapid proliferation of granulosa cells with FSH receptors, appearance and gradual increase in size of antrum. **D:** Graafian or preovulatory follicle. These follicles show effects of several days of stimulation by FSH. Very large size, ovum mature size, induction of LH receptors on surface of granulosa cells, induction of aromatase enzyme, further increase in size of antrum. Stages C and D occur only during the menstrual cycle and generally are complete within 14 days. Duration of stage D is usually 2–3 days and culminates in ovulation.

of the ovarian cycle. During this stage of follicular development, theca cells express receptors for luteinizing hormone (LH), and at some point during pre-antral growth, receptors for follicle-stimulating hormone (FSH) can be detected on granulosa cell membranes of these follicles (Fig. 6–1B). Although it is not known exactly when FSH receptors begin to be expressed, they can be seen in fairly small preantral follicles. The role of FSH during preantral growth of follicles is not well understood because preantral follicles appear to be growing in individuals with little or no circulating gonadotropin (e.g., in very young girls or in women after removal of the pituitary gland). However, it is known that this stage of follicle growth is independent of the cyclic changes in LH and FSH secretion that occur during the menstrual cycle.

As the preantral stage of follicle growth progresses, granulosa cells continue to replicate, and about 5–8 weeks after leaving the pool of primordial follicles, a small space, or "antrum," begins to develop in the granulosa cell compartment of large preantral follicles. This early antral stage of follicle development is the morphological hallmark of the onset of the *gonadotropin-dependent,* or *menstrual cycle–dependent, phase* of follicle growth. Further growth and the ultimate fate of follicles once they reach this stage of development are determined by the interplay between the pituitary gonadotropins—LH and FSH—and the gonadal hormones—estradiol, inhibin, and progesterone—which are produced by the ovarian follicle.

The Menstrual Cycle

Menstrual cycles are so named because the periodic sloughing of the endometrial lining of the uterus, termed menstruation, is the most apparent periodic event characterizing reproductive function in nonpregnant adult humans. Periodic menstruation associated with ovarian cycles is not common in nature; it accompanies ovarian cycles primarily in human and nonhuman primates—that is, in few if any other species. As a consequence, most research elucidating the mechanisms governing normal reproductive function in humans is based on extensive studies of nonhuman primates, usually *Rhesus* or *Cynomolgus macaques.* Menstruation is a single event in a sequence of changes imposed on the uterine lining (endometrium) by the cyclic secretions of the ovary. Menstrual cycles are usually about 28 days long but can vary in length substantially among individuals; cycle lengths from 24 to 33 days are considered to be in the normal range. For purposes of discussion, the menstrual cycle can be divided into three functional phases: the follicular, or proliferative, phase (~12 days); the periovulatory phase (48 hr); and the luteal, or secretory, phase (~14 days).

Follicular Phase of the Menstrual Cycle. The onset of menstruation is considered to be day 1 of the menstrual cycle. At that time, the secretion of ovarian steroids, estradiol and progesterone, is very low, and the two gonadotropic hormones, LH and particularly FSH, are elevated in the serum. In response to LH, theca cells in antral follicles secrete two androgens, androstendione and testosterone, which diffuse across the basement membrane into the granulosa compartment of the follicle. The elevation in serum FSH concentrations that occurs at the beginning of the menstrual cycle initiates FSH-dependent follicle growth in all follicles that have reached the early antral stage (Fig. 6–1C). Overall, FSH acts as the primary growth hormone to support follicular development. In this regard, FSH stimulates granulosa cell division, so the antral follicles continue to increase in size, and the open space, or antrum, in these follicles also becomes larger. The basement membrane surrounding the granulosa compartment remains intact, so the interior of the follicle is without blood supply; the antral fluid that fills the space is an exudate of plasma and is secreted by the granulosa cells. The rapidly proliferating granulosa cells all have FSH receptors, thus one consequence of the FSH-stimulated growth is an overall increase in the mass of tissue expressing FSH receptors. Under the continued stimulus of FSH, synthesis of cytochrome P450 aromatase is induced in the granulosa cells. This enzyme catalyzes the synthesis of estradiol from androstenedione and testosterone. Thus, the growing follicles begin to secrete increasing quantities of estradiol into the bloodstream. At present, it seems that primate ovaries do not express estradiol receptors, and the estradiol produced by the growing follicles does not appear to have an effect inside the follicle. However, the rising titers of estradiol in blood exert systemic effects, one of which is to feedback at the pituitary and inhibit FSH secretion. The effect of this fall in FSH concentrations on the growing follicles depends on the degree to which the follicles have responded to the several days of FSH stimulation as discussed below.

Further actions of FSH on granulosa cells are to induce the synthesis and secretion of the peptide hormone inhibin, and most importantly, to induce the synthesis of LH receptors on granulosa cell surface membranes. Preantral and early antral follicles express LH receptors only in the theca cells, whereas after several days of stimulation by FSH, large follicles begin to express granulosa cell LH receptors as well as increased numbers of FSH receptors (Fig. 6–1D). This acquisition of LH receptors has two critical effects on the follicle. First, it gives the follicle the ability to respond to the ovulatory stimulus, the LH surge. Second, acquisition of LH receptors most probably protects the largest follicles against the effects of the decreasing levels of FSH, which are falling in response to the rising titers of estradiol from the growing follicles. Inhibin also exerts negative feedback on FSH, but in higher primates and humans, the primary regulator of FSH secretion is estradiol.

To understand the protective effect of the induction of LH receptors in large follicles, one must consider the intracellular signaling cascade activated by the binding of FSH to its granulosa cell receptor. The FSH receptor is a

G-protein-linked receptor. Binding of FSH to its receptor stimulates the activity of adenylate cyclase, causing an increase in intracellular cyclic adenosine monophosphate (cAMP). This elevation of cAMP protects the granulosa cells and supports their continued growth and physiological functions, including aromatase activity. Binding of LH to its receptor also results in a stimulation of intracellular cAMP, thus a cell possessing both LH and FSH receptors continues to increase cAMP in response to LH, even though FSH is decreasing from the estradiol being secreted by this large follicle. In primates, usually only one follicle (sometimes two) has acquired enough LH receptor to protect the follicle from the mid-follicular phase decline in FSH. Thus, when FSH falls at this time, any growing follicle that has reached the gonadotropin-dependent phase of development, yet has not acquired sufficient numbers of LH receptors, will die (become atretic), whereas follicles that have both LH and FSH receptors will continue to grow in response to ambient LH and FSH (Fig. 6–1D).

Ovulation. The acquisition of LH receptors and the subsequent rapid growth of one or two follicles represents the beginning of the periovulatory period of the ovarian cycle. The rapid and sustained rise in plasma estradiol concentrations from this preovulatory follicle causes a radical change in gonadotropin secretion from the pituitary, which will be discussed later in this chapter. Estradiol concentrations surpassing 250 pg/ml and which remain at that level for ~48 hours are the direct cause of a very large secretion of LH during which, over a 24-hour period, LH rises rapidly in plasma to levels several-fold higher than those found during the basal secretion of LH that is typical of the rest of the ovarian cycle. A lesser increase in FSH from the pituitary and a small burst in ovarian progesterone secretion also occur at the time of the LH surge. This large release of LH is called the preovulatory surge of LH because this pattern of LH secretion is directly responsible for the rupture of the mature ovarian follicle and release of the ovum to the oviduct, or ovulation. The high levels of LH attained during the surge have several sequelae in the ovary. LH receptors are massively stimulated and thus decrease in number (down-regulate). The decrease in LH receptors on theca cells stops thecal androgen production, thus causing a rapid fall in estradiol secretion. During this time, follicular fluid increases rapidly in volume, but intrafollicular pressure does not increase. Rather, another effect of this LH surge is to induce increased quantities of proteolytic enzymes in the follicle wall, leading to the breakdown and eventual rupture of the follicle, thus releasing the ovum with its surrounding cells into the vicinity of the oviduct. The events mediated by the LH surge take time, and ovulation usually occurs about 36 hours after the peak of the LH surge. In addition to causing release of the ovum from the mature follicle, the LH surge also causes a breakdown of the basement membrane between the theca and granulosa cells of the ovulating follicle. Although the granulosa cells immediately surrounding the ovum (the corona radiata) leave the ovary during ovulation, the granulosa and theca cells in the wall of the follicle remain behind. With the breakdown of the basement membrane in the follicle, vascularization of the granulosa cells begins, and critical organizing events occur, during which the follicle evolves into a different endocrine gland called the corpus luteum.

Luteal Phase of the Menstrual Cycle. During the 96 hours following the LH surge, progesterone and estradiol production by the newly formed corpus luteum rise rapidly. During the first few days of luteal function, progesterone synthesis is limited by the rate of development of the vasculature of the corpus luteum. Thus, while the enzyme machinery for luteal steroid secretion is in place within hours of the LH surge, steroid production does not reach maximal output until days 4–5 after the LH surge when the new vascular supply is completed. The cells of the corpus luteum are capable of de novo synthesis of progesterone from cholesterol which is delivered to the cells from the plasma; these cells also retain the ability to synthesize estradiol from androgen precursors. Steroid secretion by the corpus luteum rises for the first 4–6 days after the LH surge, persists on a plateau for days 6–10, then decreases over the ensuing days 12–15. Progesterone levels in plasma from a functional corpus luteum are around 10 ng/ml, while estradiol is also secreted in large quantities with plasma levels in mid-luteal phase as high as 160 pg/ml.

At all phases of its life span, steroid secretion by the corpus luteum is dependent on LH secreted from the pituitary. Interruption of LH secretion at any point during the luteal phase causes an immediate fall in progesterone to undetectable levels and if the LH deprivation lasts for more than 72 hours, luteal function cannot be restored, even if LH support is resumed. Interestingly, if LH support to the corpus luteum is restored *within* 72 hours after interruption, the functional secretion of progesterone resumes, but the total life span of the corpus luteum is not changed—i.e., the corpus luteum will still regress around day 16 (13.5 days after ovulation). This observation illustrates the phenomenon of the inherent and relatively invariant life span of the corpus luteum of the primate. Once ovulation occurs, the corpus luteum functions for about 15 days, then it regresses. With regression of the corpus luteum, estradiol, progesterone, and inhibin levels decrease to basal concentrations, signaling the end of this ovarian cycle and removing the negative feedback inhibition on the pituitary. The consequent elevation in FSH secretion then initiates the next ovarian cycle with renewed follicle growth. For more detailed discussions of follicle and corpus luteum function, see references 3 and 4.

In the event that sexual intercourse occurs around the time of ovulation and a pregnancy is initiated, the fate of the corpus luteum changes. The fertilized ovum begins to undergo cell division while it is traveling down the oviduct toward the uterine cavity. Upon arrival in the uterus about 5 days after ovulation, the conceptus is now a multicellular blastocyst capable of invading the wall of the uterus; this process is called implantation. Within 48 hours of beginning to embed itself into the uterine wall, the trophoblast (conceptus) begins to secrete a hormone unique to pregnancy: human chorionic gonadotropin (hCG). This peptide hormone binds to LH receptors in the corpus luteum, but it has much greater potency and a longer half-life than LH. The hCG, acting in essence like a huge LH stimulus, rescues the corpus luteum, thereby blocking luteal regression and supporting a steady increase in progesterone secretion. This rescued corpus luteum becomes the corpus luteum of pregnancy and provides the necessary progesterone and estradiol for maintaining a progestational uterine lining until the steroid-secreting placenta becomes established during the fourth month of pregnancy.

HYPOTHALAMIC–PITUITARY REGULATION OF THE OVARIAN CYCLE

Pituitary Function

Because of the feedback interplay between the hypothalamo-pituitary axis and the secretions of the ovary, the gonadotropins regulate ovarian function and at the same time are regulated by ovarian steroids. During the first 5 days of the menstrual cycle, the ovarian hormones, estradiol, progesterone, and inhibin, are at their lowest level because of the regression of the corpus luteum from the previous cycle and the absence of large antral follicles. As a result of these low ovarian hormone levels, there is reduced negative feedback inhibition of FSH and the plasma concentration of that hormone rises. The effects of the low steroid milieu on LH are more subtle than those on FSH, but during these first few days of the menstrual cycle, LH pulses occur at about 90-minute intervals at amplitudes lower than those of luteal-phase pulses but higher than LH pulses occurring later during the follicular phase. Under the combined influence of this early follicular-phase LH and FSH, the gonadotropin-dependent phase of follicle growth is initiated, with a stimulation of estradiol and inhibin secretion. With regard to FSH, the effect of this increase in estradiol and inhibin is unequivocal; by about day 6 of the follicular phase, concentrations of FSH begin to decrease in response to the increasing potency of the negative feedback influence of those two hormones. Although both estradiol and inhibin are known to be inhibitory to FSH secretion, in humans and higher primates, estradiol is the primary regulator of FSH secretion (Fig. 6–2).

There does not appear to be any marked change in the frequency of LH pulses during this period of rising estradiol levels, but the amplitude of LH pulses at this time decreases. When high levels of estradiol persist for 48 hours or longer, the effect of this hormone on the hypothalamo-pituitary axis changes

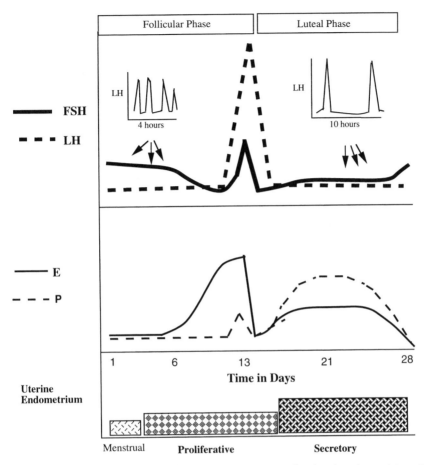

Figure 6–2. Diagram of patterns of hormone secretion correlated with endometrial cytology throughout the human menstrual cycle. The top panel shows changes in FSH (heavy solid line) and LH (dashed line) secretion in serum throughout the menstrual cycle. Small inserts in this panel show diagrams of expected patterns of detailed profiles of secretion of LH. Note the slowing of LH pulse frequency during the luteal phase. The center panel diagrams profiles of estradiol (solid line) and progesterone (dashed line) during a 28-day menstrual cycle. Patterns of inhibin levels are not shown, but they would be similar to that of estradiol. The lowest panel indicates the uterine cytology that would be expected at each phase of the menstrual cycle. Examples of each phase are shown in Figure 6–3.

from negative feedback to positive feedback. After 48 hours of the marked increase in estradiol levels in serum, LH secretion is massively stimulated and a large LH surge is secreted over a 24-hour period. This LH surge is several-fold higher than the basal LH secretion that occurs throughout the rest of the menstrual cycle and is the direct cause of ovulation of the ovum from the mature follicle. Augmented secretion of both FSH and progesterone accompany the LH surge, and after about 24 hours, all three hormones return to basal levels.

As the cells remaining in the ovary from the ovulated follicle organize into the corpus luteum under the stimulus of the LH surge, progesterone, estradiol, and inhibin levels begin to rise again, this time being secreted from the corpus luteum. The maturing corpus luteum reaches peak function about 5–6 days after the LH surge, and steroid secretion from the corpus luteum remains high for the next 5 days. The elevated levels of luteal hormones have three major effects on the hypothalamo-hypophyseal axis. First, the high estradiol and inhibin together maximally inhibit FSH, to the extent that there is virtually no gonadotropin-dependent follicle growth during the luteal phase. Second, the high concentrations of progesterone in combination with elevated estradiol inhibit LH secretion by decreasing the *frequency* of LH pulses from the follicular-phase frequency of one pulse/90 min to a luteal-phase frequency of one pulse/5–8 hr. Third, although the corpus luteum secretes estradiol in amounts comparable to that of the preovulatory follicle, the simultaneously elevated levels of progesterone block the positive feedback of the estradiol, so no LH surges are induced during the luteal phase of the ovarian cycle (Fig. 6–2).

Hypothalamic GnRH Secretion

Considering the changes in pituitary gonadotropin secretion throughout the menstrual cycle, what can be inferred about regulation of the hypothalamic peptide, gonadotropic hormone-releasing hormone (GnRH) under these changing endocrine environments? This peptide controls pituitary gonadotropin secretion yet cannot be detected in peripheral blood, largely because the portal vasculature lies between the hypothalamus and pituitary, thus measurable concentrations of GnRH are only achieved in that very small and inaccessible vascular bed. The pattern of LH secretion is therefore often used to deduce GnRH activity. The assumption underlying this approach is that all LH secretion is driven by GnRH pulses. To date, this seems to be a valid assumption in the several animal models in which it is possible to cannulate the hypothalamo-pituitary portal vasculature and to directly measure GnRH secretion. The correlation of GnRH pulses with LH pulses in those studies suggest that if an LH pulse occurs, it was preceded by a release of GnRH; thus, if LH pulse frequency increases or decreases, the number of GnRH pulses arriving at the pituitary must be increasing or decreasing.

The problem with this approach is in reaching conclusions regarding changes in GnRH pulse amplitude. If the size of an LH pulse changes, it could be because there is more or less GnRH stimulating the gonadotroph per pulse, or it could be because the pituitary release of LH in response to each pulse of GnRH has changed. The currently accepted method of addressing the issue of changes in LH pulse amplitude is to administer fixed doses of GnRH to subjects at different times during the menstrual cycle. The reasoning is that if the amount of LH released in response to a given dose of GnRH is constant (in two differing endocrine states) but the endogenous LH pulses differ in magnitude, then the amount of GnRH per pulse may well be changing. If the LH response to exogenous GnRH changes however, one can only conclude that the altered response to GnRH precludes conclusions about GnRH pulse amplitude. i.e., if LH pulse amplitude is reduced and GnRH response to a standard dose of the decapeptide is also reduced, either one or both events may be occurring. One caveat to this interpretation is that the amplitude of LH response to GnRH can be affected both by ambient steroid levels and by the interval between the artificial injection and the previous endogenous GnRH pulse.

With that as background, consider now the possible changes in GnRH secretion during the menstrual cycle. At the beginning of the menstrual cycle, LH pulses occur at a frequency of one pulse/90 min. This is the highest frequency of LH secretion in humans and occurs throughout much of the menstrual cycle. As follicular growth is stimulated, the progressive rise in serum estradiol concentrations that occurs during the second half of the follicular phase is not accompanied by any decrease in LH pulse frequency—in fact, some laboratories report a slight increase in pulse frequency at this time. While estradiol thus does not appear to exert negative feedback on the *frequency* of GnRH pulsatile secretion, the rising titers of estradiol in serum that occur during the follicular phase do alter the ability of GnRH to elicit LH secretion. Studies examining the LH response to a fixed dose of GnRH show that the pituitary response to GnRH is markedly enhanced during the second half of the follicular phase in that the LH response to a fixed dose of GnRH is much greater on days 6–10 of the follicular phase than on days 1–6. Examination of the endogenous LH secretory profile during the follicular phase of the menstrual cycle reveals, however, that LH pulses occur at a high frequency of one pulse per 60–90 min, but the amplitudes of these pulses are lower than those occurring on days 1–6 of the follicular phase or during the luteal phase. The finding of lower endogenous LH pulse amplitude at a time when the response to GnRH is known to be *increased* suggests that the GnRH pulse amplitude must be decreased at this time.

As stated above, once follicular estradiol secretion reaches a stimulatory threshold and remains there for at least 48 hours, a fundamental change occurs in the hypothalamo-hypophyseal-gonadal axis, resulting in the triggering of the ovulatory LH surge. Under the influence of elevated serum estradiol, two changes occur. The responsiveness of the gonadotrophs to GnRH stimulation continues to increase from follicular phase and becomes maximal. The best illustration of this is that in primates, even if no increment in GnRH were to occur, a surge of LH sufficient to cause ovulation will be secreted. However, in addition to the increase in GnRH responsiveness of the pituitary, the effect of estradiol on the hypothalamus changes from inhibiting amplitude of GnRH pulses to markedly stimulating amplitude and perhaps frequency of GnRH secretion. These two changes combine to produce a massive surge of LH secretion that continues for 24 hours and is the direct cause of ovulation. The most likely explanation for the termination of the GnRH–LH surge is exhaustion of readily releasable pools of the two hormones, but it is possible that either the small rise in progesterone or some unknown factor may contribute to the termination of this period of massive hormone secretion. The end of the LH surge is not caused by the abrupt decline in ovarian estradiol secretion, however, because if estradiol is artificially maintained at a surge-inducing level during and after the LH surge, the amplitude and duration of the ovulatory surge are not affected. At the end of the LH surge, LH and FSH return to basal levels, and estradiol, progesterone, and inhibin levels from the newly formed corpus luteum begin to increase.

The steroid hormones and inhibin secreted by the corpus luteum have effects on hypothalamic GnRH secretion as well as on the pituitary. During the first few days of the luteal phase, when steroid levels are relatively low, LH pulses, and thus GnRH pulses, occur at 90-minute intervals. However, with the maturation of the corpus luteum under the stimulus of LH, progesterone and estradiol secretion rises rapidly by the mid-luteal phase. This elevated concentration of progesterone exerts two effects on the hypothalamus. First, the combination of luteal-phase levels of progesterone with elevated estradiol causes a marked slowing of LH pulses because of intense negative feedback on hypothalamic GnRH secretion. If anything, the amplitude of GnRH pulses at this time either remains the same or increases because the amplitude of these slow-frequency LH pulses (one pulse/5–8 hr) is higher than at any other time in the menstrual cycle, exclusive of the LH surge. The second effect of this level of progesterone is to block the ability of estradiol to induce an LH surge. The luteal production of estradiol is comparable to levels inducing preovulatory surges during the follicular phase; however, no such surges can occur with commensurate elevation in serum progesterone levels. More detailed discussion of neural regulation of ovarian function is presented in references 1–5.

EFFECTS OF THE OVARIAN CYCLE ON THE GENITAL TRACT

In addition to the influence of ovarian steroids on the brain and pituitary gland, many tissues in the body exhibit changes in morphology or function or both during the menstrual cycle in response to cyclic changes in the levels of estradiol and progesterone (see Chapter 11). An incomplete list of organs affected is breasts, skin, vascular smooth muscle and vascular endothelium, renal function, bladder and urogenital smooth muscle, and the body temperature regulatory center in the anterior hypothalamus. The uterine endometrium and the secretion of cervical mucus exhibit ovarian cycle–dependent changes in structure and function of direct relevance to this chapter. Cyclic changes in these will be briefly reviewed below.

Uterine Endometrium[1,5]

The uterine lining, or endometrium, is a major target organ of the ovarian steroid hormones estradiol and progesterone. The waxing and waning concentrations of these hormones in the circulation are the direct cause of periodic, structural changes in the uterine lining that underlie the menstrual cycle. The uterus is a hollow organ made up of several layers. The outermost layers are uterine smooth muscle which are important for uterine contractile activity and structural integrity of the organ. The uterine lining, or endometrium, is comprised of three layers, or more accurately, regions: the basalis is the transition area between the endometrium and the muscle layers. It is largely epithelial tissue and provides the substrate for replacement and proliferation of the endometrium. The transient tissues of the uterus are the endometrial glandular tissue, the stroma, and a single cell layer of surface epithelium that lines the uterine cavity. These tissues respond to the hormonal milieu of the ovarian cycle with marked growth, differentiation, and remodeling as described below and as diagrammed in Figure 6–2.

Proliferative Phase. This phase occurs from the end of the period of menstrual bleeding through the follicular phase of the ovarian cycle and through the time of ovulation. During this interval, the endometrium, which was shed during menstruation, is repaired and replaced. The very early stages of endometrial repair may be independent of the ovarian hormones, as sealing of blood vessels and early growth of a single layer of endometrium occur in ovariectomized and postmenopausal women. However, proliferation of the uterine lining requires the growth-promoting properties of estradiol and progresses from days 5–14 of the menstrual cycle. During this period, serum titers of estradiol rise steadily because of the maturation of the preovulatory follicle. In the uterus, estradiol acts as a true growth hormone, stimulating cell division of both the endometrial glandular epithelium as well as the stroma. Both tissues demonstrate increased mitotic activity indicative of cell division under the stimulus of follicular-phase estradiol concentrations. During this period, the endometrium thickens because of growth of several elements: *(a)* proliferation and thickening of the mucosal layer (cells lining the internal surface of the uterine cavity), *(b)* epithelial glands increasing in length, and *(c)* thickening and increasing vascularity of the stroma that underlies the mucosal epithelium (Fig. 6–3A, D). By the end of the follicular phase, in the presence of maximal levels of estradiol, the uterine endometrium has grown from a single layer of epithelial cells with small, simple,

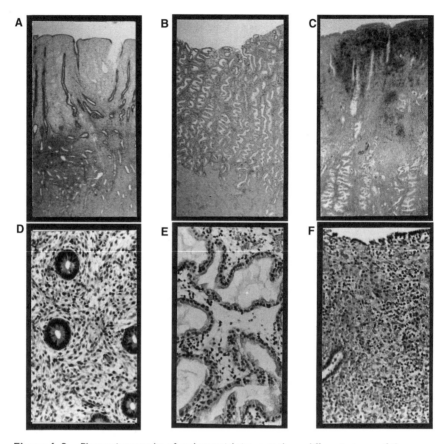

Figure 6–3. Photomicrographs of endometrial tissue at three different stages of the menstrual cycle: proliferative phase (**A, D**); secretory phase (**B, E**), and menstrual phase (**C, F**). (**A**) Low power photomicrograph of proliferative endometrium that is supported by estradiol. The basalis layer is shown just above the muscularis layer that is at the base of the panel. Long, straight grandular tissue is visible. Uterine lumen is at top of panel. (**D**) Higher power photomicrograph of tissue in A. Donut shapes are characteristic of proliferative endometrium, and are the result of the straight glands cut in cross-section. Stroma (area between "donuts") is densely packed and not edematous. (**B**) Low power photomicrograph of secretory phase endometrium induced by exposure of proliferative endometrium to progesterone. Glands have become longer and very tortuous. The muscularis layer is shown at the base of the panel on the left. Uterine lumen is at top of panel. It can be seen that the area immediately above the muscularis, called the basalis, also has responded to the progesterone. Higher power in **E** shows cross section of tortuous glands containing secretory materials. Note the edema of the stroma (nuclei farther apart than in **D**). (**C**) Low power photomicrograph of menstrual endometrium. Muscularis is not visible in this panel. Degeneration of the tissue is heaviest at lumen (top). Dark area is blood and degenerating tissue. **F** shows invasion of leukocytes to participate in removal of degenerated tissue. Breakdown of secretory endometrium results from withdrawal of hormonal support caused by luteal regression in the absence of pregnancy.

linear glandular tissue, to highly vascularized, multicellular layers of mucosa with long, straight, epithelial glands and a thickened, densely packed underlying stroma.

These proliferative changes in the uterine endometrium are driven by rising titers of ovarian estradiol, but not all of the effects of this hormone are direct. In addition to directly stimulating uterine growth, estradiol also stimulates many paracrine factors (produced by neighboring cells and diffused directly to their target without first entering the bloodstream), including growth factors that probably play a role in this epithelial build-up. In addition to the structural changes, another important effect of estradiol is that it induces the synthesis of progesterone receptor in endometrial cells. With the induction of progesterone receptors, the uterine endometrium acquires the ability to differentiate into a secretory endothelium.

Secretory Phase. The second half of the menstrual cycle, or luteal phase, is also called the post-ovulatory phase, the progestational phase, or the secretory phase. The latter two terms refer to the changes in the uterine endometrium that occur in response to the secretions of the corpus luteum. Under the influence of rising serum titers of estradiol and especially of progesterone, the mitotic activity of endometrial glandular cells and stroma continues. The glandular epithelium lengthens and the glands become tortuous or twisted and complex. The stroma becomes highly vascularized and both surface epithelium and stroma thicken. In addition, secretions of proteins and numerous growth factors markedly increase from the stimulated glandular tissue, thus giving rise to the term secretory phase (Fig. 6–3B, E). The proliferative endometrium, even at the end of the follicular phase, cannot support a conceptus. The structural changes associated with the luteal phase are essential for successful implantation and initiation of pregnancy. In particular, the effects of progesterone on the endometrium are essential, thus the term progestational phase. In fact, the steroid hormone progesterone, was named for its important role in the establishment and maintenance of pregnancy (gestation).

Menstrual Phase. If sexual intercourse resulting in fertilization of the newly ovulated ovum does not occur in the first 2–3 days following the LH surge, the corpus luteum will support the progestational endometrium for 12–14 days and then the corpus luteum will regress, causing a precipitous decline in the secretion of both estradiol and progesterone by the ovary. This event will withdraw hormonal support required by the endometrium, resulting in the breakdown and sloughing of this tissue. The fall in luteal steroids is thought to elicit an abrupt increase in prostaglandins that causes marked vasoconstriction of the uterine vasculature underlying the endometrium. This vasoconstriction of the vascular supply to the endometrium, combined with the withdrawal of steroid support, leads to degeneration of both glandular elements and stroma. These degenerative changes lead to inflammatory invasion by lymphocytes, thrombosis of the stroma, and eventual sloughing of the endometrium as menstrual flow (Fig. 6–3C, F). This flow can vary widely among individuals in volume and duration, but the average menstrual flow is 30 ml over 3–6 days. Factors influencing the volume of menstrual flow are not as yet well understood, and flow duration as short as 2 days and as long as 8 days are in the range of normal variability.

Cervical Mucus[1,5]

Both the quantity and biochemical characteristics (quality) of cervical mucus are altered by the hormonal milieu of the menstrual cycle. Under the stimulus of elevated serum concentrations of estradiol during the follicular phase, cervical secretions become copious, clear, and watery. The peak of the estradiol rise correlates with the period of maximum water content of the cervical mucus. This high water content has the effects of hydrating the mucin molecules in the cervical secretions, increasing the volume of mucus, and diluting the protein, carbohydrate, and lipid molecules that comprise this fluid. The period of maximum secretion of watery cervical mucus coincides with the periovulatory phase of the menstrual cycle. With the onset of progesterone secretion in the days following ovulation, the water content and quantity of cervical mucus decreases and the mucus becomes viscous and cloudy in appearance. These cyclic changes in the character of the cervical mucus most likely have functional significance also. The mucins in the watery, well-hydrated mucus characteristic of the periovulatory period are arrayed in parallel bundles or spindles which are aligned into molecular channels in the cervical canal. This parallel array of mucin proteins and the watery nature of the fluid are most likely permissive to the passage of sperm from the vagina into the uterus and upper genital tract. Thus, at the time of the cycle during which a newly ovulated ovum is present, cervical secretions are hospitable to sperm and may even aid in sperm transport. In contrast, the character of cervical mucus changes markedly with the onset of progesterone secretion. The overall quantity of mucus decreases in response to increasing concentrations of progesterone in circulation, and the water content of the fluid declines proportionally more than other elements. The mucus thus becomes very viscous and may form a barrier to transport of materials through the cervix. This type of cervical mucus is induced by progesterone and persists until the elevated levels of estradiol resume during the last days of the follicular phase. Besides posing a barrier to sperm transport, it is thought that nonovulatory cervical mucus may constitute an important physiological barrier to infectious agents such as bacteria or viruses, thus providing a degree of protection during much of the menstrual cycle[1] (see Chapter 12).

MENSTRUAL CYCLE: SUMMARY

The menstrual cycle can be viewed as an external manifestation of the effects of the ovarian cycle. The overall driver of the system is the hypothalamic peptide GnRH. This hormone, secreted into the pituitary portal vasculature, stimulates the secretion of both FSH and LH—the two hormones that regulate ovarian follicle growth, elicit ovulation, and support luteal function. The ovarian hormones estradiol, progesterone, and inhibin are secreted under the stimulus of FSH and LH, and the levels attained and timing of secretions of the ovarian hormones influence the hypothalamo-hypophyseal secretion of GnRH, LH, and FSH, and have direct effects on tissues of the genital tract, especially the uterine endometrium.

BEGINNING AND END OF MENSTRUAL CYCLICITY: MENARCHE AND THE MENOPAUSE

There are two periods of life during which normal, healthy individuals exhibit little or no ovarian activity, and thus have very low circulating estradiol and no reproductive potential. The first of these intervals, the childhood period of sexual immaturity, precedes adult reproductive life. The second occurs in older women who are usually 50 years of age or older, after the childbearing years of reproductive competence. Both intervals are characterized by very low estradiol levels due to low or absent ovarian follicle growth. However, the physiology underlying these two conditions is markedly different as are the sequelae of the hypoestrogenic state in each case. The following section will briefly review the mechanisms underlying menarche and the menopause, emphasizing the specific changes in the hypothalamo-hypophyseal-ovarian axis characteristic of these two normal physiologic states.

Sexual Immaturity and Onset of Menstrual Cycles

The lack of ovarian activity in immature girls can be explained by the very low levels of LH and FSH in the circulation at this time. From the age of 12 months through about 8.5–9.5 years, there is insufficient gonadotropin secretion to support ovarian function. Ovarian follicle recruitment and gonadotropin-independent growth of follicles occur, but when follicles reach the highly FSH-dependent, early antral stage, there is not enough FSH to support further growth, so atresia and death of these large, preantral follicles ensues without secretion of significant quantities of estradiol. The reason for the low gonadotropin levels in girls is that the hypothalamic peptide GnRH is not being secreted at levels high enough to elicit effective secretion of FSH and LH. This absence of stimulatory levels of GnRH secretion is the defining neuroendocrine characteristic of childhood and is the reason for the inactive ovaries and hypoestrogenic state. It has been well established in both nonhuman primates and in humans that if adult levels of GnRH are provided, pituitary and ovarian function will occur normally in immature females.

If quiescence of the GnRH system is the underlying cause of childhood immaturity, then the onset of reproductive competence must be associated with the awakening of this system. At about 9 years of age, increased activity of the GnRH system begins. This occurs first at night, during sleep, and is manifested by detectable pulses of FSH and LH secretion that occur only during sleep. At first, the period of GnRH pulses is short, with only a few LH pulses during the sleep period. Also, the rate of onset of GnRH secretion is probably highly variable among individuals, with some children showing rapid progression of increased GnRH activity and others showing sporadic or intermittent nights of GnRH activity followed by inactive, quiescent nights for several months. However, whenever GnRH pulses occur, each pulse stimulates LH and FSH secretion from the pituitary which in turn stimulates any antral follicles that may be present in the ovary at this time, causing the secretion of a small amount of estradiol. These very low levels of estradiol have systemic effects; one of the first signs of estradiol secretion is breast budding, the beginning of breast development, or thelarche. This secretion also initiates proliferative changes in the endometrium. Still another effect of augmented GnRH pulsatile activity during sexual development is maturation of the pituitary response to subsequent pulses.

When GnRH pulses first increase in occurrence, the pituitary response is a large release of FSH, with a very small LH pulse. As the pituitary receives increasing numbers of GnRH pulses each night, the proportions of LH and FSH secreted in response to each GnRH pulse gradually alter to that characteristic of adults, with a small release of FSH and a large pulse of LH. This change in pituitary response to a bolus of GnRH has been used to assess the progress of hypothalamic maturation in the early stages of puberty.

As the pubertal process progresses, the duration of the sleep-related elevation in gonadotropin secretion increases to fill the entire sleep period, driving further ovarian activity and thus greater secretion of estradiol. This augmented FSH and LH secretion can either result in steady development of a preovulatory follicle or it can remain intermittent or irregular such that follicular secretion of estradiol increases, causing further stimulation of endometrial proliferation and breast development but not progressing to full ovulation. In that case, a fall in gonadotropin levels will result in a fall in circulating estradiol levels and in the first episode of vaginal bleeding or the first menses, which is termed menarche.

Although it heralds the near approach of full reproductive function, menarche does not necessarily correlate with (nor exclude) first ovulation. For the reason illustrated above, menstrual cycles at puberty are often irregular and frequently, although not reliably, anovulatory. With continued development, GnRH pulsatile secretion gradually settles into the adult pattern of 1 pulse/

60–90 min, resulting in normal menstrual cycles occurring about every 28 days. As cycle length approaches 28 days, ovulation becomes the norm. Regular, 28-day menstrual cycles are usually established within 5 years of menarche.

The development of pubic and axillary hair, which is one of the early external indicators of impending puberty, is a consequence of a pubertal shift in adrenal secretions (adrenarche) and is beyond the scope of this chapter. However, even though adrenarche frequently occurs up to 1 year before thelarche, the developmental activation of GnRH pulsatile secretion, which is the primary event initiating puberty in humans and nonhuman primates, is not causally related to adrenarche. In fact, the physiological mechanism(s) underlying the pubertal activation of GnRH secretion is not known. It has been shown that intensive physical activities with high metabolic demand such as ballet dancing and gymnastics can delay the onset of sexual maturation. However, attempts to identify the factor or factors limiting sexual maturation have not yielded complete understanding of this important phase of reproductive life. A more complete discussion of puberty and its underlying physiology may be found in references 1, 2, 4, and 6—8.

Cessation of Menstrual Cycles: Menopause

In most women living in the Western hemisphere, the last menstrual period occurs at around 50 years of age. This cessation of monthly menstruation (men = monthly [Gr.], pause = stop) occurs because of the loss of ovarian follicles capable of responding to FSH and LH. As stated at the beginning of this chapter, all primordial follicles and thus ova available to an individual develop in the ovary in utero. From that point, the number of follicles steadily declines, primarily through atresia, and a small number is lost through ovulation. This loss of follicles begins in utero and continues throughout life until all primordial follicles are gone, a process which takes approximately 50 years in most individuals.

The primary source of circulating estradiol during the reproductive years is ovarian follicles. Approximately 8–10 years prior to the cessation of menstrual cycles, circulating concentrations of FSH begin to increase in many women. This rise in FSH levels is thought to reflect a decrease in the numbers of antral follicles present in the ovary, leading to decreased inhibin and perhaps estrogen production, although estradiol levels are not demonstrably lower at this time. Increased FSH levels in women with regular menstrual cycles is a harbinger of the approach of the menopause and has been reported by several laboratories.[1,9–11] As follicle numbers decline further, the primary tissue source of estradiol is also lost and circulating estrogen levels decline. With the cessation of ovulation and the consequent absence of corpora lutea, progesterone secretion also ceases. Because these steroids are the primary negative feedback regulators of LH, FSH, and GnRH secretion from the pituitary and hypothalamus, the cessation of cyclic ovarian function allows a reflex increase in the pituitary gonadotropins, and postmenopausal women exhibit elevated, but still pulsatile, LH and FSH. The elevated levels of gonadotropins do not appear to cause any symptoms, but the loss of circulating estradiol has system-wide effects.

In women of reproductive age, the primary estrogen is 16β-estradiol produced by the ovarian follicles, however, there are other, less potent estrogens produced from extraglandular sites as well as the ovary. After menopause, these weaker estrogens contribute to the hormonal milieu in an important fashion. The primary estrogen produced after menopause is estrone, which is derived from the aromatization of androstenedione. While functional follicles are present, circulating levels of estrone are probably not physiologically significant. However, after menopause, when ovarian estradiol is no longer available, estrone becomes the primary estrogenic factor in the circulation. Low levels of estradiol that remain in the circulation are derived from estrone.

The actual tissue source of estrone may change with increasing years after menopause. There is substantial variation in estrogen levels in the blood during the first few years after cessation of menses. Circulating steroid levels consistant with some ovarian activity have been reported in approximately 20%–40% of early postmenopausal women, limiting the utility of estrogen measurements in epidemiological studies of women in this age group. One theory is that the primary site of cellular aging in the ovary is the granulosa compartment, with relatively little degeneration of the theca cells; thus the postmenopausal ovary becomes primarily an organ of androgen secretion. This theory is supported by studies in which determinations of the ovarian-arterial gradient in postmenopausal women showed that the ovary continues to produce testosterone and androstenedione, which are also the substrates underlying ovarian estrone production. However, the postmenopausal ovary only produces ~20% of the androstenedione that is measureable in blood of these women.[1,12–14] The primary glandular source of androstenedione after menopause is the adrenal glands; the primary site of aromatization of this androgen to estrone is adipose tissue. This relationship underlies the observation that circulating levels of estrone in postmenopausal women are positively correlated with body weight and increasing age.[1,14] It is important to note, however, that even with increased conversion of androstenedione to estrone in older women, estrone is a much weaker estrogen than is estradiol, and even relatively obese postmenopausal women are hypoestrogenic compared to women in the reproductive years. This is not to say however, that the circulating estrone after menopause has no biological action. In women with no circulating estradiol, estrone binds to estradiol receptors and exerts estrogenic effects. The elevation in circulating estrone that accompanies increased percent body fat in obese women is likely a part of the mechanism whereby obesity is protective against postmenopausal osteoporosis and can also be correlated with decreased severity of many symptoms of menopause. In general, low body weight and slight body habitus after menopause is accompanied by increased severity of menopausal symptoms and disease.[14]

There are two major ways in which estradiol withdrawal after menopause acutely and negatively affects women's health. First, loss of estradiol is causally associated with a change in the dynamic of cells remodeling bone, and in the first few years after menopause there is rapid demineralization of bone particularly trabecular bone such as in the spine. The bone loss slows down somewhat after a few years, but it continues for the remainder of life. The loss of bone density is associated with significantly increased risk of fractures of the hip and spine as well as other bones, and such fractures occur with markedly higher incidence in postmenopausal women than in men of the same age. Studies among postmenopausal women have also revealed that estrogens participate in the regulation of the cardiovascular system, both in normal function and perhaps in the maintenance of general vascular tone, as estrogens affect the elasticity of the vascular wall.

Estradiol is most likely cardioprotective in that it seems to be an important player in the relatively low risk of cardiovascular disease among reproductive-age women as well as in the rapid increase in incidence of heart disease and stroke among postmenopausal women. In addition to the side effects of osteoporosis (bone weakening) and heart disease, withdrawal of estradiol is associated with episodes of inappropriate temperature regulatory activity (hot flushes). Other sequelae of a chronic hypoestrogenic state are weakening of pelvic floor muscles, leading to uterine prolapse, and/or incontinence; dryness of vagina and genital tract, leading to uncomfortable intercourse; and general loss of hydration and elasticity in skin.

MENOPAUSE AND HORMONE THERAPY

Many of the symptoms associated with menopause can be alleviated or lessened by treating postmenopausal women with exogenous hormones. There are three classes of estrogens available for hormone therapy in postmenopausal women.[13,16] Premarin, the most commonly prescribed hormone therapy, is a conjugated estrogen obtained from the urine of pregnant horses. First approved for use in 1962, by 1990 it was the fourth most prescribed drug in the United States. More recently, Premarin combined with a low dose of progesterone to prevent endometrial hyperplasia is increasing in use for women with an intact uterus. Natural estrogens and synthetic estrogens are also available although their effectiveness has not yet been established. Although postmenopausal hormonal replacement (HRT) is generally effective in reducing or eliminating most symptoms associated with menopause, clinical application of the principles of hormone replacement can be complicated, and time, effort, and commitment from both patient and physician are required to devise an effective regimen with which the patient is comfortable and is likely to continue.

In summary, although both immaturity and postmenopause are both hypoestrogenic states, there is little else in common in the two physiologic conditions. The reason for quiescent ovaries in girls is an inactive GnRH system, whereas in postmenopausal women, there is plenty of GnRH but no ovarian substrate for LH and FSH. If immaturity persists beyond the usual 14–16 years in girls, they will exhibit loss of bone density and a male-type cardiovascular risk pattern similar to that of postmenopausal women.

REFERENCES

1. Adashi EY, Rock JA, Rosenwaks Z, eds. Reproductive Endocrinology, Surgery, and Technology, Vol. 2. Philadelphia: Lippencott-Raven, 1996.

2. Ferin M, Jewelewicz R, Warren M. The Menstrual Cycle: Physiology, Reproductive Disorders, and Infertility. New York: Oxford University Press, 1993.

3. Hillier SG, Kitchener HC, Neilson JP, eds. Scientific Essentials of Reproductive Medicine. Philadelphia: WB Saunders, 1996.

4. Knobil E, Neill JD, eds. The Physiology of Reproduction, 2nd ed., Vols. 1 and 2. New York: Raven Press, 1994.

5. Yen SC, Jaffe RB, eds. Reproductive Endocrinology: Physiology, Pathophysiology and Clinical Management. Philadelphia: WB Saunders, Harcourt Brace Jovanovich, 1991.

6. Grumbach MM, Grave GD, Mayer FE, eds. The Control of the Onset of Puberty. New York: John Wiley & Sons, 1974.

7. Delemarre-van de Waal HA, Plant TM, van Rees GP, Schoemaker J, eds. Control of the Onset of Puberty III. Amsterdam: Expta Medica, 1989.

8. Plant TM, Lee PA. The Neurobiology of Puberty. Bristol: Journal of Endocrinology Limited, 1995.

9. Greendale GA, Judd HL. The menopause: Health implications and clinical management. J Am Geriatr Soc 1993; 41:426–436.

10. Samsioe G. Effect of ovarian failure on target tissues. In: Crosignani PG, Paoletti, PM, Sarrel NK, eds. Women's Health in Menopause. Amsterdam: Kluwer-Academic Publishers and Fondazione Giovanni Lorenzini, 1994, pp. 41–50.

11. Lee SJ, Lenton EA, Sexton L, Cooke ID. The effect of age on the cyclical patterns of plasma LH, FSH, oestradiol and progesterone in women with regular menstrual cycles. Hum Reprod 1988;3:851–855.

12. Lobo RA. Absorption and metabolic effects of different types of estrogens and progestogens. Obstet Gynecol Clin North Am 1987;14:143–167.

13. Gow SM, Turner EI, Glasier A. The clinical biochemistry of the menopause and hormone replacement therapy. Ann Clin Biochem 1994;31:509–528.

14. Matthews KA, Kuller LH, Wing RR, Meilahn EN, Plantinga P. Prior to use of estrogen replacement therapy, are users healthier than nonusers? Am J Epidemiol 1996; 143:971–978.

15. U.S. Congress, Office of Technology Assessment. Hormone products and prescription. In: The Menopause, Hormone Therapy, and Women's Health. OTA-BP-BA-88. Washington, DC: U.S. Government Printing Office, 1992, pp. 63–72.

7

SEX STEROID HORMONAL INFLUENCES ON CORONARY ARTERY DISEASE

Elaine Meilahn

One of the basic tenets of this book is that variations in disease frequency provide clues about disease etiology. The higher rates of coronary artery disease (CAD) in men than women, in particular during the reproductive years, points to a role for sex steroid hormones in pathogenesis. This chapter examines the commonly accepted role of sex hormones in explaining this "gender gap" as well as the interaction between risk factors and sex hormones that may influence susceptibility to CAD.

Coronary artery disease has two principal components: (*1*) atheroma, or abnormal fatty deposits in the artery wall; and (*2*) thromboembolism, or blockage of a blood vessel by a blood clot. Atherogenesis is a tissue response to injury involving chronic inflammation and repair of the vessel wall endothelium and smooth muscle cells.[1] A high circulating level of oxidized low-density lipoproteins (LDL) contributes to atherogenesis, the effects of which are partly balanced by the antioxidant activity of nitric acid in the artery wall. The clinical manifestations of CAD reflect not only narrowing of the arteries but also in some cases unstable lesions that induce thrombi (blood clots) and may lead to unstable angina or a myocardial infarction. Furthermore, even intact endothelium may be dysfunctional when vessels do not vasodilate normally, contributing to acute coronary syndromes. Thus, structural changes of vessels, hemostatic factors, and cellular function contribute to the development CAD.

Coronary artery disease reached epidemic levels in developed countries in the 1960s and 1970s and, despite declining rates, remains the major cause of death among adult men and women.[2] In the United States, for example, 1 in 9 women aged 45–64 has clinical CAD and after age 65 the figure rises to 1 in 3.[3] It is important to recognize that the epidemic of CAD is largely preventable as the major risk factors for CAD—cigarette smoking and control of hypertension and serum cholesterol—are modifiable. For example, cigarette smoking is the primary cause of over half of myocardial infarctions (heart attacks) among middle-aged women.[4]

GENDER AND CORONARY ARTERY DISEASE

Men have two to six times the risk of CAD compared with women, regardless of background national rates. In Japan, a country with very low CAD rates, the rate of CAD is 3.2 times higher in men than women aged 45–64. Similarly, the rate of CAD is 3.7 times higher among men than women in England and Wales where high rates prevail (Fig. 7–1).[5] Although gradually decreasing with age, the excess in CAD among men continues until the ninth decade of life. Other manifestations of vascular disease such as stroke and peripheral vascular disease also have a higher incidence among males than females, but the male-female rate ratios are lower than for CAD (Table 7–1).[6] The greatest disparity in cardiovascular disease rates between men and women occurs for coronary disease.

It is important to note that despite higher rates among men and a somewhat different clinical profile, CAD is the major cause of death for women after the age of 50. Thus, it is a *delay* in the onset of disease among women that is the greatest contributor to the sex difference in CAD rates; women develop CAD as often as men, but at a later age. As documented by autopsy and angiography studies, the pathophysiology of coronary atherosclerosis is similar for men and women. The later clinical onset among females is consistent with autopsy reports of increasing lipid lesions on the arterial wall among men but little increase among young women up through age 35. A striking sex difference in the clinical manifestations of CAD is the higher prevalence of syndrome X in women which consists of angina pectoris (chest pain) and positive exercise-related electrocardiographic (ECG) changes but with little or no evidence of atherosclerosis.[7] For example, in a large series of patients undergoing angiography for chest pain, over one-half of women but only 16% of men showed normal arteries, suggesting that women more often than men experience anginal pain without evidence of atherosclerotic disease.[8] After menopause, however, the proportion of women with CAD manifested as angina decreases, and rates of sudden death and myocardial infarction increase.[9]

Is the gender gap in CAD due to inherent differences between men and women or do behavioral differences account for it? Two explanations for the earlier development of CAD among males are (*1*) that men, particularly young men, engage more often than women in health-related behaviors associated with excess CAD risk, and (*2*) that women are biologically more resistant to CAD, particularly during their reproductive years.

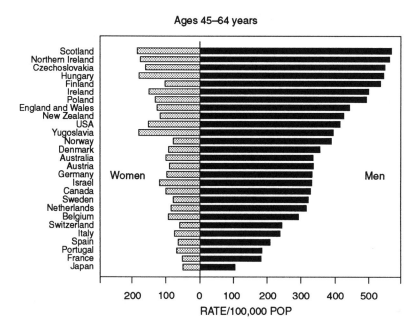

Ages 45–64 years

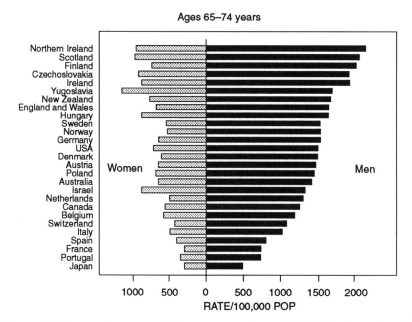

Ages 65–74 years

Figure 7–1. Heart disease mortality by country and sex, 1984–87. [Reprinted from NIH Publication No. 92-3088, Thom et al., page 17, September 1992, thanks to the National Heart, Lung, and Blood Institute[5]]

Table 7–1. Mortality Rates per 100,000 for Myocardial Infarction,
Stroke, and Other Circulatory Disease, United States, 1995

	GENDER	AGE: 35–44	45–54	55–64	65–74
Myocardial	M	15.4	67.7	194.9	437.0
infarction	F	4.1	18.8	73.7	211.1
ICD-10 270	M:F ratio	3.8	3.6	2.7	2.1
Stroke	M	6.9	19.3	53.2	155.8
ICD-10 29	F	6.1	15.7	40.3	119.2
	M:F ratio	1.1	1.2	1.3	1.3
Other circulatory	M	0.4	0.6	1.7	3.3
disease	F	0.2	0.4	1.0	2.3
ICD-10 304,	M:F ratio	2.0	1.5	1.7	1.4
305, 309					

[Reprinted from World Health Organization, page B-94, 1996[6]]

Does Behavior Explain the Sex Differential in CAD?

First, it is important to recognize that elevated levels of the well-established risk factors for CAD (cigarette smoking, blood pressure, and serum total cholesterol levels) result in about the same relative increase in risk of CAD for women as for men as shown by results of the Framingham Heart Study in Table 7–2.[10] Moreover, the fact that women in countries with high rates of CAD have higher rates of CAD mortality than men from countries with low rates of CAD (Fig. 7–1)[5] points to a strong impact of behavioral and/or environmental risk factors on both sexes. Overall, however, even after taking into account that men (particularly in middle-age) generally smoke more often than women and have higher blood pressure and serum cholesterol levels, the sex differential in CAD is reduced but not eliminated.[11] The factors responsible for the sex difference in CAD must be different from those responsible for geographic differences in CAD and for the decline in CAD mortality observed since the 1970s in most developed countries, since the decline has occurred for males and females and the sex ratio remains. Therefore, the question of why CAD is delayed in women relative to men can be explained only in part by behavioral and lifestyle factors.

Endogenous Sex Hormones and CAD

The most obvious explanation for the sex difference in the age at onset of CAD is an influence of reproductive hormones. Studies of CAD risk and endogenous sex hormones in women have traditionally focused on markers of ovarian function including surgical menopause, and age at menarche, menopause, and repro-

Table 7–2. Relative Risks for CAD in Framingham Heart Study, 1977–79, 4-year Follow-up, Comparison of 80th vs. 20th Percentile for Blood Pressure and Cholesterol Level, Smoker vs. Non-smoker

	WOMEN	MEN
Systolic blood pressure	1.4	1.6
Total cholesterol	1.4	1.4
HDL cholesterol	0.5	0.5
Cigarette smoking	1.2	1.1

[Reprinted from Journal of American Medical Association, Castelli, et al., pages 2835–2838, 1986[10]]

ductive history, and more recently they have included more direct measures of serum concentrations of hormones.

Age at Menarche and Menstrual History. Although age at onset of menses and menstrual history as markers of estrogen "exposure" during reproductive life have been evaluated with respect to risk of breast cancer and osteoporosis, only rarely have such analyses taken risk of CAD into account.[12] The two studies to date have been consistent in linking irregular menstruation with modestly increased CAD risk. LaVecchia et al.[13] found age at menarche was not related to the risk of myocardial infarction among young women, although a history of irregular menstrual cycling was linked to a relative risk of 2 compared with those reporting a history of normal menstrual cycles. Similarly, Gorgels et al.[14] found excess CAD risk among women with a history of annovulatory menstrual cycling.

Age at Natural Menopause. If premenopausal endogenous estrogen levels are cardioprotective, then that protection should be lost with the decline in ovarian function and the drop in endogenous estrogen levels that occur during the menopausal transition. However, no peak occurs in the age-specific CAD death rates around age 50–51 years for females, the median age at menopause.[15] However, any increase in rates would need to be relatively large to be detected, as rates of CAD death for women 45–55 years of age are relatively low (about 35–40 per 100,000) and the distribution of age at menopause is wide (with the 10th percentile at about 42–43 years and the 90th percentile at about age 54–55).[16]

Although national rates do not reflect a rapid pre-to postmenopause increase in risk, studies comparing pre- and postmenopausal women of the same age have found CAD (measured in various ways) to be higher in the postmenopausal group.[17] Over an 18-year follow-up, The Framingham Heart Study[9] found a relative risk of about 4 associated with postmenopausal status among women aged 40–54 at study entry. In a Dutch population of the same age, Witteman et al.[18] reported significantly greater calcification of the aorta among postmenopausal women, whether naturally or surgically postmenopausal. More recently, greater thickening of the left ventricular wall of the heart[19] has been reported among postmenopausal women than premenopausal women. However, results from two of the largest studies run counter to these findings: (1) no association of carotid artery wall thickening (measured using ultrasound) and menopausal status (or estrogen therapy use) was found among over 5,000 women aged 45–54 in the population-based Atherosclerotic Risk in Communities Study in the U.S.,[20] and (2) the Harvard Nurses' Study[21] reported no excess risk of CAD for naturally menopausal women compared with premenopausal women of the same age. Thus, vital statistics, studies of clinical endpoints, and those using subclinical measures of CAD have not been consistent in linking natural menopause with CAD for women experiencing menopause around the median age of 50–51 years. However, elevated risk of CAD has been reported for women experiencing a spontaneous menopause at a younger age than expected (less than 40–44 years)[22,23] and a decrease in CAD risk of 2% for each year's delay in menopause was estimated from a Dutch cohort study by van der Schouw et al.[24]

It is worth noting that very early spontaneous menopause prior to the age of 40 occurs in about 1% of U.S. women.[16] Causes of premature ovarian failure are largely unknown, but a subset of cases has been linked to immune dysfunction[25,26] and it is not possible to distinguish early menopause per se as a contributor to CAD risk among these women from underlying pathology associated with ovarian failure.

Age at menopause has been proposed as a marker of general aging by Snowden et al.[23] and more recently by Perls et al.,[27] who found that late age at childbearing, which is related to later onset of menopause, was linked to longevity among a group of U.S. women born in 1896.

Surgical Menopause (Oophorectomy/Hysterectomy). Surgical removal of the ovaries (oophorectomy) is associated with a sudden and complete cessation of ovarian estrogen production in contrast to the decline in estrogen levels occurring over several years or longer during the menopausal transition.[12] Oophorectomy without hormone replacement therapy has been associated with relative risk of about 2 of CAD and atherosclerosis compared with women remaining premenopausal; the excess risk appears to be eliminated by use of estrogen therapy, although only observational, rather than controlled trial, findings are available.[28]

Somewhat surprisingly, hysterectomy alone (without oophorectomy) also seems to convey an excess risk of CAD similar to that associated with oophorectomy.[29,30] The reason is unclear, although disruption of ovarian blood supply resulting in ovarian dysfunction may account for this finding.

Reproductive History and Risk of CAD. Epidemiological studies of breast cancer and osteoporosis have demonstrated the relevance of markers of duration and extent of estrogen exposure in the form of parity and age at first birth to risk of chronic disease at older ages. However, less attention appears to have been devoted to these exposures in terms of CAD. Of seven published cohort studies that examine parity and CAD, all but the Nurses' Health Study,[31] showed a relative risk of 1.2–2.5 for women with a history of five or more pregnancies compared with nulligravid women.

In contrast to breast cancer, for which early age at first birth is associated with reduced risk, CAD risk appears to be increased (two- to threefold) by giving birth at age 20 or younger as reported by case–control studies of nonfatal myocardial infarction[13,32,33] or sudden death.[34,35] While the large Harvard Nurses' Study[31] did not find this association, only 1% of study participants reported a first birth at younger than 20 years. The nurses' cohort may consist of too constrained a social class distribution; lower status is associated with high parity and early childbearing and may act as a confounder, although statistical adjustment for social class and other CAD risk factors tends to reduce but not eliminate the association between reproductive factors and CAD.[36,37]

One reason for an increased risk of CAD with high parity and early age at first birth may be the small sustained drop in HDL cholesterol found after pregnancy, along with a positive association between parity and adiposity, particularly abdominal fat.[38] Hankinson et al.[39] measured plasma estrogen levels in a sample of 216 subjects from the Harvard Nurses' Study and found plasma estrogen levels lower among women with high parity and those with young age at first birth, after controlling for body mass, alcohol consumption, and age. The lower endogenous estrogen level is consistent with lower HDL cholesterol level and with higher risk of CAD (and lower risk of breast cancer).

Serum Concentration. Among men, case–control series of myocardial infarction have shown higher estrogen levels among cases, although prospective results suggest that neither endogenous estrogen level nor testosterone predicts CAD.[40,41] Surprisingly few studies have examined endogenous hormone levels and risk of CAD among women. Among postmenopausal subjects, the one cross-sectional and one prospective study published to date found no relationship between levels of either endogenous estrogens or androgens and angiographically determined CAD or incident CAD among older women.[42,43] In the only prospective study among premenopausal women,[14] Dutch women aged 40–49 were followed for 5 to 8 years; no differences were seen for baseline urinary measures of estrone and testosterone between the 45 incident CAD cases and a group of 135 controls. Whether the single measure of sex hormone concentration used by all of these studies is sufficient to characterize "exposure" is unclear; sex hormone levels may be particularly difficult to classify during the perimenopause when intermittent ovarian production continues for some time.

The Rancho-Bernardo Study of retired men and women examined baseline dehydroepianrosterone (DHEA) (a major secretory product of the adrenal gland) and its sulfate ester (DHEAS) as predictors of ischemic heart disease death over 19 years.[43] They found a modestly reduced relative risk compared with survivors (adjusted for other risk factors) among men (relative risk = 0.79, 95% CI = 0.60–1.04) for those with values above the median for DHEAS at baseline compared with those below the median, and a slightly increased risk among women (relative risk = 1.21, 95%CI = 0.81–1.46). It is interesting that higher levels of DHEAS may be beneficial for men, but may elevate risk for women. Such opposite effects of sex hormones among men and women are consistent with the results of an intervention trial using high doses of estrogen to treat men with prostrate cancer: the treated men experienced a higher rate of cardiovascular death.[44] Additional evidence of differing responses of males and females to estrogen comes from in vitro experiments showing coronary arteries from women to be more sensitive to 17 β-estradiol, indicating greater relaxation in response to a vasoconstrictor than coronary arteries from men.[45]

Exogenous Sex Hormones and CAD

Among postmenopausal women, more than 30 studies have reported an approximate halving of the risk of coronary disease (as measured by clinical end points and by angiography) among women taking postmenopausal hormone replacement therapy (HRT) compared with nonusers; all studies were observational and most included exposure to estrogen unopposed by progestins. Only recently have epidemiological studies focused on newer forms of HRT in which estrogen is taken in combination with progestins; the largest series to date is based on only eight deaths from heart disease among users of the combined preparation[46] and shows no reduction in benefit from the addition of progestin. Controlled trial results of exogenous estrogen and CAD are not yet available, although two very large randomized trials of HRT that include CAD end points are currently underway in the U.S.[47] and the U.K.[48] and clinical trials of secondary prevention (among women with CAD) are also in progress.[49] Results from randomized trials are particularly relevant to an evaluation of the CAD risk reduction associated with HRT because of the tendency of women with favorable CAD risk-factor profiles to use HRT leading to an over estimation of the benefit of HRT for CAD risk reduction.

Taken together, the evidence consistently supports a beneficial influence of estrogen on CAD in women; moreover, excessively high androgen levels are probably linked to higher CAD risk found among women with polycystic ovary syndrome, who typically exhibit elevated androgen levels accompanied by an adverse metabolic profile, including insulin resistance.[50]

RISK FACTORS FOR CAD AND SEX HORMONES—INTERACTION?

Biological Factors

Lipoproteins. The fact that the gender difference in stroke mortality is so much smaller than in CAD provides support for a role for cholesterol in explaining this difference; while cigarette smoking and blood pressure are major risk factors for both stroke and CAD, cholesterol is strongly implicated in risk of CAD and to a much lesser degree, in risk of stroke. During the reproductive years in particular, men tend to have more adverse (in terms of CAD risk) levels of lipoprotein lipids, with higher concentrations of LDLc and lower HDLc than women.

One of the few CAD risk factors that appears to be more important among women than men is high-density lipoprotein cholesterol (HDLc) concentration—for each 0.26 mmol/liter increase in HDLc, women show a 3% and men a 2% decline in CAD risk.[51] During puberty, the protective HDLc levels decline in males but remain stable in females, resulting in women having higher life-time levels, which do not appear to decrease at menopause (Fig. 7–2).[52]

Although total serum cholesterol levels have a graded positive association with CAD mortality for both men and women,[53] the Framingham Heart Study reported that serum low-density lipoprotein cholesterol (LDLc) concentrations are better predictors of risk in men than in women.[9] Differences in predictive value for CAD of lipoproteins, including LDLc, may be due to very different lifetime patterns of exposure to lipoproteins in men and women.[54] For example, LDLc shows a later age-related increase in women than in men, resulting in a shorter exposure time to elevated LDL among women by a given age (Fig. 7–2).[52] The decline in hepatic lipase enzyme that occurs with menopause may contribute to the rise in serum LDLc level and the changes in subfractions HDL-2 and HDL-3 that have been observed in perimenopausal women.[55]

Surprisingly few studies have examined the relationship of endogenous hormone levels to lipoprotein levels in women. Elevated androgen levels among women, as evidenced by hirsutism, are associated with adverse levels of lipoproteins.[56] Barrett-Connor et al.[57] found only a very weak inverse relationship between plasma cholesterol and estrone levels, wheras Cauley et al.[58] found no association in older women. Kuller et al.[59] reported that a marked drop in serum estradiol during perimenopause was linked prospectively to an increase in LDLc in a sample of healthy middle-aged women, although cross-sectionally, serum estrogen and lipoprotein concentrations were not related. Such studies are complicated by erratic ovarian function during perimenopause.

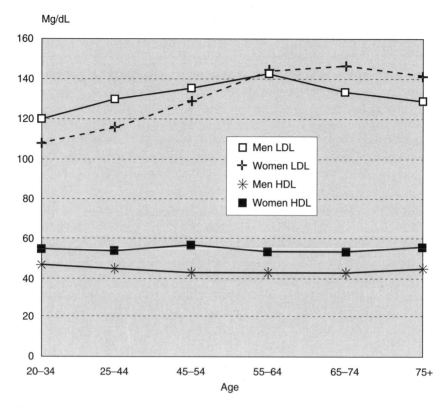

Figure 7–2. Median serum cholesterol (LDL and HDL) in milligrams/deciliter for men and women, by age, United States, 1988–91. [Reprinted with thanks to the National Cholesterol Education Program, Second Report of the Expert Panel on Detection, Evaluation and Treatment of High Blood Cholesterol in Adults, National Institutes of Health, thanks to National Heart, Lung, and Blood Institute. NIH Publication No. 93-3096, September 1993, p I A-4/5[52]]

Additional evidence that sex hormones influence lipoprotein levels comes from studies of dietary intervention showing women to exhibit less adverse lipoprotein changes in response to increased dietary fat and cholesterol than men.[60] At least among premenopausal women, the greater lipoprotein lipase and reduced hepatic lipase activity in women compared with that in men may maintain women's higher HDLc levels, even in the presence of increased dietary cholesterol and fat intake. Women's HDLc levels fall, however, if placed on a low-fat diet. Khaw and Barrett-Connor[61] proposed an interesting model in which women in low-CAD incidence populations eating a low-fat diet have low serum lipoprotein levels (including a low HDLc) accompanied by low estrogen levels; women in high-CAD incidence populations eating a high-fat diet exhibit high lipoprotein levels, including high HDLc, and they have high estrogen levels. The women in the high-risk populations are protected (in part) from the high CAD rates of men because of their higher estrogen and HDLc levels; men's HDLc remains low, possibly because of androgenic effects, and their CAD rates are high. This model accounts for the observed low CAD rates in Asian populations despite the low HDLc and low bioavailable estrogen levels observed among Japanese women.[62,63]

With respect to taking exogenous estrogen postmenopausally, beneficial effects on serum lipoproteins have been reported from a randomized clinical trial.[64] Improved blood levels of HDLc and LDLc were obtained with conjugated estrogen—unopposed and in combination with progestins—as compared with a placebo group. Little or no effect was observed on blood pressure, body weight, fat distribution, or 2-hour postload insulin levels. Recent primate experiments show oral estrogen with or without the addition of androgens reduces plasma LDL in ovariectomized monkeys via lowering arterial LDL metabolism and increasing total-body LDL catabolism (removal).[65]

Because of its effects on serum lipoprotein levels, the possible interaction of estrogen therapy with use of the lipid-lowering drug lovastatin was evaluated in the Carotid Artery Progression Study.[66] Results showed no difference in lipid-lowering effects of lovastatin between women who reported use of estrogen therapy and those who did not; among women taking a placebo, hormone use was associated with reduced progression of wall thickness of the carotid arteries to about the same degree as use of lipid-lowering therapy. Thus, estrogen therapy and lovastatin showed no synergistic effects for lipid-lowering when taken in combination, but the anti-atherogenic effects of each were approximately the same. Similar results were reported recently from a trial comparing lipid-lowering effects of estrogen plus progestin in comparison with simvastatin.[67] Results from both trials support a possible protective effect of postmenopausal hormone use via its lipid-lowering effects.

Thus, evidence for a beneficial influence of estrogen on lipoprotein levels among women is consistent, although results from studies attempting to measure endogenous hormone levels are less convincing than those from studies using indirect measures of sex hormone levels, possibly because of methodological difficulties in characterizing endogenous sex hormone levels. Reproductive markers such as menstrual patterns may better measure long-term exposure than endogenous levels measured only once.

Body Fat. Body fat is not considered a major independent CAD risk factor for women, although women have proportionally more body fat than men and obesity is linked to risk of CAD, largely via its adverse effects on blood pressure, lipoprotein levels, and carbohydrate metabolism.[69,70] Weight gain with age is common among both men and women, but the age-related pattern differs, with men gaining on average twice as much weight as women between ages 17 and

34 whereas women tend to gain weight after age 35, as reported by Yong and Kuller[68] in a prospective investigation.

Why women gain weight later in life is unknown, but endogenous estrogen levels may affect appetite. According to studies in rates, removal of the ovaries led to increased meal size, which was decreased by estadiol administration,[88] although a prospective observational study (The Healthy Women Study) found no evidence of increased food intake (measured by 24-hour dietary recall) from pre- to postmenopause.[89]

One reason that adiposity is not associated as strongly to CAD among women as it is among men may be that peripheral fat is the major source of estrogen, being the primary site of aromatization of androstenedione to estrone, in postmenopausal women; thus, fatter women tend to have higher levels of circulating estrone and less often report hot flushes at menopause than thinner women.[87] This is not true among premenopausal women in whom the ovaries are the primary source of estrogen,[90] although extremely lean premenopausal women are more likely to have extended and annovulatory menstrual cycles or become amenorrheic than normal-weight women.[91]

Because weight gain in the later reproductive years has been linked to increased waist-hip ratio,[68] The weight gain common to women in western countries may be associated with relatively increased visceral fat deposits. Where, rather than how much, fat is deposited may be relevant to CAD risk. Women who carry their fat like men do, or abdominally, have two to three times higher risk of CAD than women with peripheral fat in the "female pattern."[71] Fat distribution has been proposed as the basis for the gender difference in CAD, given that male fat pattern, independent of obesity, is linked to a complex of adverse CAD risk factors, including greater insulin resistance, higher systolic blood pressure, reduced fibrinolytic potential, and lower HDLc than female fat pattern. Lonnquist et al.[72] found that men released twice as much free fatty acid (FFA) to the liver than premenopausal women (postmenopausal women were not studied). Increased secretion of FFA by visceral fat cells and subsequent release to the liver may help to explain why abdominal (male) fat patterning is associated with adverse CAD risk in the form of glucose intolerance and dyslipidemia.

The question is whether some women exhibit a "male" fat pattern because of hormonal determinants. Cross-sectionally, a visceral (male) fat pattern is associated with increased plasma testosterone and decreased SHBG levels among premenopausal (but not postmenopausal) women,[73,74] and visceral fat increased over 3 years among female transsexuals taking testosterone.[75] In women, testosterone is associated with higher adipose tissue lipoprotein lipase and larger abdominal fat cells, which appear to be associated with a greater number or activity of androgen receptors in visceral fat.[76] In contrast, testosterone tends to be lower in men with greater visceral fat load and administration to obese men reduces visceral fat and improves insulin sensitivity.[77]

Insulin-Glucose Metabolism. Men tend to have higher insulin and insulin resistance than women, but the gender difference lessens with age. Does increased androgenicity with age lead to greater insulin resistance? Whereas higher testosterone levels are associated with reduced glucose and insulin levels among men, the converse is true for women.[73] Female rats treated with testosterone exhibit decreased insulin sensitivity,[78] and in two prospective studies, low levels of sex hormone–binding globulin (as a measure of androgenicity) were predictive of noninsulin-dependent diabetes in women.[79,80] Whether altered testosterone levels precede or result from insulin resistance is controversial. Experimental evidence shows that insulin stimulates ovarian production of androgens.[81] Female diabetics tend to resemble males in their fat deposition patterns and have nearly equal risk of CAD.[82] Reasons for the loss of "female advantage" among diabetics is unclear. The disturbed endocrine mileu of diabetic women may extend to sex hormone levels, as evidenced by the menstrual irregularity found among hyperinsulinemic Pima Indian women[83] and diabetic Danish women.[84] Although observational study results[85] suggest postmenopausal estrogen improves glucose intolerance, results of the randomized postmenopausal estrogen–progestin interventions (PEPI) trial provide little support.[64]

Blood Pressure. Apart from the case of pre-eclampsia during pregnancy, changes in blood pressure have not been consistently associated with reproductive events nor has an impact of postmenopausal therapy on blood pressure been reported in the PEPI trial.[64] In addition, the lack of a gender gap in thromboembolic stroke mortality, for which blood pressure is a major risk factor, suggests that influence of sex hormones on blood pressure is not likely to play a role in the gender difference in CAD.

Hemostatic Factors. Elevated plasma fibrinogen level has been identified as a risk factor for both men and women and is similar in magnitude to elevated serum cholesterol.[92] Evidence abounds for an influence of both menopausal status and exogenous estrogen on levels of fibrinogen and other plasma coagulation and fibrinolytic factors.[93,94] Age-related patterns for fibrinogen, factors VII and VIII, plasminogen activator inhibitor-1, and anti-thrombin III are all similar to that for LDL cholesterol, which shows lower average values for women than men up until about age 50, after which values for women exceed those for men. Postmenopausal women of the same age as premenopausal women exhibit higher plasma levels for a number of hemostatic factors including fibrinogen.[94] Moreover, exogenous estrogen has marked effects on plasma hemostatic factor levels including potentially pro- and anti-thrombotic changes. The strongest evidence for a potentially beneficial effect from exogenous estrogen comes from the PEPI trial[64] which showed a 10mg/dl average decrease in plasma fibrinogen levels with treatment compared with placebo, which is similar in magnitude to the 10–15 mg/dl increase in fibrinogen occurring around the time of menopause.

Overall, the interrelationship between male–female fat distribution and metabolic risk factors for CAD appears to be mediated by sex hormones. Gender differences in determinants of fat distribution may underlie the CAD risk difference.[82]

Behavioral Factors

Stress. Higher CAD rates among men than women have been attributed in part to the stress men experience at work. When women began to work outside the home in large numbers, it was feared that their CAD rates would rise as they adopted behavioral patterns more similar to those of men. Not only do working women not experience higher CAD rates, their CAD risk factors tend to be more favorable than those of homemakers.[95] In fact, impact of psychosocial factors on CAD appear to be modified by estrogen status,[96] with females' higher estrogen levels possibly affording "protection" from acute effects of stress. In primate experiments, stress has been shown to lead to increased cortisol and lower lutenizing hormone (LH) secretion when monkeys were in the luteal as opposed to follicular stage of their menstrual cycle; cortisol levels are higher in young women during a cold pressor (stress) test taken during the luteal (lower estrogen) phase of their menstrual cycle than during the follicular phase.[97] Sex hormones appear to modify response to psychological stressors. Whether postmenopausal women therefore exhibit increased cardiovascular response to stress compared with premenopausal women is currently under investigation.

Health Behaviors. What women consume in the form of tobacco, food, and alcohol influences their risk of CAD. The effects of these risk factors may be due in part to modification of serum sex hormone levels. Although cigarette smoking has not been associated with reduced serum estrogen levels in pre- or postmenopausal women,[98] it is linked to increased hepatic metabolism of estrogens[99] and elevated concentrations of androgens[61,98] and follicle-stimulating hormone.[100] Moreover, nonsmoking premenopausal women reporting passive exposure to cigarette smoke had FSH levels that were 39% higher than in unexposed nonsmokers.[98] These findings are consistent with the 1- to 2-years earlier menopause experienced by smokers than by nonsmokers.[101]

Diet influences total and bioavilable estrogen levels in women. Caloric restriction, independent of weight loss, appears to influence menstrual cycling.[102] and may be linked to an earlier menopause.[103] In times of famine, reproductive potential drops in female mammals; food deprivation affects reproduction via change in activity of gonadotropic-releasing hormone (GnRH) neurons in the forebrain.[104] Most epidemiological research has centered on diet and risk of breast cancer and, in general, has found that high dietary fat intake is associated with higher estrogen levels, while high intake of fiber and, possibly isoflavinoids is associated with lower levels.[105] Interestingly, soy protein (containing isoflavinoids) in combination with estrogen treatment had an interactive effect (greater than would be expected by simple additive effects of both) on improving serum lipids and reducing arterial lipid content in an experiment with ovariectomized monkeys,[106] which suggests a dietary impact on vascular effects of estrogen. Moreover, treatment with a low-fat diet may lead to a decrease in estradiol levels in postmenopausal women.[107] Whether dietary effect on estrogen differs for pre- compared with postmenopausal women is unclear, although the increased risk of breast cancer with high dietary fat appears to be largely confined to postmenopausal women;[108] dietary influence on sex hormone levels may be relatively low during the reproductive years when ovarian production of estrogen is high. The bioavailability of estrogen as well as its concentration may be influenced by diet: release of free fatty acids leads to a higher insulin level, resulting in decreased sex hormone–binding globulin (SHBG) which in turn increases the proportion of unbound (bioavailable) estrogen.

Moderate alcohol consumption (1–2 drinks per day) among healthy pre- or postmenopausal women appears to have little impact on endogenous estrogen levels.[109,110] Recently, however, an interaction between postmenopausal estrogen therapy and alcohol was reported in an experimental study[111]; among women taking therapy, drinking about three alcoholic drinks acutely raised serum estradiol to a level three times higher than that attained with estrogen therapy alone. Although both estrogen therapy and moderate alcohol intake have been linked to reduced risk of CAD, it is unknown whether the mechanism involves elevation of endogenous estrogen.

Exercise is another behavioral factor linked to risk of CAD. It appears to modify estrogen levels in that vigorous, sustained exercise patterns can alter menstrual patterns so that they are consistent with annovulatory cycling and lower estrogen exposure.[91] Such high-intensity exercise patterns are uncommon, however, among older women, and it is important to note the benefits of exercise in terms of CAD risk. Cardiovascular fitness has been linked prospectively to lower mortality in women[112]; those who exercise even moderately have more favorable serum lipid levels than sedentary women.

In light of these relationships, it is tempting to speculate that the higher compliance and long-term usage of postmenopausal estrogen among women who exercise heavily and have a high dietary intake of fiber[87] is linked to their (initially) lower endogenous estrogen levels. A hypothesis by Wade et al.[104] proposes that glucose and fatty acid metabolism, rather than body fat per se, regulates reproductive physiology. This is consistent with the increased infertility observed among women with eating disorders, uncontrolled diabetes, and strenuous exercise patterns, and among women living in times of famine.

Possible Mechanisms for an Effect of Sex Hormones on CAD Risk

Sex steroid hormones appear to influence CAD via a number of potential pathways including circulating levels of atherogenic risk factors as well as direct endothelial and possibly coronary effects. Underpinning the development of atherosclerotic disease in the coronary arterial bed are adverse serum levels of lipoproteins, high LDLc, and/or low HDLc. Reproductive-related events in a woman's life—menarche, menstruation, pregnancy, and menopause—as well as use of exogenous estrogen result in alterations in serum lipoprotein patterns. Beneficial effects of postmenopausal estrogen on serum lipids have been well documented by observational, experimental, and controlled trial results. Furthermore, estrogen may reduce oxidation of LDL cholesterol, thereby rendering it less atherogenic.[65]

Anti-atherogenic effects of β-estradiol have been attributed not only to improved blood lipid levels but also to effects on the vascular endothelium, including reduced production of vasoconstrictive endothelin-1[113] as well as increased release of nitric oxide (endothelium-derived relaxation factor)[114]; this response is diminished, however, with addition of progestins to estrogen. Similarly, experimental evidence largely from studies of primates shows the coronary atherosclerosis induced by a high-cholesterol diet is prevented by estrogen therapy alone, but not when administered in combination with progestins,[115] despite improved lipid levels. These recent findings are potentially very important because nearly all of the observational evidence that postmenopausal estrogen therapy reduces CAD risk is derived largely from populations using estrogen unopposed by progestins, although current prescribing practice indicates combined therapy for women with an intact uterus. The cardioprotective effects of estrogen, however, are not likely confined to attenuation of atherogenesis but appear to include enhancement of vessel endothelial wall response to vasoconstriction. The improvement in response may be lost in the presence of advanced lesions however.[116]

Evidence largely from animal experiments shows that exposure to 17β-estradiol enhances basal nitric oxide production, resulting in increased vessel wall distensibility[117] but without altering blood pressure.[118] Experiments on healthy postmenopausal women and those with elevated risk of CAD showed improved vasomotor function in forearm arteries, but the effect was greater for women at high risk.[119] Similarly, 17β-estradiol prevented acetylcholine-induced coronary artery vasoconstriction in postmenopausal women with CAD but had no effect in men.[120] Whether adding progestin attenuates the beneficial effect of estrogen on vasomotion is not clear—some findings support[114] reduced benefit while others have reported no diminuation of estrogenic effect on arterial endothial function with the addition of progestins.[121]

Limited data from clinical studies have shown that both endogenous and exogenous estrogen may affect cardiovascular response. Results from a small study of 13 premenopausal, normally cycling women with occasional fast heart rate (paroxysmal suopraventricular tachycardia) showed that episodes of tachycardia increased when plasma progesterone levels were highest and, conversely, the number of episodes were lowest when plasma estradiol levels were high.[122] This suggests that sex hormone levels influence the occurrence of arrhythmia. Results of a small, double-blind, placebo-controlled trial ($n = 25$) of treatment with 17β-estradiol (administered via skin patches) for women with syndrome X (chest pain with normal angiography findings) showed a reduction of about one-half in reported episodes of chest pain but no difference in treadmill exercise duration.[123]

Taken together, results of many types of studies consistently show multiple potentially beneficial effects of exogenous oral estrogen on CAD risk, for women as shown in Table 7–3. Although it is not clear whether the same benefits are attained when estrogen is administered in combination with progestins, progesterone has recently been reported[124] to inhibit smooth muscle cell proliferation (as found in atherogenesis), which is consistent with the reported protective effect of combination postmenopausal therapy. In addition, nearly all of the evidence on CAD risk and estrogen has come from studies of oral prepara-

Table 7–3. Possible Mechanisms for an Effect
of Estrogen on Coronary Artery Disease

MECHANISM	MODE OF ACTION	TYPES OF STUDIES	EVIDENCE
Improved serum lipoproteins	Hepatic enzymes, ↓ LDLc, ↑HDLc, ↑ triglycerides	Exp, Obs, RCT	+++
Lipid oxidation	↓Oxidation of LDLc	Exp	++
Carbohydrate metabolism		Exp, Obs, RCT	+
Cardioreactivity		Exp	+
Blood flow/vessel wall distensibility	↑Nitric oxide production Calcium antagonism	Exp	++
Plasma hemostatic factors	Hepatic, ↓ fibrinogen, improved fibrinolysis	Exp, Obs, RCT	+++
Endothelial function		Exp	++
Smooth muscle cell proliferation	Inhibited	Exp	+

Exp, controlled experiment; obs, observational study; RCT, Randomized clinical trial. Strength of evidence showing an effect: +++ strong/consistent; ++ modest; + limited or weak evidence.

tions; whether other forms of administration such as the "skin patch" have similar effects is not known. Therefore, the optimal route and dose of exogenous sex hormones for CAD risk reduction have not been determined nor do we understand how to identify women who are likely to benefit from taking postmenopausal hormone therapy and those who will not benefit.

STUDY DESIGN CONSIDERATIONS IN ASSESSING THE ASSOCIATION BETWEEN SEX STEROID HORMONES AND CORONARY ARTERY DISEASE

Development of Theoretical Models

Knowledge of how sex hormones influence CAD risk has been limited because of the following research constraints:

1. Until recently, studies of CAD have been restricted to men.
2. Measurement of endogenous sex hormones to characterize individual levels is extremely difficult in epidemiological studies because of the cyclical variation among premenopausal women and the very low levels among postmenopausal women requiring highly sensitive assays.
3. Animal models of natural menopause do not exist; experiments rely on ovariectomy, which results in a sudden marked drop in testosterone and estrogen levels.[125] Only since the 1980s have prospective studies begun of CAD risk factor change through natural menopause among human subjects.
4. Clinical CAD is an "end-stage" disease that is normally detected only after a long period of disease progression and it usually occurs among older women. As techniques to measure subclinical disease improve, studies will be able to examine the relationship between sex hormones and disease progression well before the situation is complicated by co-morbidities and medications use.
5. With respect to a relationship between exogenous estrogen and CAD, only observational evidence is available, apart from one very small clinical trial by Nachtigall et al.[126] Observational studies of postmenopausal estrogen therapy and CAD may be plagued by confounding or bias.

Confounding. In epidemiological terms, confounding is a form of bias providing an alternative explanation for an observed effect of exposure on outcome due to a confounding factor associated with exposure and outcome of interest. Women who elect to take postmenopausal therapy tend to be thinner, better educated, drink more alcohol, exercise more, have lower blood pressure and fasting insulin levels, and higher HDL cholesterol than women who don't take therapy.[127] Thus, a better CAD risk factor profile among estrogen users than nonusers could bias results of observational studies that have consistently shown a markedly reduced risk of CAD among users.[128] Furthermore, women with a history of chronic disease, including breast cancer, diabetes mellitus, or heart disease, are less likely to be prescribed HRT than women without a history of these conditions.[129] As a consequence, HRT use is linked to a lower risk of these conditions.

Compliance Bias. The Nurses Health Study,[130] for example, has shown reduced CAD risk (RR) among current (RR = 0.5) but not past (RR = 0.9) users; either the benefit is lost following cessation of use or long-term users have an underlying lower risk of CAD than short-term users, which suggests that compliance is a marker for lower risk. Evidence in support of "compliance bias" comes from results of randomized trials of lipid-lowering treatment, which showed consistently that among the placebo group, compliers had about the same reduction in mortality relative to noncompliers as that found for reduced CAD among users of estrogen therapy.[128] A large proportion of women who begin postmenopausal therapy stop using it. Even in the carefully monitored trial, PEPI, about one-third of women with an intact uterus who had been assigned to the therapy stopped taking it by the end of the 3-year study.[64]

Measurement of Study Outcomes and Exposures. Measurement of both CAD and many of the relevant exposures have been developed for studies in men. Are they appropriate for use in studies of women? Physical activity measures, for example, are largely based on uptake of sports and leisure-time activity, whereas a major source of activity for many women is housework. This is not typically included in commonly used activity assessments such as the Paffenbarger Activity Questionnaire, which was developed for use in men.[131] An example of gender specific differences in CAD measures is the Rose Questionnaire,[132] which was developed using male subjects to assess angina pectoris (chest pain). When validated against exercise thallium-201 scintigraphy (to measure myocardial ischemia) in men and women,[133] the ability of the questionnaire to positively predict ischemia in women was much worse than for men (positive predictive value was 26% for females and 73% for males). The Rose Questionnaire commonly has been used to measure prevalence of chest pain in population studies and to assess treatment effects in clinical trials; yet it clearly does not detect ischemia as well among females as males.

To date, measures of body fat and its distribution have been relatively crude; increasing use of methods that provide greater discrimination between fat and lean body mass, such as computerized tomography and dual energy X-ray absorptiometry (DEXA), is likely to improve understanding of the relationship between body fat and sex hormone metabolism.

It should be noted that most experiments have utilized 17β-estradiol, the predominant estrogen in reproductive-age women; the most commonly utilized postmenopausal estrogen therapy is conjugated equine estrogen, which circulates largely in the form of estrone sulfate. Therefore, the extent to which results from experiments using estradiol can be extrapolated to postmenopausal women is unclear.

A further point to be made about progress in understanding the role of exogenous estrogen in CAD risk relates to the fact that experimental research has relied on dietary cholesterol-loading of subjects. In a departure from this practice, Wagner et al[134] placed ovariectomized monkeys on a lipid-lowering diet with or without estrogen treatment and found that monkeys on estrogen exhibited no additional reduction in atherosclerosis over 30 months, relative to diet-only monkeys—despite lower body weight and less abdominal fat among the estrogen-fed monkeys. The point that, in the absence of a high-cholesterol diet, CAD progression may be much less dramatic and pharmacological therapies such as estrogen may not be required, should not be lost. Rates of CAD among Japanese women, who tend to eat a much lower fat/cholesterol diet than Western women, are among the lowest in the world, even though they have relatively low endogenous estrogen levels. Conversely, treatment for elevated serum cholesterol levels, even among women with diagnosed CAD, falls well below recommendations; only about one-third of women patients attain the treatment goal of 130 mg/dl or lower of LDLc.[49] Thus it appears that even among high-risk patients, desirable lipid levels are not generally achieved.

CONCLUSIONS

Primary prevention of CAD can be population based, which then includes low-risk healthy individuals, or it can target only those at high risk. General recommendations for postmenopausal women to take estrogen supplementation to prevent CAD involves mass pharmacological treatment of healthy individuals, most of whom will not benefit from this. An important difference between men and women when considering use of drug therapy to attain reduction in risk factors is the risk–benefit balance. The benefit from cholesterol lowering, for example, is less in absolute terms among women because of their lower rates of CAD. Thus, on average, more women than men need to be treated to prevent one heart disease death, particularly among the young and middle-aged; this results in a potentially different risk–benefit balance for pharmacologic interventions like estrogen for women.[135]

True prevention on a population basis is an attempt to deal with underlying causes.[136] The protection from CAD associated with use of postmenopausal estrogen therapy occurs in a high-risk milieu in which a high proportion of women eat a high fat diet, smoke cigarettes, and are hypertensive.

Although sex hormones have an impact on CAD risk and contribute to the gender gap in CAD, behavioral factors must play an even greater role, as evidenced by the higher CAD rates among women in high-incidence countries relative to rates among men in low-incidence countries (Fig. 7–1).[5] Thus, healthy behaviors, a diet high in fruits and vegetables and low in fat, exercise, and avoidance of tobacco have a beneficial impact on CAD for both men and women and should form the foundation of CAD prevention.[137] In particular, subgroups of women who are likely to be at excess risk of CAD because of endocrine disturbance leading to androgen excess, those with irregular menses or a male fat pattern, and possibly diabetic women should adopt healthy behaviors to minimize CAD risk; whether these groups would benefit from estrogen therapy is not yet clear. Finally, studies of CAD in women should not consider hormonal influences on risk in isolation from behavioral and environmental risk factors, given the evidence for potentially important interactive effects.

REFERENCES

1. Libby P. Atheroma, more than mush. Lancet (Suppl I) 1996;348:1–31.

2. Wenger NK. Coronary heart disease: An older woman's major health risk. BMJ 1997;315:1085–1090.

3. Wenger NK, Speroff L, Packard B. Cardiovascular health and disease in women. N Engl J Med 1993;329:247–256.

4. Willett W, Green A, Stampfer MJ, et al. Relative and absolute excess risks of coronary heart disease among women who smoke cigarettes. N Engl J Med 1987;317: 1303–1309.

5. Thom TJ, Epstein FH, Feldman JJ, Leaverton PE, Wolz M. Total mortality and mortality from heart disease, cancer, and stroke from 1950 to 1987 in 27 countries. Washington, DC: U.S. Dept. Health Human Services, Public Health Service, Natl. Inst. Health, NIH Publ. No. 92–3088, Sept. 1992, p. 17.

6. World Health Organization, World Health Statistics, Annual 1995. Geneva: WHO, 1996, Table B-1, p. B-94.

7. Editorial. Syndrome X. Lancet 1987;ii:1247–1248.

8. Pearson TA. Coronary arteriography in women: Advantages in the study of the etiology and natural history of coronary artery disease. In: Eaker ED, Packard B, Wenger NK, Clarkson TB, Tyroler HA, eds. New York: Haymarket Doyma, 1987; pp. 144–150.

9. Kannel WB, Wilson PWF. Risk factors that attenuate the female coronary disease advantage. Arch Intern Med 1995;155:57–61.

10. Castelli WP, Garrison RJ, Wilson PWF, Abbott RD, Kalousdia S, Kannel WB. Incidence of coronary heart disease and lipoprotein levels. The Framingham Study. JAMA 1986;256:2835–2838.

11. Wingard DL. The sex differential in morbidity, mortality, and lifestyle. Annu Rev Public Health 1984;5:433–458.

12. Harlow SD, Ephross SA. Epidemiology of menstruation and its relevance to women's health. Epidemiol Rev 1995;17:265–286.

13. La Vecchia C, Decarli A, Franceschi S, et al. Menstrual and reproductive factors and the risk of myocardial infarction in women under fifty-five years of age. Am J Obstet Gynecol 1987;157:1108–1112.

14. Gorgels WJMJ, Graaf YVD, Blankenstein MA, Collette HJA, Erkelens DW, Banga JD. Urinary sex hormone excretions in premenopausal women and coronary heart disease risk: A nested case–referent study in the DOM-cohort. Clin Epidemiol 1997;50: 275–281.

15. Heller RF, Jacobs HS. Coronary heart disease in relation to age, sex, and the menopause. Br Med J 1978;1:472–474.

16. MacMahon B, Worcester J. Age at menopause: United States. In: U.S. Vital and Health Statistics 1960–62. Washington DC: National Health Service, Government Printing Office, PHS Publ. No. 1000, Series 11, No. 19, 1966, pp. 1–20

17. Sowers MF, La Pietra MT. Menopause: Its epidemiology and potential association with chronic diseases. Epidemiol Rev 1995;17:287–301.

18. Witteman JCM, Grobbee DE, Kok FJ, Hofman A, Valkenburg HA. Increased risk of atherosclerosis in women after the menopause. BMJ 1989;298:642–644.

19. Pines A, Fisman EZ, Levo Y, et al. Menopause-induced changes in left ventricular wall thickness. Am J Cardiol 1993;72:240–241.

20. Nabulsi AA, Folsom AR, Szklo M, White A, Higgins M, Heiss G. No association of menopause and hormone replacement therapy with carotid artery intima-media thickness. Circulation 1996;94:1857–1863.

21. Colditz GA, Willett WC, Stampfer MJ, Rosner B, Speizer FE, Hennekens CH. Menopause and the risk of coronary heart disease in women. N Engl J Med 1987;316: 1105–1110.

22. Jacobsen BK, Nilssen S, Heuch I, Kvale G. Does age at natural menopause affect mortality for ischemic heart disease? Clin Epidemiol 1997;50:475–479.

23. Snowdon DA, Kane RL, Beeson WL, et al. Is early menopause a biologic marker of health and aging? Am J Public Health 1989;79:709–714.

24. van der Schouw YT, van der Graaf Y, Steyerberg EW, Eijkemans MJC, Banga JD. Age at menopause as a risk factor for cardiovascular mortality. Lancet 1996;347:714–718.

25. Naz RK, Thurston D, Santoro N. Circulating tumor necrosis factor (TNF)-α in normally cycling women and patients with premature ovarian failure and polycystic ovaries. Am J Reprod Immunol 1995;34:170–175.

26. Hoek A, van Kasteren Y, de Hann-Meulman M, Hooijkaas H, Schoemaker J, Drexhage HA. Analysis of peripheral blood lymphocyte subsets, NK cells, and delayed type hypersensitivity skin test in patients with premature ovarian failure. Am J Reprod Immunol 1995;33:495–502.

27. Perls TT, Alpert L, Fretts RC. Middle-aged mothers live longer. Nature 1997; 389:133.

28. Stampfer MJ, Colditz GA, Willett WC. Menopause and heart disease. A review. Ann NY Acad Sci 1990;592:193–203.

29. Ritterband AB, Jaffe IA, Densen PM, Magagna JF, Reed E. Gonadal function and the development of coronary heart disease. Circulation 1963;26:237–251.

30. Novak ER, Williams TJ. Autopsy comparison of cardiovascular changes in castrated and normal women. Am J Obstet Gynecol 1966; 80:863–872.

31. Coldtiz GA, Willett WC, Stampfer MJ, Rosner B, Speizer FE, Hennekens CH. A prospective study of age at menarche, parity, age at first birth, and coronary heart disease in women. Am J Epidemiol 1987;126:861–870.

32. Palmer JR, Rosenberg L, Shapiro S. Reproductive factors and risk of myocardial infarction. Am J Epidemiol 1992;136:408–416.

33. Rosenberg L, Miller DR, Kaufman DW, et al. Myocardial infarction in women under 50 years of age. JAMA 1983;250:2801–2806.

34. Talbot EO, Kuller LH, Detre K, et al. Reproductive history of women dying of sudden cardiac death: A case–control study. Int J Epidemiol 1989;18:589–594.

35. Beard CM, Fuster V, Annegers JF. Reproductive history in women with coronary heart disease: A case–control study. Am J Epidemiol 1984;120:108–114.

36. Ness RB, Schotland HM, Flegal KM, Shofer FS. Reproductive history and coronary heart disease risk in women. Epidemiol Rev 1994;16:298–314.

37. Kvale G, Heuch I, Nilssen S. Parity in relation to mortality and cancer incidence, a prospective study of Norwegian women. Int J Epidemiol 1994;23: 691–699.

38. Kaye, SA, Folsom AR, Prineas RJ, Potter JD, Gapstur SM. The association of body fat distribution with lifestyle and reproductive factors in a population study of postmenopausal women. Int J Obesity 1990;14:583–591.

39. Hankinson SE, Colditz GA, Hunter DJ, et al. Reproductive factors and family history of breast cancer in relation to plasma estrogen and prolactin levels in postmenopausal women in the Nurses' Health Study (United States). Cancer Causes Control 1995;6:217–224.

40. Cauley JA, Gutai JP, Kuller LH, Dai WS. Usefulness of sex steroid hormone levels in predicting coronary artery disease in men. Am J Cardiology 1987;60:771–777.

41. Barrett-Connor E, Khaw KT. Endogenous sex hormones and cardiovascular disease in men: A prospective population-based study. Circulation 1988;78:539–545.

42. Cauley JA, Gutai JP, Glynn NW, Paternostro-Bales M, Cottington E. Kuller LH. Serum estrone concentrations and coronary artery disease in postmenopausal women. Arterioscler Thromb 1994;14:14–18.

43. Barrett-Connor E, Goodman-Gruen D. The epidemiology of DHEAS and cardiovascular disease. Ann NY Acad Sci 1995;774:259–270.

44. Henriksson P, Johansson S-E. Prediction of cardiovascular complications in patients with prostatic cancer treated with estrogen. Am J Epidemiol 1987;125:970–978.

45. Chester AH, Jiang C, Borland JA, Yacoub MH, Collins P. Oestrogen relaxes human epicardial coronary arteries through non-endothelium-dependent mechanisms. Coron Artery Dis 1995;6:417–422.

46. Grodstein F, Stampfer MF, Manson JE, Colditz GA, Willett WC, Rosner B, Speizer FE, Hennekens CH. Postmenopausal estrogen and progestin use and the risk of cardiovascular disease. N Engl J Med 1996;335:453–456.

47. Finnegan LP. The NIH Women's Health Initiative: Its evolution and expected contributions to to women's health. Am J Prev Med 1996;12:292–293.

48. Vickers MR, Meade TW, Wilkes HC. Hormone replacement therapy and cardiovascular disease: the case for a randomized controlled trial. CIBA Found Symp 1995;191:150–160.

49. Schrott HG, Bittner V, Bittinghoff E, Herrington DM, Hulley S for the HERS Research Group. Adherence to National Cholesterol Education Program treatment goals in postmenopausal women with heart disease. JAMA 1997;277:1281–1286.

50. Birdsall MA, Farquhar CM, White HD. Association between polycystic ovaries and extent of coronary artery disease in women having cardiac catheterization. Ann Intern Med 1997;126:32–35.

51. Gordon DJ, Probstfield JL, Garrison RF, et al. High-density lipoprotein cholesterol and cardiovascular disease: Four prospective studies. Circulation 1989;79:8–15.

52. National Cholesterol Education Program. Second Report of the Expert Panel on Detection, Evaluation, and Treatment of High Blood Cholesterol in Adults. National Institutes of Health, National Heart, Lung, and Blood Institute. NIH Publication No. 93–3095, September, 1993.

53. Verschuren WMM, Kromhout D. Total cholesterol concentration and mortality at a relatively young age: Do men and women differ? BMJ 1995;311:779–783.

54. Kuller LH, Meilahn EN. Risk factors for cardiovascular disease among women. Curr Opin Lipidol 1996;7:203–208.

55. Matthews KA, Meilahn E, Kuller LH, Kelsey SF, Caggiula AW, Wing RR. Menopause and risk factors for coronary heart disease. N Engl J Med 1989;321: 641–646.

56. Castelo-Branco C, Casals E, de Osaba MJM, Sanllehy C, Fortuny A. Plasma lipids, lipoproteins and apolipoproteins in hirsute women. Acta Obstet Gynecol Scand 1996;75:261–265.

57. Barrett-Connor E, Goodman-Gruen D. Prospective study of endogenous sex hormones and fatal cardiovascular disease in postmenopausal women. Brit Med J 1995; 311:1193–1196.

58. Cauley JA, Gutai JP, Kuller LH, Powell JG. The relation of endogenous sex steroid hormone concentrations to serum lipid and lipoprotein levels in postmenopausal women. Am J Epidemiol 1991;132:884–894.

59. Kuller LH, Gutai JP, Meilahn EN, Matthews KA, Plantinga P. Relationship of endogenous sex steroid hormones to lipids and apoproteins in postmenopausal women. Arteriosclerosis 1990;10:1058–1066.

60. Clifton PM, Nestel PJ. Influence of gender, body mass index, and age on response of plasma lipids to dietary fat plus cholesterol. Arterioscler Thromb 1992;12: 955–962.

61. Khaw K-T, Barrett-Connor E. Sex differences, hormones, and coronary heart disease. In: Marmot M, Elliott P, eds. Coronary Heart Disease Epidemiology. From Aetiology to Public Health, New York: Oxford University Press, 1992, pp. 274–286.

62. Key TJA, Chen J, Wang DY, Pike MC, Boreham J. Sex hormones in women in rural China and in Britain. Br J Cancer 1990;62:631–636.

63. Moore JW, Clark GM, Takatani O, Wakabayashi Y, Hayward JL, Bulbrook RD. Distribution of 17β-estradiol in the sera of normal British and Japanese women. J Natl Cancer Inst 1983;71:749–754.

64. Writing Group for the PEPI Trial. Effects of estrogen or estrogen/progestin regimens on heart disease risk factors in postmenopausal women. JAMA 1995;273: 199–208.

65. Wagner JD, Schwenke DC, Zhang L, Applebaum-Bowden D, Badgage JD, Adams MR. Effects of short-term hormone replacement therapies on low-density lipoprotein metabolism in cynomolgus monkeys. Arterio Thromb Vascular Biol 1997;17: 1128–1134.

66. Espeland MA, Applegate W, Furberg CD, et al. Estrogen replacement therapy and progression of intimal-medial thickness in the carotid arteries of postmenopausal women. Am J Epidemiol 1995;142:1011–1019.

67. Darling GM, Johns JA, McCloud PI, Davis SR. Estrogen and progestin compared with simvastatin for hypercholesterolemia in postmenopausal women. N Engl J Med 1997;337:595–601.

68. Yong L-C, Kuller LH. Tracking of blood pressure from adolescence to middleage: The Dormont High School Study. Prev Med 1994;23:418–426.

69. Denke MA, Sempos CT, Grundy SM. Excess body weight. An under-recognized contributor to dyslipidemia in white American women. Arch Intern Med 1994;154: 401–410.

70. Mosca L, Manson JE, Sutherland SE, Langer RD, Manolio T, Barrett-Connor E. Cardiovascular disease in women. A statement for healthcare professionals from the American Heart Association. Circulation 1997;96:2468–2482.

71. Folsom AR, Prineas RJ, Kaye SA, Soler JT. Body fat distribution and self-reported prevalence of hypertension, heart attack, and other heart disease in older women. Int J Epidemiol 1989;18:361–368.

72. Lonnqvist F, Thorne A, Large V, Arner P. Sex differences in visceral fat lipolysis and metabolic complications of obesity. Arterioscler Thromb Vasc Biol 1997;17: 1472–1480.

73. Haffner SM. Sex hormone–binding protein, hyperinsulinemia, insulin resistance and noninsulin-dependent diabetes. Horm Res 1996;45:233–237.

74. DePergola G, DeMitrio V, Perricci A, et al. Influence of free testosterone on antigen levels of plasminogen activator inhibitor-1 in premenopausal women with central obesity. Metabolism 1992;41:131–134.

75. Elbers JMH, Asscheman H, Seidell JC, Gooren LIG. Increased accumulation of visceral fat after long-term androgen administration in women. Int J Obes [Abstract]1995;19:25.

76. Zamboni M, Armellini F, Milani MP, et al. Body fat distribution in pre- and postmenopausal women: Metabolic and anthropometric variables and their interrelationships. Int J Obes Relat Metab Discord 1992;16:495–504.

77. Marin P, Holmang A. The effects of testosterone treatment on body composition and metabolism in middle-aged obese men. Int J Obesity 1992;16:991–997.

78. Holmang A, Svedberg J, Jennische E, Bjorntorp P. Effects of testosterone on muscle insulin sensitivity and morphology in female rats. Am J Physiol 1990;259: E555–E560.

79. Lindstedt G, Lundberg PA, Lapidus L, Lundgren H, Bengtsson C, Bjorntorp P. Low sex hormone–binding globulin concentration as independent risk factor for development of NIDDM: 12-year follow-up of population study of women in Gothenburg, Sweden. Diabetes 1991;40:123–128.

80. Haffner SM, Valdez RA, Morales PA, Hazuda HP, Stern MP. Decreased sex hormone–binding globulin predicts non-insulin dependent diabetes mellitus in women but not in men. J Clin Endocrinol Metab 1993;77:56–60.

81. Barbieri RL, Ryan KJ. Hyperandrogenism, insulin resistance and acanthosis nigricans syndrome: A common endocrinopathy with distinct pathophysiologic features. Am J Obstet Gynecol 1983;147:90–101.

82. Barrett-Connor E. Sex differences in coronary heart disease. Why are women so superior? The 1995 Ancel Keys Lecture. Circulation 1997;95:252–264.

83. Weiss DJ, Charles MA, Dunaif A, et al. Hyperinsulinemia is associated with menstrual irregularity and altered serum androgens in Pima Indian women. Metabolism 1994;43:803–807.

84. Kjaer K, Hagen C, Sando SH, et al. Epidemiology of menarche and menstrual disturbances in an unselected group of women with insulin-dependent diabetes mellitus compared to controls. J Clin Endocrinol Metab 1992;75:524–529.

85. Barrett-Connor E, Laakso M. Ischemic heart disease risk in postmenopausal women: Effects of estrogen use on glucose and insulin levels. Arteriosclerosis 1990; 10:531–534.

86. Espeland MA, Stefanick ML, Kritz-Silverstein D, et al. Effect of postmenopausal hormone therapy on body weight and waist and hip girths. Postmenopausal estrogen–progestin interventions study investigators. J Clin Endocrinol Metab 1997;82: 1549–1556.

87. Persson I, Bergkvist L, Londgren C, Yuen J. Hormone replacement therapy and major risk factors for reproductive cancers, osteoporosis, and cardiovascular diseases: Evidence of confounding by exposure characteristics. J Clin Epidemiol 1997;50: 611–618.

88. Hrupka BJ, Smith GP, Geary N. Ovariectomy and estradiol affect postingestive controls of sucrose licking. Physiol Behav 1997;61:243–247.

89. Meilahn EN, Kuller LH, Wing RR, Matthews KA, Nowalk MP. Menopausal changes in lipids and weight—relationship to diet. In: Angle A, et al., eds. Progress in Obesity Research 94. London: John Libbey, 1995, pp. 419–422.

90. Potischman N, Swanson CA, Siiteri P, Hoover RN. Reversal of relation between body mass and endogenous estrogen concentrations with menopausal status. J Natl Cancer Inst 1996;88:756–758.

91. Cooper GS, Sandler DP, Whelan EA, Smith KR. Association of physical and behavioral characteristics with menstrual cycle patterns in women age 29–31 years. Epidemiology 1996;7:624–628.

92. Kannel WB, D'Agostino RB, Belanger AJ. Fibrinogen, cigarette smoking and risk of cardiovascular disease: Insights from the Framingham Study. Am Heart J 1987; 113:1106–1110.

93. Meilahn EN, Cauley JA, Tracy RP, Macy EO, Gutai JP, Kuller LH. Association of sex hormones and adiposity with plasma levels of fibrinogen and PAI-1 in postmenopausal women. Am J Epidemiol 1996;143:159–66.

94. Meilahn EN, Kuller LH, Matthews KA, Kiss JE. Hemostatic factors according to menopausal status and use of hormone replacement therapy. Ann Epidemiol 1992;2: 445–455.

95. Haertel U, Heiss G, Filipiak B, Doering A. Cross-sectional and longitudinal associations between high density lipoprotein cholesterol and women's employment. Am J Epidemiol 1992;135:68–78.

96. Kaplan JR, Adams MR, Clarkson TB, Manuck SB, Shively CA, Williams JK. Psychosocial factors, sex differences, and atherosclerosis: Lessons from animal models. Psychosom Med 1997;58:598–611.

97. Tersman Z, Collins A, Eneroth P. Cardiovascular responses to psychological and physiological stressors during the menstrual cycle. Psychosom Med 1991;53: 185–197.

98. Cooper GS, Baird DD, Hulka BS, Weinberg CR, Savitz DA, Hughes CL Jr. Follicle-stimulating hormone concentrations in relation to active and passive smoking. Obstet Gynecol 1995;85:407–411.

99. Jensen J, Christiansen C, Rodbro P. Cigarette smoking, serum estrogens, and bone loss during hormone-replacement therapy early after menopause. N Engl J Med 1985;313:973–975.

100. Hopper JL, Seeman E. The bone density of female twins discordant for tobacco use. N Engl J Med 1994;330:387–392.

101. McKinlay SM, Bifano NL, McKinlay JB. Smoking and age at menopause. Ann Int Med 1985;103:350–356.

102. Harlow SD, Matanoski GM. The association between weight, physical activity, and stress and variation in the length of the menstrual cycle. Am J Epidemiol 1991;133:38–49.

103. Bromberger JT, Matthews KA, Kuller LH, Wing RR, Meilahn EN, Plantinga P. Prospective study of the determinants of age at menopause. Am J Epidemiol 1997;145:124–133.

104. Wade GN, Schneider JE, Li HY. Control of fertility by metabolic cues. Am J Physiol 1996;270(1 Pt 1):E1–19.

105. Kuller LH. The etiology of breast cancer—from epidemiology to prevention. Public Health Rev 1995;23:157–213.

106. Wagner JD, Cefalu WT, Anthony MS, Litwak KN, Zhang L, Clarkson TB. Dietary soy protein and estrogen replacement therapy improve cardiovascular risk factors and decrease aortic cholesteryl ester content in ovariectomized cynomolgus monkeys. Metabolism 1997;46:698–705.

107. Prentice R, Thompson D, Clifford C, Gorbach S, Goldin B, Byar D. Dietary fat reduction and plasma estradiol concentration in healthy postmenopausal women. J Natl Cancer Inst 1990;82:129–134.

108. Howe GR. Dietary fat and breast cancer risks. An epidemiologic perspective. Cancer 1994;74(3 Suppl):1078–1084.

109. Cauley JA, Gutai JP, Kuller LH, Le Donne D, Powell JG. The epidemiology of serum sex hormones in postmenopausal women. Am J Epidemiol 1989;129:1120–1131.

110. London S, Willett W, Longcope C, McKinlay S. Alcohol and other dietary factors in relation to serum hormone concentrations in women at climacteric. Am J Clin Nutr 1991;53:166–171.

111. Brett KM, Madans JH. Use of postmenopausal hormone replacement therapy: Estimates from a nationally representative cohort study. Am J Epidemiol 1997;145: 536–545.

112. Blair SN, Kohl HW, Paffenbarger RS, et al. Physical fitness and all-cause mortality. A prospective study of healthy men and women. JAMA 1989;262:2395–2401.

113. Akishita M, Ouchi Y, Miyoshi H, et al. Estrogen inhibits endothelin-1 production and c-*fos* gene expression in rat aorta. Arterosclerosis 1996;125:27–38.

114. Imthurn B, Rosselli M, Jaeger AW, Keller PJ, Dubey RK. Differential effects of hormone-replacement therapy on endogenous nitric oxide (nitrite/nitrate) levels in postmenopausal women substituted with 17 beta-estradiol valerate and cyproterone acetate or medroxy-progesterone acetate. J Clin Endocrinol Metab 1997;82:388–394.

115. Adams MR, Register TC, Golden DL, Wagner JD, Williams JK. Medroxyprogesterone acetate antagonizes inhibitory effects of conjugated equine estrogen on coronary artery atherosclerosis. Arterioscler Thromb Vasc Biol 1997;17:217–221.

116. Honore EK, Williams JK, Washburn SA, Herrrington DM. The effects of disease severity and sex on coronary endothelium-dependent vasomotor function in an atherosclerotic primate model. Coron Artery Dis 1996;7:579–585.

117. Wellman GC, Bonev AD, Nelson MT, Brayden JE. Gender differences in coronary artery diameter involve estrogen, nitric oxide, and Ca^+-dependent K^+ channels. Circ Res 1996;79:1024–1030.

118. Volterrani M, Rosano G, Coats A, Beale C, Collins P. Estrogen acutely increases peripheral blood flow in postmenopausal women. Am J Med 1995;99:119–122.

119. Gilligan DM, Badar DM, Panza JA, Quyyumi AA, Cannon RO. Acute vascular effects of estrogen in postmenopausal women. Circulation 1994;90:786–791.

120. Collins P, Rosano GMC, Sarrel PM, et al. 17β-estradiol attenuates acetyl-choline-induced coronary arterial constriction in women but not men with coronary heart disease. Circulation 1995;92:24–30.

121. McCrohon JA, Adams MR, McCredie RJ, et al. Hormone replacement therapy is associated with improved arterial physiology in healthy postmenopausal women. Clin Endocrinol Oxf 1996;45:435–441.

122. Rosano GM, Leonardo F, Sarrel PM, Beale CM, DeLuca F, Collins P. Cyclical variation in paroxysmal supraventricular tachycardia in women. Lancet 1996;347: 786–788.

123. Rosano GM, Peters NS, Lefroy D, et al. 17β-estradiol therapy lessens angina in postmenopausal women with syndrome X. J Am Coll Cardiol 1996;28:1500–1505.

124. Lee W-S, Harder JA, Yoshizumi M, Lee M-E, Haber E. Progesterone inhibits arterial smooth muscle cell proliferation. Nature Med 1997;9:1005–1008.

125. Judd HL. Hormonal dynamics associated with the menopause. Clin Obstet Gynecol 1976;19:775.

126. Nachtigall LE, Nachtigall RH, Nachtigall RD, Beckman EM. Estrogen replacement therapy II: A prospective in the relationship to carcinoma and cardiovascular and metabolic problems. Obstet Gynecol 1979;54:74–79.

127. Matthews KA, Kuller LH, Wing RR, Meilahn EN, Plantinga P. Prior to use of estrogen replacement therapy, are users healthier than nonusers? Am J Epidemiol 1996; 143:971–978.

128. Petitti DB. Coronary heart disease and estrogen replacement therapy. Can compliance bias explain the results of observational studies? Ann Epidemiol 1994;4: 115–118.

129. Moorhead T, Hannaford P, Warskyj M. Prevalence and characteristics associated with use of hormone replacement therapy in Britain. Br J Obstet Gynaecol 1997; 104:290–297.

130. Stampfer MJ, Willett WC, Colditz GA, Rosner B, Speizer FE, Hennekens CH. A prospective study of postmenopausal estrogen therapy and coronary heart disease. N Engl J Med 1985;313:1044–1049.

131. Paffenbarger RS Jr, Wing AL, Hyde RT. Physical activity as an index of heart attack risk in college alumni. Am J Epidemiol 1978;108:161–175.

132. Rose GA. Chest pain questionnaire. Milbank Mem Fund Q 1965;43:32–39.

133. Garber CE, Carleton RA, Heller GV. Comparison of 'Rose questionnaire angina' to exercise thallium scintigraphy: Different findings in males and females. J Clin Epidemiol 1992;45:715–720.

134. Wagner JD, Martino MA, Jayo MJ, Anthony MS, Clarkson TB, Cefalu WT. The effects of hormone replacement therapy on carbohydrate metabolism and cardiovascular risk factors in surgically postmenopausal cynomolgus monkeys. Metabolism 1996; 45:1254–1262.

135. Khaw K-T. Gender and cardiovascular risk. J Hum Hypertens 1996;10: 403–407.

136. Rose GA. Strategies of prevention: The individual and the population. In: Marmot M, Elliot P, eds. Coronary Heart Disease Epidemiology. From Aetiology to Public Health. Oxford: Oxford University Press, 1992, pp. 311–324.

137. Meilahn E, Becker RC, Corrao JM. Primary prevention of coronary heart disease in women. Cardiology 1995;86:286–298.

8

HORMONAL INFLUENCES ON OSTEOPOROSIS AND FRACTURES: AN EPIDEMIOLOGIC PERSPECTIVE

Jane A. Cauley and Frances Leslie Lucas

Osteoporosis is a systemic skeletal disease characterized by low bone mass and microarchitectural deterioration of bone tissue with a consequent increase in bone fragility and fractures after minimal trauma.[1] An expert panel convened by the World Health Organization (WHO) developed a definition of osteoporosis based on bone densitometry: *osteopenia* is a bone mineral density (BMD) measurement of the hip, spine, or distal forearm of >1.0 but ≤2.5 standard deviations (SD) below the young normal mean; *osteoporosis* is a BMD at one of the three sites of >2.5 SD below the young normal mean.[2] The purpose of this operational definition of osteoporosis was to estimate the worldwide prevalence of the disease. It is currently used clinically to identify women in need of treatment or prevention of osteoporosis. Although the WHO definition relies solely on BMD measurements, with no consideration of the "microarchitectural" deterioration in bone tissue that accompanies the loss of bone mass, it is believed that BMD measurements do provide some information on the microarchitectural properties of bone, especially if the problems are severe.[3]

PUBLIC HEALTH IMPACT

Osteoporosis is a major public health problem. Of the 1.3 million fractures that occur in the United States each year, 70% of all fractures among individuals age 45 and over are attributable to osteoporosis.[4] The three most common fractures associated with osteoporosis are hip, vertebral, and distal forearm but recent data from the Study of Osteoporotic Fractures have shown that most fractures, at least among women 65 years or older, are indeed due to osteoporosis.[5] In the United States, 250,000 individuals over age 65 fracture their hip each year; by 2040, over 650,000 hip fractures will occur each year.[6,7] One in six (17.5%) white women will fracture a hip in her lifetime. The lifetime risk of hip fracture in men is estimated at 6%.[8] Hip fractures have major consequences, including an 18%–33% mortality within the first year of the hip fracture.[9,10] Among survivors, only 21% regained their prefracture functioning in six instrumental activities of daily living.[11] Hip fractures are a major cause of institutionalism, given that 45% of those who were living independently in their community were discharged to a nursing home after their hip fracture hospitalization and 15%–25% remain institutionalized for a year after their fracture.[12] The direct and indirect cost of osteoporosis in the United States in 1995 approached $14 billion annually.[13]

The lifetime risk of clinical vertebral fractures approaches that of hip fractures: 15.6% among women and 5.0% among men.[8] Only one-third of vertebral fractures reach clinical attention and recent estimates of vertebral fracture prevalence that rely on morphometric definitions (measurement of vertebral heights) suggest that the overall prevalence of vertebral fractures is actually much higher (about 20%) and similar in men and women.[14,15] Up until recently, it was not believed that vertebral fractures were associated with a significant mortality. However, data from the Mayo Clinic demonstrated almost a 20% decreased survival 5 years after the diagnosis, especially among individuals over age 75 years.[16]

Vertebral fractures also have an important impact on the quality of life and functional status of older individuals. Among elderly women ages 65 to 70, the most severe vertebral deformities were associated with moderate to severe back pain (odds ratio [OR]= 1.9, 95% confidence intervals [CI], 1.5–2.4) and a higher risk of disability involving the back (OR = 2.6; CI, 1.7–3.9).[17]

The lifetime risk of distal forearm fractures is 2.5% in men and 16% in women.[8] Although there is no excess mortality risk associated with distal forearm fractures, about 50% of subjects reported fair or poor functional status 6 months after the fracture.[18]

In summary, osteoporotic fractures are relatively common events. Forty percent of women and 13% of men will experience a hip, vertebral, or distal forearm fracture in their lifetime.[8] Although hip fracture incidence rates have stabilized in the United States, the number of fractures will increase because of the relative increase in the number of persons over age 65. The impact of hip fracture on mortality and morbidity is likely to increase since the fastest growing segment of our older population is those individuals age 85 and over. It is these individuals who are most likely to die or become institutionalized or disabled from their hip fracture.

TYPE I AND TYPE II OSTEOPOROSIS

Riggs and Melton have proposed a model for involutional osteporosis that distinguishes two types: type I (postmenopausal) osteoporosis and type II (age-related) osteoporosis.[19] Type I osteoporosis primarily affects postmenopausal women aged 51–75 at six times the rate of men, and it is associated with accelerated rates of bone loss due to estrogen deficiency. There is a disproportionate loss of trabecular bone. It is characterized by fractures in sites that are predominately trabecular, such as distal forearm fractures and vertebral crush fractures. Type II osteoporosis primarily affects individuals after age 70, with a female-to-male ratio of 2:1. It is characterized by a slow rate of bone loss that begins around age 40 in both men and women. Both cortical and trabecular bone loss occurs, resulting in hip and verebral (multiple wedge) fractures.

Although this theory is not univerisally accepted, it is interesting to epidemiologists because the theory stemmed from examination of the epidemiology of fractures and patterns of bone loss with age. Wrist fractures occur primarily in young postmenopausal women, increasing rapidly until age 70. After age 70, the rate of wrist fractures plateaus. Hip fractures on the other hand, increase slowly up to about age 75, when an exponential increase in hip fractures occurs and continues into the tenth decade.[20] Thus, epidemiologic observations have led to important hypotheses about the etiology of osteoporotic fractures.

DESCRIPTIVE EPIDEMIOLOGY: MEN VS. WOMEN

Bone mass in infants is similar in boys and girls and gender differences in bone mass do not become manifest until puberty.[21] Studies have shown that men experience greater gains in BMD and bone size (width, cross-sectional area) in adolescence than women. This difference is primarily observed in areal density measures, e.g., BMD and volumetric density (g/cm^3).[22] After puberty, BMD is greater in men than women and the rate of decline in BMD with age in men appears to be slower.[23]

As indicated earlier in the chapter, lifetime risks of hip, vertebral and distal forearm fractures are lower in men than women.[8] Up until age 45, fracture incidence rates are actually higher in men.[24] The cross-over in rates occurs around the time of menopause in women. After age 50, hip fractures tend to occur about 5–10 years later in men. For vertebral fractures, recent data relying on morphometric definition have shown that the prevalence of fractures is similar in men and women but the proportionate increase with age is greater for women than men.[14,15]

Although there are marked differences in hip fracture rates in African-American and Caucasian women, African-American and Caucasian men have similar rates.[25] This suggests that there may be some interaction between gender and race. In certain geographical areas where, in general, hip fracture rates are low, such as Hong Kong, gender differences are not apparent.[26] Nevertheless, in most countries, the primary victim of osteoporosis is the older white female; this reflects her lower peak bone mass, her accelerated bone loss with menopause, and her longer life expectancy.

ENDOGENOUS ESTROGENS, BONE MASS, AND FRACTURE

The primary source of circulating estrogens in premenopausal women is the direct secretion from the ovaries. Levels of estradiol and estrone vary across the menstrual cycle but are considerably higher than the concentrations observed in postmenopausal women.[27] For postmenopausal women, the principle source of estrogens is the aromatization of an adrenal hormone, androstenedione, to estrone. Estrone can be further reduced to estradiol. Testosterone is also a precursor to estradiol. In general, the average level of estrone in postmenopausal women is about 35 pg/ml and estradiol, approximately 13 pg/ml.[28] Serum levels of estrone and estradiol after administration of exogenous estrogen range from 51 to 300 pg/ml estrone and 19 to 120 pg/ml estradiol.[29]

Most of the research on endogenous sex steroid hormones and osteoporotic fractures have been retrospective case–control studies of women with fracture(s) in comparison with controls. These retrospective studies have a number of important limitations. Sample sizes were generally small, limiting statistical power. The subjects tended to be restricted to convenient samples of patients recruited from clinic populations. Changes in behavior after the fracture and treatment for the fracture could also influence hormone levels. Most studies did not include adjustment for important confounding factors. Only a few studies assessed estrogen binding and metabolism and their availability to target tissues. There is not sufficient information to draw conclusions about these issues. Prospective studies are needed to assess whether endogenous hormone levels predict fracture risk.

Studies of serum estrogens in women with a vertebral fracture compared with controls have in general reported mixed results. Marshall et al. reported a lower serum estrone concentration in women with vertebral fracture (28.3 pg/ml) compared to women with menopausal symptoms (38.6 pg/ml), women with back pain (34.3 pg/ml), or women who had recently undergone a bilateral oophorectomy (30.8 pg/ml).[30] A similar finding was reported by Aloia et al. in 1985.[31] Other studies have not shown a difference in serum estrone between cases and controls.[32,33] In two studies, estradiol concentrations were actually higher among the cases[34,35] than controls. Women with an "osteoporotic fracture" and control women had similar serum estrogen concentrations.[36,37]

There is only one population-based case control study of vertebral fractures and endogenous hormones.[38] Women with incident vertebral fractures ($n =$ 62) were compared with 620 community controls. Results showed no difference between cases and controls for estrone (cases, 41.0 pg/ml; controls, 38.0 pg/ml) or estradiol (cases, 8.0 pg/ml; controls, 7.7 pg/ml).

Estrone and estradiol have also been found to be similar in a small case–control study of hip fractures and controls.[39] Free estradiol levels and the percentage of free estradiol were lower among the cases (1.5 pg/ml and 0.17%) than controls (1.77 pg/ml and 0.21%). In a subgroup analysis of 12 pairs matched on age and weight, however, there were no differences in any estrogen measure.

In summary, these retrospective studies have not provided strong evidence that serum estrogens differ in women with and without osteoporosis. Nevertheless, the limitations of these studies may have biased their results.

There is only one prospective study of serum estrogens and hip and vertebral fracture. As part of the Study of Osteoporotic Fractures (SOF), a case–cohort study was done to compare baseline levels of hormones in women who went on to suffer a hip or vertebral fracture with levels in randomly selected controls.[40] The risk of hip and vertebral fracture was elevated among women with estradiol levels below the sensitivity of the assay (<5 pg/ml) compared with the control: the age- and body weight–adjusted relative risk of hip fracture was 2.48 (1.35 to 4.55); and vertebral fracture, 2.46 (1.43 to 4.22). There appeared to be a threshold decrease in risk associated with estradiol concentrations. These results provide the strongest evidence to date that individual measurements of estradiol may identify high-risk women. These results need to be replicated in other groups of women, including women of other racial groups.

ENDOGENOUS HORMONES, RACE, AND BONE MASS

Incidence rates for hip fractures[25] and all fractures[41] are consistently lower in black women compared with white women. This difference has been attributed to the higher bone mass in blacks compared with whites.[42] Blacks may have higher bone mass than whites because of higher concentrations of endogenous sex hormones. Racial differences in trabecular bone mass became manifested around puberty,[43] although higher bone mass has been reported for very young black children.[44,45] The influence of puberty on bone mass could be due to sex hormones, growth hormones, or gonadotropins. In postmenopausal women, the aromatization of androstenedione to estrone primarily occurs in fat tissue[46–48] and the degree of obesity is a major determinant of serum estrone and estradiol in postmenopausal women.[49] The association of obesity with bone mass of non-weight-bearing bones, such as the radius,[50] suggest that systemic factors, e.g., sex hormones, contribute to level of bone mass. The greater degree of obesity in blacks, and hence, possible higher levels of endogenous hormones, could influence bone mass.

To test the hypothesis that racial differences in serum hormones contribute to racial differences in bone mass and fracture,[51] we compared serum hormones in two samples of elderly women: 86 African-American women recruited from the Monongahela Valley, near Pittsburgh, PA and Baltimore County, MD, and an age-stratified random sample of 273 white women participating in the Study of Osteoporotic Fractures at the Pittsburgh Clinic. All of the women were at least 65 years of age at entry to the study; white women were of mean age 73.6 ± 5.8 years; African-American women, mean age 71.4 ± 4.9 years, P <0.002. The African-American women were on average about 10 kg heavier than the Caucasian women.

Bone mineral density declined with age but the effect was more apparent in white women. Estrone concentrations also decreased with age in white women but not in African-American women (Fig. 8–1). These data suggest that age-related declines in serum estrone may contribute to the decline in BMD with age among white women.

Bone mineral density increased linearly with increasing degree of obesity in both white and African-American women. This may reflect increasing levels of estrogen with increasing obesity. As shown in Figure 8–2, estrone concentrations were greatest among women with the greatest body mass index (BMI) in both racial groups. There was also a linear increase in radial bone mineral density in both black and white women with increasing concentrations of estrone, even after adjustment for age and degree of obesity (Fig. 8–3). There was no

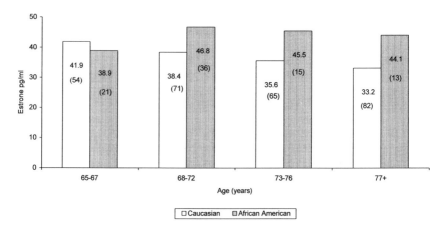

Figure 8–1. Estrone concentration (pg/ml) by age in Caucasian and African-American women, Number of women shown in parentheses. *African Americans, **P** = 0.46; **Caucasians, **P** <0.001

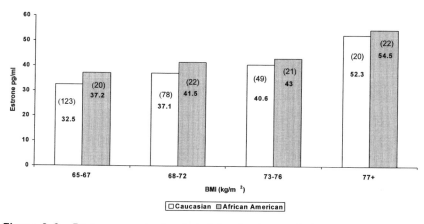

Figure 8–2. Estrone concentration (pg/ml) by the degree of obesity in Caucasian and African-American women, Number of women shown in parentheses.

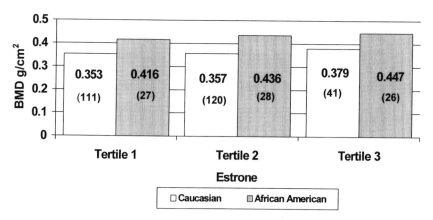

Figure 8–3. Distal radius bone mineral density (BMD) (g/cm²) by tertile of estrone in Caucasian and African-American elderly women, estrone tertile: <32.1; 32.1 −48.4; >48.4 pg/ml + age and BMI adjusted BMD.

significant interaction between race and estrone on BMD, suggesting similar effects of estrone on BMD within each race.

Within each age, BMI, or estrone stratum, African-American women had significantly higher bone mineral density. We controlled for several important confounding factors and in every analysis the BMD was greatest among the African-American women. There may be other factors which we did not measure in our study that could contribute to racial differences in BMD. Nevertheless, the role of genetics in explaining these racial differences is not known. Molecular epidemiologic studies are needed to determine whether racial differences in the expression of gene(s) important to osteoporosis differ by race.

EXOGENOUS ESTROGEN

Estrogen replacement therapy (ERT) is the cornerstone of pharmacologic therapy for osteoporosis. The pooled effect of estrogen on hip fracture is estimated to be a 25% reduction among women who have ever used estrogen.[52] The overall protective effect of estrogen on hip fractures is greatest among current users, approaching a relative risk of approximately 0.50.[53] Estrogen also reduces the risk of all fractures, with estimates ranging from a 35%[53] to 50%[54] reduction.

Epidemiologic studies have played major roles in furthering our understanding of estrogen effects on fracture reduction. Clinical trials have demonstrated improvements or maintenance of BMD among women randomized to estrogen treatment. Clinical studies of the effect of withdrawal of treatment on BMD have also been carried out. Finally, clinical trials have shown a reduction in the risk of vertebral fractures associated with ERT.[55] However, there has been no clinical trial of the effect of estrogen on hip fractures. All of the data on ERT and hip fractures have been accumulated from case–control studies or observational cohort studies, such as Framingham[56] or SOF.[53] Important questions about the timing of therapy initiation with respect to menopause or identification of the minimum duration of estrogen therapy can best be answered by observational epidemiologic studies. It is obviously impractical and unethical to randomize women at the onset of menopause to estrogen or a placebo and follow them for 30 or more years for the occurrence of hip fractures.

Duration of Use and Timing of ERT with Respect to Menopause

While ERT is an established means of prevention and treatment for osteoporosis and fracture, several important issues remain. The minimum duration of estrogen therapy for the prevention of fractures and bone loss has not been established, but most studies have shown that long duration is more beneficial in reducing fractures than short duration.[53,57,58] However, duration of use is correlated with age at initiation of use. Women who initiate use early in the menopausal transition and continue to use it will by definition be "long" duration users. Few authors have attempted to differentiate the effects of timing of initiation from duration of use.

Schneider and colleagues have recently made an important observation.[59] They compared women who reported current ERT use at entry into the study and who initiated use before or after age 60 with past users and never-users. The BMD was highest among current users who initiated use before age 60. It is important to note, however, that current users who initiated use after age 60 had significantly greater BMD than women who had never used ERT. These data suggest that ERT could be started much later after menopause and still be beneficial. This observation, if true, is important, since the overall duration would be shorter, thereby reducing the possible risk that long-duration ERT use among older women may contribute to breast cancer.

These data conflict with an earlier publication from the Study of Osteo-porotic Fractures.[53] The risk of suffering any nonspinal fracture was examined among current long-term users (10 or more years of estrogen use)—those women who initiated use early with respect to menopause (<5 years) and those who started ERT late with respect to menopause (≥5 years) (Fig. 8–4). Early initiation among long-term users was associated with a 50% reduction in the risk for all nonspinal fracture but no effect was noted if estrogen was initiated late, even among women who used ERT for ≥10 years (Fig. 8–4). These results suggest that for *optimal* protection against fractures, the primary clinical indica-tion of osteoporosis, estrogen should be initiated soon after menopause and con-tinued indefinitely.

Additional data with sufficient statistical power to examine the effect of timing of ERT on fracture risk are needed. Large cohort observational studies such as the Women's Health Initiative could provide this information.

Estrogen Replacement Therapy in Combination with Other Therapies

Estrogen therapy is often given with other medications, e.g., progestin and cal-cium supplements. Thiazide diuretics are also commonly prescribed for hyper-tension and may have independent effects on the risk of fracture. Sample sizes required in a clinical trial for an intention to treat analysis of the effect of the combination therapies compared with estrogen alone would preclude these studies from being carried out. Hence, observational epidemiologic studies can provide useful descriptive information on whether the combination of therapies are indeed more beneficial than the effect of exogenous estrogens alone.

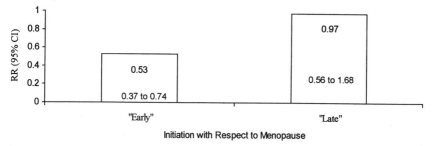

Figure 8–4. Relative risk of nonspinal fractures among current long-term users of estro-gen (≥10 yeas) compared with never-users by initiation with respect to menopause. "Early," 2 years before menopause to 5 years after menopause; "Late," >5 years after menopause.

PROGESTINS

Women with intact uteri are given estrogen in combination with a progestin to prevent estrogen-associated endometrial hyperplasia. Most epidemiologic studies have examined the relation of unopposed estrogen and fracture. A prospective cohort study from Sweden that included about 30% of participants reporting estrogen plus progestin found that the combination therapy was effective in reducing the risk of hip fracture.[60] This study did not, however, compare the relative risks separately for unopposed and combination therapy. In the SOF, we found no difference in the effect of unopposed therapy and combination therapy on the risk of wrist fracture or all nonspinal fractures.[53]

Progestins given alone have been shown to reduce bone loss, particularly loss of cortical bone,[61] and there may be additive or synergistic effects on bone associated with combination therapy. Riis et al. reported that monotherapy and combination therapy had similar effects on BMD.[62] On the other hand, Grey and colleagues demonstrated that after 1 year of therapy, lumbar spine BMD increased almost 7% among women randomized to the combination therapy compared with a 4% increase among women randomized to unopposed therapy.[63] The difference between groups reached statistical significance. An accompanying editorial suggests that the observed differences may reflect different rates of bone turnover in hysterectomized women and nonhysterectomized women.[64]

Results from the Postmenopausal Estrogen/Progestin Interventions (PEPI) trial demonstrated that women assigned to the conjugated equine estrogen (0.625 mg/day) plus continuous medroxyprogesterone acetate (MPA) (2.5 mg/d) had significantly greater increases in spinal BMD (increase of 5%) than those assigned to the other three active regimens, one of which was unopposed estrogen (average increase 3.8%).[65] However, when they limited their analyses to adherent women, there were no differences in BMD changes across the four active treatment groups. These PEPI results provide the strongest evidence to date that addition of a progestin does not enhance the BMD responsiveness to estrogen therapy, at least to the hormone regimens commonly given in the United States.

CALCIUM SUPPLEMENTS

Calcium supplements are now widely recommended for the prevention and treatment of osteoporosis, especially among women with dietary intakes less than the current recommendation of 1200 to 1500 mg/day. An early paper by Ettinger et al. suggested that a lower dose of estrogen could be used if calcium supplements were given in combination.[66] Fractional calcium absorption declines across menopause and improves with estrogen treatment.[67] Hence, it is possible that women on estrogen who continue their calcium supplements could

Table 8–1.   Radial BMD by Calcium Supplements
and Estrogen Replacement Therapy

	N	DISTAL RADIUS MEAN (SD)	PROXIMAL RADIUS MEAN (SD)
Calcium + ERT	967	0.40 (0.09)	0.68 (0.10)
Calcium alone	2616	0.35 (0.08)	0.61 (0.10)
ERT alone	280	0.42 (0.09)	0.70 (0.09)
Neither calcium nor ERT	2623	0.35 (0.08)	0.62 (0.10)
P interaction, ERT × calcium		0.02	0.15

Data from the Study of Osteoporotic Fractures. BMD (gm/cm2) adjusted for age and body weight.

have a higher net absorption of calcium. This higher absorption could lead to a positive impact on BMD above and beyond the effects of their estrogen.

The effect of estrogen on BMD was examined separately among women currently taking calcium supplements and those not taking calcium supplements in the SOF cohort. Past users were excluded from these analysis. There was no evidence of an additive effect on BMD among women taking both calcium and ERT (Table 8–1). Since the mean baseline calcium intake in the SOF was moderate at 714 mg/day, it is possible that calcium supplements could enhance ERT among women with very low dietary intakes of calcium.

THIAZIDE DIURETICS

Thiazide diuretics have been shown to preserve bone mass and reduce the risk of fractures.[68] Among women enrolled in the Hawaiian Osteoporosis Study, women who were on both ERT and thiazide had significantly greater BMD and fewer vertebral fractures than women on either therapy alone.[69] In the SOF, we examined BMD among current users of ERT and thiazide diuretics with women who had never used either therapy (Table 8–2). Past users were excluded from these analyses. The BMD of women on ERT and thiazide diuretics was not significantly different from the BMD of women on ERT alone. There was no consistent pattern showing an additive effect of thiazide diuretic use and unopposed or combination estrogen.

RESPONSE TO TREATMENT OF ESTROGEN BY INITIAL BMD

Recent studies have demonstrated that ERT is effective in reducing bone loss in women with established osteoporosis[55] and in elderly women.[53] It has also been shown that obese women and those with lower vertebral BMD may respond better to ERT than slender women with higher BMD.[70] To test the hypothesis that there may be a differential effect of ERT on fracture risk by BMD, women

Table 8–2. Radial BMD by Thiazide Diuretic Use and ERT Among
Women Enrolled in the Study of Osteoporotic Fractures

	(N)	DISTAL RADIUS MEAN (SD)	PROXIMAL RADIUS MEAN (SD)
Thiazide diuretic + ERT	362	0.40 (0.09)	0.69 (0.10)
ERT alone	984	0.40 (0.09)	0.68 (0.10)
Thiazide diuretic alone	1495	0.36 (0.09)	0.64 (0.11)
Neither	4169	0.35 (0.08)	0.61 (0.10)
P (thiazide × ERT)		0.06	0.02

BMD (g/cm²) adjusted for age and body weight.

Table 8–3. Effect of ERT on Fractures by BMD
Level in the Study of Osteoporotic Fractures

	LOW BMD (N = 1498)[a]		HIGH BMD (N = 8096)[b]	
	NO. OF FRACTURES	RR (95% CI)	NO. OF FRACTURES	RR (95% CI)
Wrist	(58)	0.38 (0.09, 1.55)	(164)	0.49 (0.30, 0.79)
Osteoporosis	(216)	0.82 (0.68, 1.64)	(577)	0.72 (0.58, 0.91)

[a]Low BMD: distal radius BMD <1 SD below mean, >0.2777 (g/cm²).
[b]High BMD: distal radius BMD, ≥0.2777 g/cm²

with "low" BMD (defined as <1 SD below the mean radius distal BMD, <0.277 g/cm²) were compared with women with "high" BMD (≥0.277 g/cm² distal radius BMD). As shown in Table 8–3, ERT was effective in reducing the risk of wrist and osteoporotic fractures among both groups of women, suggesting that the response to ERT is independent of BMD.

ESTROGENS AND BONE METABOLISM

Estrogens could directly influence the skeleton through several mechanisms. Estrogen can decrease the number of activated bone remodeling units, thereby decreasing bone turnover.[71] Several cytokines including interleuken (IL)-1, IL-6, IL-11, tumor necrosis factor (TNF), macrophage colony-stimulating factors (M-CSF), and granulocyte-macrophage stimulating factor (GM-CSF) have been identified and shown to increase cytoclast formation.[72] IL-1 and TNF are also potent stimulants of bone resorption and inhibitors of bone formulation. Estrogen has been shown to decrease the production of IL-1 and TNF and to decrease osteoclast activation.[72]

Estrogen may also antagonize parathyroid hormones stimulation of bone resorption.[73] Fractional calcium absorption improves with estrogen replacement, which suggests an additional mechanism.[67]

Finally, estrogen could influence neuromuscular function and muscle strength, thereby reducing the risk of falls. In a small study, ERT users had greater grip strength and exhibited a slower decline in strength with age.[74] However, in the SOF cohort as well as other studies, there was no evidence that estrogen therapy influences muscle strength or the risk of falls.[75,76]

LIMITATIONS TO EPIDEMIOLOGIC STUDIES OF ESTROGEN AND OSTEOPOROSIS

The major limitation to epidemiologic studies of estrogen replacement is the selection bias for ERT use. Women who use hormones are different from women who don't use hormones. For example, they are less obese, more likely to participate in physical activities, less likely to smoke, better educated, and obviously have access to medical care.[77] Thus, hormone therapy may be a marker of socioeconomic, clinical, or lifestyle variables that place users at a lower risk of fractures.

Secondly, "long-term" users of estrogen are by definition "compliant" women. Hence, at least part of the benefits observed with ERT may reflect a compliance bias.[78] Third, epidemiologic studies rely primarily on self-report of medication use, including historical information on age at initiation of use and duration of use. There may be a recall bias associated with this information, but inaccurate recall of use would bias our results towards no association and recall accuracy for estrogen use has been found to be quite high.[79] Only a randomized trial can provide conclusive evidence of the effects of estrogen on BMD and fractures.

Because of issues of cost and feasibility, most studies of endogenous hormones and osteoporosis rely on a single measurement of endogenous hormones. This is a major limitation to the epidemiologic approach. Interpretation of these studies is difficult since measurement of hormones at a discrete point in time may not reflect a woman's long-term exposure to estrogen. In addition, endogenous estrogens, specifically estradiol concentrations, are low in postmenopausal women; thus, there is a greater possibility of laboratory error. Finally, circulating estrogen levels in the blood may not relate to biological effects in tissue such as breast cancer.

SUMMARY

Epidemiologic studies produced important evidence that one of the major etiologic factors of osteoporosis is an estrogen deficiency. Development of the theory of types I and II osteoporosis relied heavily on epidemiologic data on patterns of bone loss and fractures with age. Descriptive epidemiologic studies of gender differences in the patterns of fractures and bone mass have also provided important information on the role of estrogen in osteoporosis. Specific studies of endogenous hormones and estrogen replacement therapy and the risk of osteoporosis have helped establish a basis for the prevention and treatment of osteoporosis.

REFERENCES

1. Christiansen C. Consensus development conference on osteoporosis. Am J Med 1993:95.

2. Kanis JA, Melton J, Christiansen C, Johnston CC, Khaltaev N. The diagnosis of osteoporosis. J Bone Min Res 1994;9:1137–1141.

3. Marcus R. The nature of osteoporosis. In: Marcus R, Feldman D, Kelsey J, eds. Osteoporosis. San Diego, CA: Academic Press, 1996, pp. 647–659.

4. Iskrant AP, Smith RW. Osteoporosis in women 45 years and over related to subsequent fractures. Public Health Rep 1969;84:33–38.

5. Seeley DG, Browner WS, Nevitt MC, Genant HK, Scott JC, Cummings SR. Which fractures are associated with low appendicular bone mass in elderly women? The Study of Osteoporotic Fractures Research Group. Ann Intern Med 1991;155(11): 837–842.

6. Gullberg B, Johnell O, Kanis JA. World-wide projections for hip fracture. Osteoporos Int 1997;7:407–413.

7. Schneider EL, Guralnik JM. The aging of America—Impact of health care costs. JAMA 1990;263:2335–2340.

8. Melton LJ, Chrischilles EA, Cooper C, Lane AW, Riggs BL. How many women have osteoporosis? J Bone Min Res 1992;7:1005–1010.

9. Magaziner J, Simonsick EM, Kashner M, Hebel JR, Kenzora JE. Survival experience of aged hip fracture patients. Am J Public Health 1989;79:274–278.

10. Jacobsen SJ, Goldberg J, Milist P, Brody JA, Stiers W, Rimm AA. Race and sex differences in mortality following fracture of the hip. Am J Public Health 1992;82: 1147–1150.

11. Jette AM, Harris BA, Cleary PD, Campion EW. Functional recovery after hip fracture. Arch Phys Med Rehabil 1987;68:735–740.

12. Magaziner J, Simonsick EM, Kashner TM, Hebel JR, Kenzora JE. Predictors of functional recovery one year following hospital discharge for hip fracture: A prospective study. J Gerontol Med Sci 1990;45:M101–M107.

13. Ray NF, Chan JK, Thaner M, Melton LJ. Medical expenditures for the treatment of osteoporotic fractures in the United States in 1995: Report from the National Osteoporosis Foundation. J Bone Miner Res 1997;12:24–35.

14. O'Neill TW, Felsenberg D, Varlow J, Cooper C, Kanis JA, Silman AJ. The prevalence of vertebral deformity in European men and women: The European vertebral osteoporosis study. J Bone Miner Res 1997;11:1010–1018.

15. Davies KM, Stegman MR, Heaney RP, Recker RR. Prevalence and severity of vertebral fracture: The Saunders County Bone Quality Study. Osteoporosis Int 1996;6: 160–165.

16. Cooper C, Alkinson EJ, Jacobsen SJ, O'Fallon WM, Melton LJ. Population based study of survival following osteoporotic fractures. Am J Epidemiol 1993;137: 1001–1005.

17. Ettinger B, Black DM, Nevitt MC, et al. Contribution of vertebral deformities to chronic back pain. J Bone Miner Res 1992;7:449–456.

18. Kaukonen JP, Karaharju EO, Porras M, Luthje P, Jakobsson A. Functional recovery after fractures of the distal forearm. Ann Chir Gynaecol 1988;77:27–31.

19. Riggs BL, Melton LJ. Evidence for two distinct syndromes of involutional osteoporosis. Am J Med 1983;75:899–901.

20. Kassem M, Melton J, Riggs BL. The type I/type II model for involutional osteoporosis. In: Marcus R, Feldman D, Kelsey J, eds. Osteoporosis. San Diego, CA: Academic Press, 1996, pp. 691–713.

21. Bachrach LK. Osteopenia in childhood and adolescence. In: Marcus R, Feldman D, Kelsey J, eds. Osteoporosis. San Diego, CA: Academic Press, 1996, pp. 785–800.

22. Gilsanz V, Boechat I, Roe TF, Loro ML, Sayre JW, Goodman WG. Gender differences in vertebral body sizes in children and adolescents. Radiology 1994;190: 673–677.

23. Looker AC, Wahner HW, Dunn WL, et al. Proximal femur bone mineral levels of U.S. adults. Osteoporosis Int 1995;5:389–409.

24. Donaldson LJ, Cook A, Thomson RG. Incidence of fractures in a geographically defined population. J Epidemiol Community Health 1990;44:241–245.

25. Farmer ME, White LR, Brody JA, Bailey KR. Role and sex differences in hip fracture incidence. Am J Public Health 1984;74:1374–1380.

26. Melton LJ. Epidemiology of fractures. In: Riggs BL, Melton LJ, eds. Osteoporosis: Etiology, Diagnosis and Management. New York: Lippincott-Raven Press, 1995, pp. 225–247.

27. Yen SSC. The biology of menopause. Reprod Med 1977;18:287.

28. Jaffe RB. The menopause and perimenopausal period. In: Yen SSC, Jaffe RB, eds. Reproductive Endocrinology. Philadelphia: W.B. Saunders, 1986, pp. 406–423.

29. O'Connell MB. Pharmacokinetic and pharmacologic variation between different estrogen products. J Clin Pharmacol 1995;35:18S–24S.

30. Marshall DH, Crilly RG, Nordin BEC. Plasma androstenedione and oestrone levels in normal and osteoporotic post-menopausal women. Br Med J 1977;2: 1177–1179.

31. Aloia JF, Cohn SF, Vaswani A, et al. Risk factors for postmenopausal osteoporosis. Am J Med 1985;78:95–100.

32. Riggs BL, Ryan RJ, Wahner HW, et al. Serum concentrations of estrogen, testosterone and gonadotropins in osteoporotic and nonosteoporotic postmenopausal women. J Clin Endrocrinol Metab 1973;36:1097–1099.

33. Bartizal FJ, Coulam CB, Gaffey TA, et al. Impaired binding of estradiol to vaginal mucosal cells in postmenopausal osteoporosis. Gynecol Invest 1976;7:330–336.

34. Davidson BJ, Rigg BL, Wahner HW, et al. Endogenous cortisol and sex steroids in patients with osteoporotic spinal fractures. Obstet Gynecol 1983;61:275–278.

35. Longcope C, Baker RS, Hur SL, et al. Androgen and estrogen dynamics in women with vertebral crush fractures. Maturitas 1984;6:309–318.

36. Riis BJ, Christiansen C, Deftos LJ, et al. The role of serum concentrations of estrogens on postmenopausal osteoporosis and bone turnover. In: Christiansen C, ed. Osteoporosis: Aalborg. Stifsbogtrykkeri Printers, 1984, pp. 333–336.

37. Riis BJ, Rodbro P, Christiansen C. The role of serum concentrations of sex steroids and bone turnover in the development and occurrence of postmenopausal osteoporosis. Calcif Tissue Int 1986;38:318–322.

38. van Hemert AM, Birkenhager JC, De Jong FH, et al. Sex hormone binding globulin in postmenopausal women: A predictor of osteoporosis superior to endogenous oestrogens. Clin Endocrinol 1989;31:499–509.

39. Davidson BJ, Ross RK, Paganini-Hill A, et al. Total and free estrogens and androgens in postmenopausal women with hip fractures. J Clin Endocrinol Metab 1982;54:115–120.

40. Cummings SR, Browner WS, Bauer D, et al. Endogenous sex and calciotropic hormones and the risk of hip and vertebral fractures in older women: The study of osteoporotic fractures. N Engl J Med 1998 (in press).

41. Griffin MR, Ray WA, Fought RL, et al. Black–white differences in fracture rates. Am J Epidemiol 1992;136:1378–1385.

42. DeSimone DP, Stevens J, Edwards J, et al. Influence of body habitus and race on bone mineral density of the midradius, hip and spine in aging women. J Bone Miner Res 1989;4:827–830.

43. Gilsanz V, Roe TF, Mora S, et al. Changes in vertebral bone density in black girls and white girls during childhood and puberty. N Engl J Med 1991;325:1597–1600.

44. Li JY, Specker BL, Ho ML, et al. Bone mineral content in black and white children 1 to 6 years of age: early appearance of race and sex differences. Am J Dis Child 1989;143:1346–1349.

45. Bell NH, Shary J, Stevens J, et al. Demonstration that bone mass is greater in black than in white children. J Bone Miner Res 1991;6:719–723.

46. Siiteri PK, Murai JT, Hammond GL, et al. The serum transport of steroid hormones. Recent Prog Horm Res 1982;38:457–510.

47. MacDonald PC, Edman CD, Hemsell DL, et al. Effect of obesity on conversion of plasma androstenedione to estrone in postmenopausal women with and without endometrial cancer. Am J Obstet Gynecol 1978;130:448–455.

48. Kirschner MA, Schneider G, Ertel NH, et al. Obesity, androgens, and cancer risk. Cancer Res 1982;42(8 suppl):3281s–3285s.

49. Cauley JA, Gutai JP, Kuller LH, et al. The epidemiology of serum sex hormones in postmenopausal women. Am J Epidemiol 1989;129:1120–1131.

50. Bauer DC, Browner WS, Cauley JA, et al. Factors associated with appendicular bone mass in older women: The Study of Osteoporotic Fractures Research Group. Ann Intern Med 1993;118:657–665.

51. Cauley JA, Gutai JP, Kuller LH, Scott J, Nevitt MC. Black–white differences in serum sex hormones and bone mineral density. Am J Epidemiol 1994;139:1035–1046.

52. Grady D, Rubin SM, Petitti DB, et al. Hormone therapy to prevent disease and prolong life in postmenopausal women. Ann Intern Med 1992;117:1016–1037.

53. Cauley JA, Seeley DG, Ensrud K, et al. Estrogen replacement therapy and fractures in older women. Ann Intern Med 1995;122:9–16.

54. Hammond CB, Jelovsek FR, Lee KL, Creasman WT, Parker RT. Effects of long-term estrogen replacement therapy. Am J Obstet Gyncol 1979;122:525–536.

55. Lufkin EG, Wahner HW, O'Fallon WM, et al. Treatment of postmenopausal osteoporosis with transdermal oestrogen. Ann Intern Med 1992;117:1–9.

56. Kiel DP, Felson DT, Anderson JJ, Wilson PW, Moskowitz MA. Hip fracture and the use of estrogens in post-menopausal women. The Framingham Study. N Engl J Med 1987;317:1169–1174.

57. Paganini-Hill A, Ross RK, Gerkins VR, et al. Menopausal estrogen therapy and hip fractures. Ann Intern Med 1981;95:28–31.

58. Weiss NS, Ure Cl, Ballard JH, Williams AR, Daling JR. Decreased risk of frac-

ture of the hip and lower forearm with postmenopausal use of estrogen. N Engl J Med 1980;303:1195–1198.

59. Schneider DL, Barrett-Connor EL, Morton DJ. Timing of postmenopausal estrogen for optimal bone mineral density. The Rancho Bernardo Study. JAMA 1997;277: 543–547.

60. Naessen T, Persson I, Adama HO, Bergstrom R, Bergkvist L. Hormone replacement therapy and the risk for the first hip fracture. A prospective, population-based cohort study. Ann Intern Med 1990:113:95–103.

61. Gallagher JC, Kable WT, Goldgard D. Effect of progestin therapy on cortical and trabecular bone: comparison with estrogen. Am J Med 1991;90:171–178.

62. Riis BJ, Thomsen K, Strom V, Christiansen C. The effect of percutaneous estradiol and natural progesterone on postmenopausal bone loss. Am J Obstet Gynecol 1987;156:61–65.

63. Grey A, Cundy T, Evans M, Reid I. Medroxyprogesterone acetate enhances the spinal bone mineral density response to oestrogen in late post-menopausal women. Clin Endocrinol 1996;44:293–296.

64. Kanis JA. Medroxyprogesterone and bone mineral density response to oestrogen. Clin Endocrinol 1996;44:297–298.

65. The Writing Group for the PEPI Trial. Effects of hormone therapy on bone mineral density. JAMA 1996;276:1389–1396.

66. Ettinger B, Genant HK, Cann CE. Postmenopausal bone loss is prevented by treatment with low dosage estrogen with calcium. Ann Intern Med 1987;106:40–45.

67. Heaney RP, Recker RR, Stegman MR, Moy AJ. Calcium absorption in women: Relationships to calcium intake, estrogen status, and age. J Bone Miner Res 1989;4(4): 469–475.

68. Cauley JA, Cummings SR, Seeley DG, et al. Effects of thiazide diuretic therapy on bone mass, fractures, and falls. Ann Intern Med 1993;118:666–673.

69. Wasnich RD, Philip RD, Heilbrun LK, et al. Differential effects of thiazide and estrogen upon bone mineral content and fracture prevalence. Obstet Gynecol 1986;67: 457–462.

70. Armamento-Villareal R, Civitelli R. Estrogen action on the bone mass of postmenopausal women is dependent on body mass and initial bone density. J Clin Endocrinol Metab 1995;80:776–782.

71. Vaananen HK, Harkonen PL. Estrogen and bone metabolism. Maturitas 1996; 23:S65–S69.

72. Pacifici R. Estrogen, cytokines, and pathogenesis of postmenopausal osteoporosis. J Bone Miner Res 1996;11:1043–1051.

73. Cosman F, Shen V, Xie F, et al. Estrogen protection against bone resorbing effects of parathyroid hormone infusion: assessment by use of biochemical markers. Ann Intern Med 1993;118:337–343.

74. Cauley JA, Petrini AM, LaPorte RE, et al. The decline of grip strength in the menopause: Relationship to physical activity, estrogen use and anthropometric factors. J Chron Dis 1987;40:115–120.

75. Seeley DG, Cauley JA, Grady D, Browner WS, Nevitt MC, Cummings SR. Is postmenopausal estrogen therapy associated with neuromuscular function or falling in elderly women? Arch Intern Med 1995;155:293–299.

76. Brown M, Birge SJ, Kohrt WM. Hormone replacement therapy does not augment gains in muscle strength or fat-free mass in response to weight-bearing exercise. J Gerontol 1997;52a:B166–B170.

77. Cauley JA, Cummings SR, Black DM, Mascioli SR, Seeley DG. Prevalence and determinants of estrogen replacement therapy in elderly women. Am J Obstet 1990;163: 1438–1444.

78. Petitti DB. Coronary heart disease and estrogen replacement therapy: Can compliance bias explain the results of an observational study. Ann Epidemiol 1994;4: 115–118.

79. West S, Savitz D, Koch G, et al. Recall accuracy for prescription medication: Self-report compared with database information. Am J Epidemiol 1995;142:1103–1112.

9

EPIDEMIOLOGY OF BREAST CANCER

Lewis H. Kuller

Breast cancer is the second most common malignancy among women. There were an estimated 182,000 new cases and 46,000 deaths in 1994 in the United States. Breast cancer incidence rates increase with age; approximately three-fourths of breast cancer cases occur among women who are postmenopausal and over the age of 50.[1,2] From 1973 to 1991 the incidence of invasive breast cancer in the United States increased 25.8% in whites and 30.3% in blacks.[3] This increase proceeded slowly until the recent widespread introduction of mammography resulted in a steeper reported rate of increase, especially among postmenopausal women.

In women under age 45 there is a higher incidence of breast cancer in blacks; in women over age 45, incidence is higher in whites. Based on data from 1983 to 1990 in the United States, the 5-year relative survival rate of breast cancer was 81.6% for white women and 65.8% for black women in the United States.[3,4] For other ethnic and racial groups such as Asian Americans, Native Americans, and Mexican-American populations, breast cancer rates remain lower, although they are increasing.[4]

Incidence of and mortality due to breast cancer have generally been higher in upper socioeconomic groups.[5] The follow-up from the National Health and Nutrition Examination Survey I Epidemiologic Follow-up Study, 1971–1992, reported that women in the United States with greater than 16 years of education had a 2.3- (1.3–4.2) fold increased risk of breast cancer compared with women having less than 12 years of education. Level of income was also related to risk of breast cancer: women reporting family income greater than $50,000 had about a 1.7-fold increased risk compared with those with less than a $7,000 income, adjusted for age. The study related these differences to variations in the risk factors for breast cancer that are associated with education level, especially height, age at first pregnancy, age at menarche, and age at menopause.

Variations in the distribution of breast cancer among countries suggest that lifestyle is one determinant of breast cancer.[6] Japan, for example, which has had low death rates and incidence of breast cancer in the past, has experienced a gradual increase in breast cancer, but its rates remain much lower than those in the United States and many countries in Europe.[7] Women migrating to the United States from Japan and other low-incidence countries (China) have an increase in their rates of breast cancer mortality even within the first generation.[8] The increase is related in part to age at migration: the younger the age, the greater the risk.[8] There is a substantial increase in both body weight and height among Japanese migrants in the United States. Evidence suggests that increase in weight, perhaps secondary to changes in diet and exercise patterns, may be a major factor in the increase of breast cancer among Japanese migrants in the United States. The increase in body size, height, and weight of this population, over time or following migration, may contribute to early age at menarche and thus to increased risk of breast cancer.

The evidence suggests that prevention of breast cancer depends on the identification of the key mitogens (especially early in life), the determinants of the higher estrogen or hormone levels in the breast, and the identification of major genes (i.e., genetic polymorphisms) which are associated with susceptibility.[9] After discussing how cancers are classified, we will consider this model in detail.

CLASSIFICATION OF BREAST CANCER

Breast cancer is usually classified into two broad categories: invasive breast cancer and noninvasive cancer (or carcinoma in situ) where the disease is confined to the ducts or lobules without microscopic invasion into the surrounding breast stroma. The noninvasive types of breast cancer are further subdivided into ductal carcinoma in situ (DCIS), or intraductal carcinoma, and lobular carcinoma in situ (LCIS).[10] Each of these types of noninvasive breast cancer has specific clinical features. Lobular carcinoma in situ is often detected as an incidental finding at breast biopsy for a suspicious or benign "lump,"[11] thus its frequency depends on the prevalence of clinical examination and breast biopsies.[11] Some epidemiological studies exclude lobular carcinoma in situ from analysis to reduce potential ascertainment biases. The risk of developing invasive breast cancer is substantially increased among women who have lobular carcinoma in situ, probably a risk of about 1% per year, or about seven- to ten-fold above the average risk.[11]

Ductal carcinoma in situ is often diagnosed by mammography and may account for 50% of all of the breast cancers detected by mammography.[12] The reported frequency of ductal carcinoma in situ is a function of the prevalence of mammography in the community. The percentage of women in a community having mammograms is reflected in the estimated incidence of breast cancer and the characteristics of women at risk of breast cancer, especially ductal carcinoma in situ. For example, it has been suggested that women on hormone replacement therapy (HRT) may have more frequent mammographic evaluations and thus have a greater likelihood of the diagnosis of ductal carcinoma in situ. Therefore, it is very important to "adjust" for the prevalence of mammography and probably for the quality of the mammograms. Some, but not all, ductal carcinoma in situ may progress to invasive breast cancer. The histopathology of breast lesions can possibly be further utilized for etiological research. It has been suggested, for example, that estrogen stimulates the progression from ductal hyperplasia to ductal carcinoma in situ.[13-16]

Infiltrating ductal carcinoma is the most common invasive mammary tumor, accounting for about two-thirds of all invasive breast cancer. Infiltrating lobular carcinoma accounts for 5%–10% and other histopathologic types of breast cancer account for less than 1%. The epidemiology and natural history can differ by histopathological type of breast cancer.[14-16] The classification of breast cancer further includes size of the tumor, presence of cancer in regional lymph nodes, and distal metastasis. The number of positive axillary lymph nodes is directly related to survival. The presence or absence of estrogen and progesterone receptors has also been evaluated within epidemiological studies for their role in survival.

ETIOLOGY OF BREAST CANCER

The most plausible parsimonious model to explain the etiology of breast cancer is as follows.[17] First, mutagens, especially exposures fairly early in life or even in utero, are the primary cause of the initial neoplastic changes that occur within oncogenes or suppressor genes. Second, higher levels of estrogens—primarily estradiol or its metabolite—are a major stimulus for increased mitotic activity of the luminal mammary epithelial cells. This increased activity is determined directly through estrogen receptors and post-translational DNA synthesis or indirectly by the effects of estrogens on growth factors, both autocrine and paracrine, in the breast.[18] Recent studies also show that there may be different types of "estrogen receptors" with varying post-translational effects.[19] Third, the probability of developing breast cancer is related to host susceptibility, which in turn could be related to specific oncogenes, tumor suppressor genes, metastasis suppressor genes, DNA repair genes, or genes affecting carcinogen metabolism (i.e., cytochrome P-450, etc.)[9] or hormone metabolism. Major gene effects such as mutations *BRCA1* and *BRCA2* account for a very small percentage of all breast cancers.[20,21] It is very unlikely that a major gene will be found to account for most breast cancer cases. Rather, polymorphism (i.e., frequency >1%) in the population is associated with moderate increases in risk of breast cancer in relation to environmental mutagens.[9,22] Therefore, the basic approach to studying breast cancer etiology remains assessment of the interaction between host (genetic), agent (mutagens), and environment (hormone).

MUTAGENS

Initiation of Breast Tumors—Risk Factors

The chemicals associated with cancer—chemical carcinogens—are small lipophilic molecules that often undergo conversion to more electrophilic chemicals. The level of exposure to a chemical carcinogen, the site of exposure, and the rate of metabolism of the carcinogen have a direct effect on the potential for mutagenesis.[23] Metabolism of these environmental carcinogens probably plays an important role in protection against their deleterious effects.[24] Although animal studies have suggested that even a single dose of a chemical carcinogen may be sufficient to cause a cancer, it is likely that multiple exposures, the multi-hit theory of carcinogenesis, is necessary for the development of the cancer and subsequent metastasis.

Breast ductal epithelial cells are exposed to many environmental agents that may be potential carcinogens.[25] Current models of breast cancer assume that the earlier the age of mutagenic exposure, the greater the risk of breast cancer.[26] The time between menarche or even before menarche and first full-term pregnancy could be the most critical period for the initiation of changes in the DNA of the breast cells (i.e., mutation or activation of oncogenes or suppressor genes and the development of neoplasia).[18]

Critical support for these hypotheses comes from the following epidemiologic observations: *(1)* early age at first pregnancy reduces the risk of breast cancer among pre- and postmenopausal women[27] (i.e., this appears to have some lifetime effect); and *(2)* environmental exposures, such as radiation, increase the risk of breast cancer, primarily when exposure occurs at a younger age (usually before the age of 30).[28,29] In fact, at the present time, radiation exposure to the breast is the only identified major environmental risk factor for breast cancer. For instance, there is a linear relationship between exposure and the risk of breast cancer among survivors of the atomic bombing of Hiroshima.[29] The interrelationship between risk factors for breast cancer, such as age at first pregnancy and risk of breast cancer following radiation exposure,[28] produces varying rates of risk for breast cancer.

Environmental exposure, detoxification, and bioactivation play important roles in the development of cancer. Repair genes and suppressor genes affect the cycling of cells that serve to protect the organism from the adverse effects of environmental carcinogens.[30] A variety of metabolic enzymes also protect against environmental carcinogens. Genetic polymorphisms of metabolizing enzymes may be important in the metabolism of environmental carcinogens and increased risk of breast cancer.[31] Other chemicals (especially drugs) may also induce or activate these metabolizing genes, resulting in higher levels of the proteins important in carcinogenic metabolism.

Among the chemicals under investigation are polychlorinated pesticides such as DDT, which are considered xeno estrogens.[32,33] Xeno estrogens are chemicals that have estrogen-like activity and may bind to estrogen receptor(s). There is considerable interest in whether these xeno estrogens as well as potential carcinogenic metabolites[17,34–36] or variants of natural estrogens such as DES (diethylstibesterol) are human breast carcinogens.[37] Clusters of high rates of breast cancer in communities on Long Island in New York state and at Cape Cod, Massachusetts, have been attributed to prior exposure to pesticides in these areas. There is, however, little evidence of major geographic variation for breast cancer within the United States in general.[38,39] Current ongoing studies are evaluating the relationship between prior pesticide exposures and risk of breast cancer. The evidence to date strongly shows that levels in nonoccupationally exposed women are not related to risk of breast cancer.[33]

By using a technique pioneered by Petrakis et al., in San Francisco,[25,40] breast secretions (not breast milk) can be evaluated for potential carcinogens especially among premenopausal women.[41,42] Many potential carcinogens have been identified in breast secretions; however, there have been no studies to date linking any specific environmental carcinogens identified in breast secretions to higher rates of breast cancer.

In addition to environmental carcinogens, exposure to pharmacological agents can be identified in breast tissue. Although these might be mutagens, there are currently no consistent data to suggest that any specific class of drugs is associated with an increased risk of breast cancer, except hormonal exposures.[43,44] However, women who receive anti-neoplastic drug treatment in childhood and as young adults for diseases such as Hodgkin's[45] disease or leukemia, may be at risk due to early carcinogenic exposure. There is an increasing population of long-term survivors who have been exposed to potent carcinogenic drugs. More recently, the use of these drugs for the treatment of lupus and rheumatoid arthritis may provide an even larger population of women at potential risk of breast cancer.

Growth of Breast Cancer Cells—Estrogens and Mitogenesis

The growth of breast cancer cells is encouraged by a high-estrogen environment. Estrogen and progesterone receptors were identified in the 1960s.[46] The estrogen receptor content in both breast and metastatic lesions is related to the probability of survival and the responses to hormone therapy. Approximately 70%–80% of patients with breast cancer have estrogen-responsive tumors. Women with estrogen receptor–positive tumors are older and have slower growing tumors and a better prognosis. The estrogen receptors are part of the steroid hormone nuclear receptor superfamily that includes both steroids, thyroid, vitamin D, and vitamin A receptors. Epidemiological studies have recently focused on the interrelationship between vitamin D and vitamin A as they may relate to the etiology and treatment of breast cancer.[47,48] Genetic variations in the receptors have also been of great interest with regard to the etiology of steroid-related cancers.

Recently, it has become possible to evaluate the various autocrine and paracrine growth factors in the breast and their interrelationship with estrogens, other hormones, and risk factors. The epidermal growth factor receptor (EGF-R) is a member of the tyrosine kinase family of cell membrane receptors. Several growth factors (i.e., ligands) for the EGF-R have been identified, including epidermal growth factor (EGF) and transforming growth factor alpha (TGF-α), both of which have been found to increase the growth rate of normal and breast cancer cells. Estrogens increase the expression of the EGF-R.[49–51] The insulin-like growth factors (IGF) may also play an important role in the development of breast cancer.[52,53] IGF-I and -II are found much less frequently in breast cancer cells and cell cultures than TGF-α and EGF.[54] Fibroblast growth factors have also been identified in breast cancer cell lines.

Overall, an inflammatory response to breast carcinoma may result in greater cytokine activity and levels of growth factors. The potential role of growth factors as determinants (both genetic and environmental) in breast cancer may be important in understanding its etiology. The measurement of autocrine and paracrine effects of growth factors and inhibitors at the breast is extremely difficult, however, in epidemiological studies.

The increase in reported incidence of carcinoma in situ over time associated with greater use of mammography suggests that there is probably a very large number of women who have undetected small in situ carcinomas of breast cancer that have varying growth rates (latency periods) prior to clinical presentation.[12] Breast cancer is probably similar to prostate cancer in that a very high proportion of women have breast cancer but only a relatively small percentage develop clinical breast cancer and an even smaller percentage, advanced disease, as measured by the growth rate (i.e., mitotic activity of the breast cancer cells) and length of survival of the woman. The rate of growth of the breast cancer is primarily dependent on estrogens and other growth factors.[55–57]

Influence of Estrogen. The growth of breast neoplasms is faster in a high-estrogen environment, that is, faster among premenopausal women than post-menopausal women[27]; it is also faster during the early than the late postmenopausal period. This observation may account for the observed slowing of the rate of increased incidence of breast cancer among older women. The initial mutagenic effects may in part determine the growth rate of the neoplasm, given a specific exposure to estrogens and other growth factors. Thus the balance between a specific oncogene and suppressor genes may determine the susceptibility of the neoplastic cells to the effects of estrogens or other growth factors.[56] A second mutagenic event in breast epithelial cells results in greater mitotic activity, which may result in a more virulent phenotype and metastatic disease.[58]

There have been many epidemiologic studies of the relationship between endogenous sex steroid hormones and risk of breast cancer. Traditional studies measured markers of high estrogen exposure and risk of breast cancer. Early age at menarche and later age at menopause are associated with a longer exposure to high estrogen levels and increased risk of breast cancer.[59,60] Studies have documented that the earlier the age at artificial menopause, the lower the risk of breast cancer, and this protection continues to some degree into older ages.[60] Postmenopausal oophorectomy, which would have no effect on estrogen levels, is not associated with a reduction in risk of breast cancer.[60]

Some widely used hormone therapies affect the estrogen environment. Tamoxifen, an anti-estrogen (at least at the breast), reduces mortality and morbidity among women who have breast cancer. This effect may be either direct (by its effect on the estrogen receptor) or indirect (by modification of growth factors).[61] Oral contraceptives do not substantially change estrogen and progesterone levels as measured in comparison to those in women not on oral contraceptives. There has been some suggestion that oral contraceptive exposure prior to age at first pregnancy or early in life might be associated with an increased risk of breast cancer. However, most studies suggest that the increased risk, if present at all, is very modest.[62] Long-term use of estrogen replacement therapy among postmenopausal women has been associated with an increase in the risk of breast cancer.[43,44] Women who have been on estrogen therapy for longer periods of time at older ages appear to be at higher risk.[43]

Factors that modulate the hypothalamic–pituitary ovarian axis could either increase or decrease the risk of breast cancer by modifying the production and secretion of estrogens by the ovary. Very high levels of exercise affect hypothalamic pituitary function, resulting in amenorrhea and, probably, a reduction of breast cancer risk.[63,64] Moderate exercise levels may also affect the hypothalamic–pituitary axis. Several observational studies have suggested a reduced risk of breast cancer with moderate exercise, primarily in premenopausal women.[65–67]

Obesity is also associated with a reduced risk of premenopausal breast cancer[68] because it is related to lower levels of peak estrogen in premenopausal women from anovulatory menstrual cycling. Obesity produces a decrease in sex hormone–binding globulin (SHBG) and promotes more rapid clearing of estrogen from the blood.[69]

Estradiol, synthetic estrogen, is bound to SHBG. This binding, however, is much weaker than that for testosterone and, especially for dihydro-testosterone.[70] Estrone and progesterone are not bound to SHBG. The levels of SHBG are dramatically decreased by obesity, higher testosterone levels, and insulin levels, whereas they are increased by estradiol. The non-sex hormone–binding globulin, estradiol, is partially bound to albumin. More free estradiol is rapidly cleared from the circulation, possibly resulting in decreased estrogen exposure at the breast.[69]

Weight. Obesity is associated with irregular menstrual cycling in a linear dose–response pattern.[71,72] Irregular menstrual cycling in turn marks anovulation and reduced peak estradiol levels.[71] Irregular menses are also related to reduced breast cancer risk.[72] It is important to recognize that progesterone, as well as estrogen, stimulates mitotic activity of breast glandular tissue.[73] Lack of progesterone due to anovulation may therefore decrease rather than increase the risk of breast cancer (i.e., unopposed estrogens during the premenopausal years may not be a major risk factor for breast cancer).

African-American women, who have higher estrogen levels (both pre- and postmenopausal) than Caucasian women,[74] also have a higher occurrence of obesity, especially early-age obesity.[75] Premenopausal African-American women have higher breast cancer rates than Caucasian women, whereas the rates of breast cancer among postmenopausal African-American and Caucasian women are very similar.[3–5]

Very low body weight may also be associated with amenorrhea and premature menopause, reducing the risk of breast cancer. Thus in populations with very low caloric intake, infertility, anovulation, and premature menopause may be associated with lower risk of breast cancer.

Breast-Feeding. Finally, breast feeding after a pregnancy has been associated with a small decrease in the risk of premenopausal, but not consistently postmenopausal, breast cancer.[76] One likely explanation is that breast feeding is associated with a decrease in peak estrogen levels (i.e., anovulatory periods), resulting in a decrease in the risk of breast cancer. Changes in breast epithelial cells during breast feeding may also contribute to a decrease in the risk of breast cancer. It has been suggested that breast-feeding is associated with a reduction in breast exposure to environmental carcinogens (i.e., removed in the breast milk), accounting for a decrease in the risk of breast cancer. However, it is likely that this decrease in breast cancer risk would continue into the postmenopausal years if reduction in environmental exposures were the primary factor related to the decrease in the of breast cancer.

DETECTION OF CANCER BY MEASUREMENT OF HORMONES

Direct Measures

The determinants of high levels of estrogen or other hormones in the breast is the second element in the model we are considering. Their measurement in plasma, urine, or breast tissue is complex.[77] The evaluation of hormone levels among premenopausal women is difficult because of the substantial variation in hormone levels (estrogen, progesterone) during the menstrual cycles.[78,79] It has not been determined whether the peak level of estrogen or of estrone and progesterone, the average level over a cycle, or some integrated measure of level and duration of exposure is related to risk of breast cancer. The within-woman variability of hormone levels over time, especially early in the premenopause and in the perimenopause, further limits epidemiological studies. There is relatively little long-term data describing stability of hormone levels in women during their premenopausal years.

The determinants of risk of breast cancer among women during the first 5 years after menopause are also probably different from those among women 5+ years postmenopause. The development of breast cancer during the early menopausal years is likely a function of perimenopausal hormone levels, as well as early postmenopausal levels, whereas later postmenopausal breast cancer may be primarily related to postmenopausal hormone levels. Studies of endogenous hormones and breast cancer should focus on time since menopause in the analysis and probably not combine early and late menopausal breast cancer.

Estrogen levels in the breast measured in breast secretions have been shown to be substantially higher than those in plasma,[42] especially in premenopausal women. The differences in these levels have continued to limit the interpretation of epidemiological studies of estrogen levels in plasma since it is still unclear whether estrogen levels in the breast and in plasma are correlated. The levels of estrogen in the breast are determined by the levels of precursors, including androstenedione (an adrenal androgen in postmenopausal women) and estrone sulfate. The conversion of androstenedione to estrone in stromal fat cells, are estrone sulfatase to estrone by sulfatase activity and estrone to estradiol by hydroxylases may play a key role in etiology of breast cancer.[80] Moreover, it is possible that the local production of estrogen in breast tissue (especially after development of subclinical breast cancer) is the "cause" of higher blood levels of estradiol in older women with breast cancer is possible.[80]

In recent years it has become apparent that hormones can have an indirect effect on the growth of breast cancer cells by modifying various growth factors (both passive and active). These in turn can have effects on DNA and protein synthesis[9] similar to those of estradiol by aromatase. One prominent hypothesis is that increased aromatase activity in breast stromal fat tissue converts androstenedione to estrone, which is then converted into estradiol by 17-hydroxy-lase enzymes. The interaction of estradiol with the receptor can stimulate growth factors, which then results in an increase in aromatase activity and further production of estrogens (autocrine and paracrine effects). There is some evidence that estrogen production in the breast (in proximity to a breast tumor) is greater than in tissue at a distance from the breast cancer, which suggests a paracrine loop, and this results in an increase in the growth of breast cancer cells. Glucocorticoids and cytokines, being inflammatory response elements, may play an important role in increasing aromatase activity in breast stromal fat tissue.[80,81]

It is very difficult in epidemiological studies to measure local paracrine and autocrine growth factor levels. It has been possible in recent years to perform multiple needle biopsies in breast tissue in women at high risk of breast cancer to measure the amount of RNA, or mutations in DNA in either suppressor genes or oncogenes that may be related to various growth factors.[82]

An important methodologic caveat is timing the measurement of metabolic changes in relation to the development of breast cancer. The incubation period of breast cancer from the initial environmental exposure to breast cancer is fairly long. The changes in activity of metabolizing enzymes in breast tissue at the time of the diagnosis of breast cancer may be relevant to the etiology of breast cancer or, alternatively, may be secondary to the initial development of breast cancer. A breast cancer could be considered a "foreign body" or an altered cell in the breast. The secondary "inflammatory response" by stromal cells may therefore be a response to aberrant cells, not the cause of the breast cancer.

Since postmenopausal breast cancer develops in a much lower estrogen environment than premenopausal breast cancer, the risk factors related to breast cancer during the early postmenopausal years are probably a function of the pre-, peri-, and postmenopausal hormonal environment. Some studies report that late age at menopause is a risk factor for postmenopausal breast cancer.[59] The later the age of menopause, the greater the continued exposure to higher levels of estrogens and progestins during the perimenopausal period. It is important to recognize, however, that defining the menopause as a time of cessation of menses is not accurate, especially with regard to hormonal levels. There are substantial variations in hormone levels during the long perimenopausal period prior to the cessation of menses.[83] The frequency of irregular cycling and changes in hormone levels during the perimenopausal period may play an important role in the development of breast cancer during the early postmenopausal years. Thus it may be important to focus on the changes in menstrual cycling patterns and hormone levels during the peri- to postmenopause.

Variations Related to Weight

As women age a higher percentage of their total body composition becomes fat. At this time there is also an increase in body weight and perhaps an increase in intra-abdominal fat.[84,85] Premenopausal obesity is associated with a higher frequency of anovulatory or irregular menstrual cycling and a lower estrogen environment, whereas postmenopausal obesity is associated with more estrogens and a greater risk of breast cancer. Women who may be at highest risk of breast cancer are those who gain weight (i.e., become overweight or obese postmenopausal) from the peri- to the postmenopausal years.[68] Obese women have substantially higher postmenopausal estradiol and estrone levels due to greater aromatization in stromal fat cells of androstenedione to estrone.[86–88] Aromatase activity also increases with age.[69,89] Obese postmenopausal women tend to have higher estrone and estradiol levels, lower sex hormone–binding globulin, and therefore higher levels of free or non-sex hormone–binding estradiol levels. The contribution of increasing percentage of body fat to the development of postmenopausal breast cancer, as well as the distribution of body fat, needs further investigation.[90]

Weight gain among postmenopausal women may result in a greater accumulation of intra-abdominal fat than subcutaneous or thigh fat. Aromatase activity is greater in thigh fat,[91] however, the increase in intra-abdominal fat may be associated with increased insulin levels[92] as well as free fatty acid flux to the liver and an associated decrease in sex hormone–binding globulin.[69] Increased insulin levels or activity may be a risk factor for breast cancer, especially among older women.[17] Insulin could increase the levels of growth factors in the breast, possibly through insulin-like growth factor receptors.[80] The relation among insulin levels, insulin resistance, and breast cancer has not been evaluated in epidemiologic studies. Newer methods of measuring intra-abdominal fat, such as computerized tomography and magnetic resonance imaging (MRI), as well as of total body fat and fat distribution using dual energy X-ray absorptiometry (DEXA), may provide better methods of measuring the relationship between the distribution of body fat, total body fat, obesity, and subsequent risks of breast cancer.

Higher body mass index also has an adverse effect on the life expectancy of women with breast cancer.[93] This effect is usually greater in postmenopausal women and may be related to greater production of estrogen in the breast tissue of fatter women and stimulation of the growth of breast cancer cells.

Several major longitudinal studies have documented that higher postmenopausal blood levels of estradiol, total and nonprotein-bound testosterone, and free testosterone levels are risk factors for postmenopausal breast cancer.[94–96] The association tends to be linear and independent of other risk factors.

The possible sources of higher estrogen and testosterone at the breast—such as adrenal androgens and stromal fat (i.e., aromatization of androstenedione), ovarian production of androgens, and production directly in breast tissue—need to be considered.

Increased levels of adrenal androgen (i.e., androstenedione, DHEA, DHEAS, and metabolites) as a probable risk factor for postmenopausal breast cancer is the focus of recent epidemiological studies.[97,98] Although the variables that determine production of androstenedione in the adrenal gland in postmenopausal women have not been determined,[99] there is considerable controversy about the role of adrenal cortical tropic hormone (ACTH).[100] There does not appear to be any relationship between obesity and the production of androstenedione by the adrenal gland, but increased alcohol intake may stimulate adrenal androgen production and psychosocial "stress" may be a risk factor for higher androstenedione levels. The production of androstenedione by the adrenal gland decreases from pre- to postmenopause and during the postmenopause, in part because of the reduction in production of androstenedione from the ovary the adrenal gland.[101] This has sometimes been referred to as the adrenopause. Whether the determinants of change in adrenal androgen production in postmenopausal women are important risk factors for breast cancer has not been determined. Postmenopausal women with lower androstenedione production would be at lower risk of breast cancer because of lower estradiol levels.

Also being studied is the possibility that the ovaries of some postmenopausal women continue to produce large amounts of testosterone.[89] The increased testosterone could be converted to estradiol or be directly related to risk of breast cancer (through increased mitotic activity). Removal of postmenopausal ovaries apparently does not reduce the risks of breast cancer but does decrease testosterone levels. However, the reason for removal of the ovaries may confound or bias these analyses.

Indirect Measures

Higher estrogen exposure is associated with higher bone mineral density in both pre- and postmenopausal women.[102] Other factors can determine bone mineral density, but sex steroid hormones, estrogens in particular, are a primary determinant. Women who have an oophorectomy (artificial menopause) and thus a drop in estrogen level have lower bone mineral density. Women have a substantial reduction in trabecular bone density, especially in the spine, peri- to postmenopause. Estrogen therapy, however, can prevent bone loss. Bone mineral density can therefore be considered a surrogate for long-term estrogen levels. Recent studies have documented that higher bone mineral density is associated with an increased risk of breast cancer.[103,104] Several studies have also documented that women with fractures (i.e., probably related to lower bone mineral density) have a lower risk of breast cancer.[103]

Breast density is also related to higher estrogen exposure.[105] Thus premenopausal women tend to have higher breast density than postmenopausal women, and women on hormone replacement therapy have higher breast density than those not on HRT. Oophorectomy is also associated with a reduction in breast density. There is strong evidence that greater breast density may be a risk factor for both pre- and postmenopausal breast cancer.[106–108]

The density of the breast tissue on a mammogram may be a marker for local estrogen synthesis. Since stroma fat cells are the major source of aromatase activity, production of estrogens from androstenedione, the distribution of fat cells, and breast density within the breast could be important determinants of the risk of breast cancer. Women with dense breasts, especially premenopausal women, have a substantially increased risk of clinical breast cancer, which appears to be independent of the greater difficulty of diagnosing breast cancer by mammography among women with dense breasts.

Hormone replacement therapy is clearly associated with an increase in both bone and breast density whereas, as noted, oophorectomy and postmenopause result in decreased breast and bone density. Breast density may serve as a surrogate marker for local estrogen activity at the breast while bone mineral density probably serves as a surrogate marker for total production of estrogens. Estrogen, however, may affect similar growth factors in both breast and bone, so measurement of breast and bone density may also provide some estimate of estrogen effect at the breast.

The metabolites of estrogen, usually measured in the urine, may be more specific risk factors for breast cancer. The absolute levels of these metabolites as determined by their ratio to estrogen have been studied. The 16-αhydroxy and the 4-hydroxy estrone metabolites have been linked to greater estrogenic activity and possibly to a higher risk of breast cancer than the 2-hydroxy metabolites in the urine.[109] Most studies to date that have linked estrogen metabolites to risk of breast cancer have been either small longitudinal studies with short-term follow-up or more frequently case–control studies.[110] The estrogen metabolites are probably determined by both genetic (i.e., metabolism in p-450 enzymes) and environmental factors (such as obesity, physical activity, and specific dietary factors).

Diet and Breast Cancer

The marked geographic variation in breast cancer mortality among countries suggests that variations in dietary intake probably play an important role in the etiology of postmenopausal and most likely, premenopausal breast cancer. The question whether higher dietary fat or total caloric intake is associated with an increased risk of breast cancer has been the most widely studied diet issue.[117–120]

The international variations in breast cancer rates in relation to population dietary fat intake are not necessarily linear and suggest that dietary fat intake may have to be reduced to 20%–25% of total fat to see any substantial impact on breast cancer rates. Furthermore, many of the longitudinal and case–control observational studies of dietary fat and breast cancer have failed to demonstrate a strong association between reported dietary fat intake and subsequent risk of breast cancer.[121,122] There are two basic problems with these studies. The first is our inability to accurately measure fat intake in relatively homogeneous populations.[117,123–125] The second is that the percentage of women in the United States consuming relatively low fat diets (i.e., 25% or so of calories from fat) is small. Most women may have a dietary fat consumption above the threshold for substantially reducing risk of breast cancer.

Studies conducted under controlled dietary conditions (i.e., in metabolic units) have found that a lower fat intake, which is usually associated with a higher fiber intake, results in reductions in estrone, estradiol, and testosterone.[126,127] Diets higher in total fat may also be associated with greater risks of obesity, higher estrogen levels, and risk of breast cancer in postmenopausal women. Hyperinsulinemia secondary to obesity or high-fat diet may also act synergistically with estrogens to increase the amount of breast glandular epithelial cells, mitotic activity, and growth of breast cancer cells.[125,128]

Estrogens are excreted in the urine and bile with some reabsorption in the small intestine, or they are excreted in the feces. High-fiber diets may increase estrogen excretion in the feces and could therefore lower blood estrogen levels. Experimental evidence supports the association of high-fiber diets with a decrease in blood estrogen levels. Thus, some populations with high fiber intake may have lower risks of breast cancer, secondary to greater excretion of estrogens in the feces.[129,130]

Many vegetables (and other plants) contain isoflavines and lignins, which may be converted in the bowel into weak estrogens that would then compete with estradiol for target binding sites. Lignins and isoflavinoids may stimulate the production of sex hormone–binding globulin and could be important[131,132] physiological regulators of SHBG. Lignins and isoflavinoids are diphenolic compounds and are found in high concentrations in soy.[133] The current dietary levels, as measured by concentrations in the urine, are fairly high in humans. Intake of isoflavinoids is higher among vegetarians and individuals who consume large amounts of whole grain products. The excretion of isoflavinoids is also higher in Japan because of higher intake of soy products. But vegetarians, who consumed the highest amounts of fiber and thus of lignins and isoflavinoids, are at only slightly lower risk of breast cancer than those who are not vegetarians.[134] Breast cancer rates are very low in Asian populations that have relatively low soy intake.[134]

Oxidative damage due to normal metabolism, especially of dietary fruits and vegetables or by chemicals, may be a major cause of mutagenesis and risk of breast cancer. There are numerous antioxidant defenses.[135] Several of the vitamins, especially vitamins E, C, and A, as well as substances such as selenium, are also important antioxidants.[136,137] There is little evidence that the average intake of vitamins from dietary sources is related to the risk of breast cancer. Pharmacological doses of vitamins, especially vitamin E and possibly vitamin D, could be associated with a decrease in the risk of breast cancer.[138] High levels of vitamin D may prevent mutagenic changes in breast cancer neoplastic cells as well as in other cancer cells (i.e., in the prostate) and therefore could be associated with a reduced risk of breast cancer. Trials evaluating the relation of vitamins A, E and D to risk of breast cancer are under way.

Several ongoing clinical trials are evaluating the effects of reduced fat intake on both primary and secondary prevention of breast cancer morbidity and mortality. Additional studies are assessing the effect of phytoestrogens on sex steroid hormone metabolism, on changes in menstrual cycling among premenopausal women, and on hormone levels in postmenopausal women. The impact of increased exercise on hormone metabolism, breast and bone density, and possible risk of breast cancer is also being studied. Finally, estrogen receptor mediators, such as tamoxifen and raloxifene, are being tested in clinical trials of high-risk women to determine their possible contribution to primary prevention of breast cancer by reducing the effects of estrogens on breast glandular epithelial cells. The activity of these drugs may be independent of their competitive binding to the estrogen receptor.

HOST SUSCEPTIBILITY

Genetic Determinants

The familial aggregation of breast cancer can be due to shared environmental exposures or lifestyles and/or genetic attributes. The genotypic determinants of breast cancer must be separated from somatic mutations that are part of the developmental pathology from normal cellular composition to neoplasia to metastasis.[111] Many epidemiological studies have documented at least a two-fold increased risk of breast cancer among first degree relatives of index breast cancer cases.[111] The risk is greater if the index case was diagnosed in the affected, premenopausal period, if there are multiple first degree relatives (i.e., sister and mother), and if the index case has bilateral breast cancer. Probably 10%–15%

of all breast cancer cases have a first degree relative with a history of breast cancer.[112]

The risk of breast cancer is increased in identical twins but the degree of concordance is relatively low. In a recent detailed study of 570 twin pairs in an older cohort from Sweden born between 1886 and 1925, 35 twin pairs were concordant, including 17 of 197 monozygotic and 18 of 372 dizygotic twin pairs. In the younger cohort born between 1926 and 1958, there were 222 twin pairs; 5 of 81 monozygotic and 5 of 141 dizygotic pairs were concordant. The risk of breast cancer increased among both the sisters of index dizygotic and of monozygotic breast cancer cases.[113]

The genetic determinants of breast cancer could be due either to major genotypes of relatively low prevalence (i.e., *BRCA1* and *BRCA2*) but associated with a very high risk of breast cancer, or to genetic polymorphisms with a frequency of >1% in the population but with only a moderate increased risk of breast cancer. There are also families in which different types of cancer (ovary, colon, prostate) are inherited together within the same family.[114,115] Development of new genetic molecular approaches have made it possible to study the specific genotypic abnormalities rather than to focus, as in the past, primarily on phenotype (i.e., breast cancer cases in a family). The breast cancer–associated gene I (*BRCA1* on chromosome 17_Q 21) is associated with a marked increased risk of both breast and ovarian cancer.[115]

An inherited copy of a mutant allele causes the familial predisposition to cancer, with somatic mutation of the other paired allele occurring later in life and resulting in subsequent development of malignancy. It is possible that in certain cases, sporadic mutations in both the *BRCA1* genes are associated with cancer. *BRCA1* could account for up to 45% of very early-onset familial breast cancer (i.e., less than 35 years of age) and perhaps 80% of very early familial breast cancer in which there was a history of both breast and ovarian cancer.[111] Women who have *BRCA1* mutations have a cumulative risk increasing from about 3% by age 30 to about 50% by age 50 for breast cancer and from about 25% at age 50 to almost 65% by age 70 for ovarian cancer. *BRCA2* has been identified and is also associated with a high risk of breast cancer but not ovarian cancer. It is also associated with an increased risk of breast cancer in both men and women.[116]

Genetic polymorphisms, the genes that affect enzymes involved in sex steroid hormone metabolism, hormone receptors, and post-translational effects, could also be associated with an increased risk of breast cancer.[9] Similarly, as noted, genes that affect the metabolism of potential environmental carcinogens (both type 1 and type 2 enzymes) may also contribute to the risk of breast cancer. It is very likely that these genetic polymorphisms are only associated with a modest increased risk of breast cancer and are important in association with specific environmental exposures.

CONCLUSION

The epidemiology of breast cancer fits a coherent model of host, agent, and environment. Host susceptibility can be attributed to major genetic influences (i.e., *BRCA1* and *BRCA2*) or to polymorphisms related to hormone metabolism, environmental mutagens, metabolizing effects, and breast glandular and stromal tissue sensitivity (e.g., suppressor and oncogenes). Host susceptibility is also related to lifestyle factors that determine the sensitivity of breast tissue to environmental carcinogens (or agents). Age at first pregnancy and number and spacing of pregnancies are probably important determinants of susceptibility. Most of the agents that cause breast cancer—the mutagens—have not been identified. Radiation is the only consistently identified environmental agent. Cigarette smoking may be a risk factor in a subset of susceptible women, given the metabolism of carcinogens in cigarette smoke.

The future search for "agents" (or mutagens) causing breast cancer should probably focus on exposure to mutagens at younger ages. Newer approaches such as measurement of breast secretions[40] and early changes in breast tissue (i.e., atypical hyperplasia, oncogenes, suppressor genes and growth factor changes) also need to be developed. The most important variable in the development of breast cancer is probably the hormonal environment during the pre- and postmenopause. Most risk factors, such as demographics (age at menarche and menopause), nutrition (obesity, weight gain), alcohol, and exercise, affect the hormone environment. The effects of hormone therapies on breat cancer risk are also part of the increased environmental exposure hypothesis.

The next major step in understanding how the hormone environment affects breast cancer is to understand the determinants of higher or lower sex steroid hormone levels during the pre- to postmenopause as well as variations in metabolism of the hormones. Many future studies may depend on both short-term clinical laboratory studies and clinical trials in which the key environmental determinants of hormone levels (diet, obesity, etc.) can be modified. These studies may also require a better definition of the genetic, or host, susceptibility.

The interrelationship among hormone environment and local breast tissue responses, growth factors, and immune responses must also be considered in future epidemiological studies of breast cancer. Given the complexities of the interrelationship among host, agent, and environmental determinants of breast cancer, experimental clinical trials that test the efficacy of specific interventions without defining each piece of the pathophysiology of breast cancer may lead to a reduction in breast cancer morbidity and mortality.

REFERENCES

1. Feuer EJ, Wun LM, Boring CC, Flanders WD, Timmel MJ, Tong. The lifetime risk of developing breast cancer. J Natl Cancer Inst 1993;85:892–897.

2. Campbell MK, Feuer EJ, Wun LM. Cohort-specific risks of developing breast cancer to age 85 in Connecticut. Epidemiology 1994;5:290–296.

3. Chu KC, Tarone RE, Kessler LG, Ries LAG, Hankey BF, Miller BA, Edwards BK. Recent trends in the U.S. breast cancer incidence, survival, and mortality rates. J Natl Cancer Inst 1996;88:1571–1579.

4. Hankey BF. Breast. In: Miller BA, Ries LAG, Hankey BF, et al., eds. Cancer Statistics Review: 1973–1989. Bethesda, MD: National Cancer Institute, 1992 (NIH publication no. 92–2789).

5. Heck KE, Pamuk ER. Explaining the relation between education and post-menopausal breast cancer. Am J Epidemiol 1997;145:366–372.

6. Levi F. Breast cancer mortality in Europe. J Natl Cancer Inst 1996;88:21.

7. Hoel DG, Davis DL, Miller AB, Sondik EJ, Swerdlow AJ. Trends in cancer mortality in 15 industrialized countries, 1969–1986. J Natl Cancer Inst 1992;84: 313–320.

8. Ziegler RG, Hoover RN, Pike MC, et al. Migration patterns and breast cancer risk in Asian-American women. J Natl Cancer Inst 1993;85:1819–1827.

9. Feigelson HS, Ross RK, Yu MC, Coetzee GA, Reichardt JKV, Henderson BE. Genetic susceptibility to cancer from exogenous and endogenous exposures. J Cell Biochem 1996;25S:15–22.

10. Wazer DE, Gage I, Homer MJ, Krosnick SH, Schmid C. Age-related differences in patients with nonpalpable breast carcinomas. Cancer 1996;781:1432–1437.

11. Bodian CA, Perzin KH, Lattes R. Lobular neoplasia. Long term risk of breast cancer and relation to other factors. Cancer 1996;78:1024–1034.

12. Ernster VL, Barclay J, Kerlikowske K, Grady D, Henderson C. Incidence of and treatment for ductal carcinoma in situ of the breast. JAMA 1996;275:913–918.

13. Longnecker MP, Bernstein L, Paganini-Hill A, Enger SM, Ross RK. Risk factors for in situ breast cancer. Cancer Epidemiol Biomarkers Prev 1996;5:961–965.

14. Page DL, Jensen RA. [Editorial] Ductal carcinoma in situ of the breast: Understanding the misunderstood stepchild. JAMA 1996;275:948–949.

15. Page DL, Dupont WD. Indicators of increased breast cancer risk in humans. J Cell Biochem 1992;16G:175–182.

16. Hayes DF. Ductal carcinoma in situ of the breast: A new model. J Natl Cancer Inst 1997;89:991–993.

17. Kuller LH. The etiology of breast cancer—from epidemiology to prevention. Public Health Rev 1995;23:157–213.

18. Pike MC, Spicer DV, Dalmoush L, Press MF. Estrogens, progesterones, normal breast cell proliferation, and breast cancer risk. Epidemiol Rev 1993;15:17–35.

19. Gustafsson JA. Estrogen receptor β—getting in on the action? Nature Med 1997;3:493–494.

20. Struewing JP, Hartge P, Wacholder S, et al. The risk of cancer associated with specific mutations of BRCA1 and BRCA2 among Ashkenazi Jews. N Engl J Med 1997; 336:1401–1408.

21. Krainer M, Silva-Arrieta S, FitzGerald MG, et al. Differential contributions of BRCA1 and BRCA2 to early-onset breast cancer. N Engl J Med 1997;336: 1416–1421.

22. Kastan M. Clinical implications of basic research. Ataxia-telangiectasia—broad implications for a rare disorder. N Engl J Med 1995;333:662–663.

23. Smith CAD, Smith G, Wolf CR. Genetic polymorphisms in xenobiotic metabolism. Eur J Cancer 1994;30A:1921–1935.

24. Ambrosone CB, Freudenheim JL, Graham S, et al. Cytochrome P4501A1 and glutathione S-transferase (M1) genetic polymorphisms and postmenopausal breast cancer risk. Cancer Res 1995;55:3483–3485.

25. Petrakis NL. Epidemiologic studies of mutagenicity of breast fluids—relevance to breast cancer risk. In: Pike MC, Sisiteri PK, Welsch CW, eds. Banbury Report 8: Hormones and Breast Cancer. Cold Spring Harbor, NY: Cold Spring Harbor Laboratory, 1981, pp. 243–255.

26. Krieger N. Exposure, susceptibility, and breast cancer risk: A hypothesis regarding exogenous carcinogens, breast tissue development, and social gradients, including black/white differences, in breast cancer incidence. Breast Cancer Res Treat 1989; 13:205–223.

27. Pathak DR, Whittemore AS. Combined effects of body size, parity, and menstrual events on breast cancer incidence in seven countries. Am J Epidemiol 1992;135: 153–168.

28. Land CE, Hayakawa N, Machado SG, et al. A case–control interview study of breast cancer among Japanese A-bomb survivors. II. Interactions with radiation dose. Cancer Causes Control 1994;5:167–176.

29. Tokunaga M, Land CE, Yamamoto T, et al. Incidence of female breast cancer among atomic bomb survivors, Hiroshima and Nagasaki, 1950–1980. Radiat Res 1987; 112:243–272.

30. Whitlock JP, Okino ST, Dong L, Ko HP, Clarke-Katzenberg R, Ma Q, Li H. Induction of cytochrome P4501A1: A model of analyzing mammalian gene transcription. FASEB J 1996;10:809–818.

31. Rebbeck TR, Rosvold EA, Duggan DJ, Zhang J, Buetow KH. Genetics of *CYP1A1*: Coamplification of specific alleles by polymerase chain reaction and association with breast cancer. Cancer Epidemiol Biomarkers Prev 1994;3:511–514.

32. Davis DL, Telang NT, Osborne MP, Bradlow HL. Medical hypothesis: Bifunctional genetic–hormonal pathways to breast cancer. Environ Health Perspect 1997;105: 571–576.

33. Hunter DJ, Hankinson SE, Laden F, et al. Plasma organochlorine levels and the risk of breast cancer. New Engl J Med 1997;337:1253–1258.

34. Stone R. Environmental estrogens stir debate. Science 1994;265:308–310.

35. Wolff MS, Toniolo PG, Lee EW, Rivera M, Dubin N. Blood levels of organochlorine residues and risk of breast cancer. J Natl Cancer Inst 1993;85:648–652.

36. Krieger N, Wolff MS, Hiatt RA, et al. Breast cancer and serum organochlorines: A prospective study among White, Black, and Asian women. J Natl Cancer Inst 1994;86:589–599.

37. Colton T, Greenberg R, Noller K, et al. Breast cancer in mothers prescribed diethylstilbestrol in pregnancy. Further follow-up. JAMA 1993;269:2096–2100.

38. Laden F, Spiegelman D, Neas LM, et al. Geographic variation in breast cancer incidence rates in a cohort of U.S. women. J Natl Cancer Inst 1997;89:1373–1378.

39. Kulldorff M, Feuer EJ, Miller BA, Freedman LS. Breast cancer clusters in the Northeast United States: A geographic analysis. Am J Epidemiol 19997;146:161–170.

40. Petrakis NL, Gruenke LD, Craig JC. Cholesterol and cholesterol epoxides in nipple aspirates of human breast fluid. Cancer Res 1981;41:2563–2565.

41. Petrakis NL, Gruenke LD, Beelen TC, et al. Nicotine in breast fluid of nonlactating women. Science 1978;199:303–304.

42. Petrakis NL. Nipple aspirate fluid in epidemiologic studies of breast disease. Epidemiol Rev 1993;15:188–195.

43. Collaborative Group on Hormonal Factors in Breast Cancer. Breast cancer and hormone replacement therapy: Collaborative reanalysis of data from 51 epidemiological studies of 52,705 women with breast cancer and 108,411 women without breast cancer. Lancet 1997;350:1047–1059.

44. Colditz GA, Hankinson SE, Hunter DJ, et al. The use of estrogens and progestins and the risk of breast cancer in postmenopausal women. N Engl J Med 1995;332: 1589–1593.

45. Bhatia S, Robison LL, Oberlin O, et al. Breast cancer and other second neoplasms after childhood Hodgkin's disease. N Engl J Med 1996;334;745–751.

46. Jensen EV. History of the estrogen receptor concept and its relation to antiestrogens. In: Lindsay R, Dempster DW, Jordon VC, eds. Estrogens and Antiestrogens. Philadelphia: Lippincott-Raven, 1997; pp. 3–28.

47. Eisman JA, Frampton RJ, Sher E, Suva LJ, Martin TJ. Presence and role of 1, 25-dihydroxyvitamin D receptors in human cancer cells. In: Meyskens FL, Prasad KN, eds. Modulation and Mediation of Cancer by Vitamins. Basel: Karger, 1983, pp. 282–286.

48. Daxenbichler G, Widschwendter M, Marth C. Sensitivity of breast and ovarian cancer cells for interferons (IFNs) and retinoids. In: Castagnetta L, Nenci I, Bradlow HL, eds. Basis for Cancer Management. Ann NY Acad Sci 1996;784:294–303.

49. Clarke R, Dickson RB, Lippman ME. Hormonal aspects of breast cancer. Growth factors, drugs and stromal interactions. Crit Rev Oncol/Hematol 1992;12:1–23.

50. Lippman ME. Growth factors, receptors, and breast cancer. J NIH Res 1991;3: 59–62.

51. Wilding G, Lippman ME, Dickson RB. The cellular response of human breast cancer to estrogen. In: Hankins WD, Puett D, eds. Hormones, Cell Biology, and Cancer: Perspectives and Potentials. New York: Alan R. Liss 1988, pp. 181–196.

52. LeRoith D, Adamo M, Werner H, Roberts CT Jr. Insulin-like growth factors and their receptors as growth regulators in normal physiology and pathological states. Trends Endocrinol Metab 1991;2:134.

53. Russo IH, Calaf G, Russo J. Hormones and proliferative activity in breast tissue. In: Stoll BA, ed. Approaches to Breast Cancer Prevention. Dordrecht, Netherlands: Kluwer Academic Publishers, 1991, pp. 35–51.

54. Raiol MJ, Smitten KV, Pekonen F. The prognostic value of insulin-like growth factor-I in breast cancer patients. Results of a follow-up study on 126 patients. Eur J Cancer 1994;30A:307–311.

55. Spicer DV, Pike MC. Sex steroids and breast cancer prevention. Monogr Natl Cancer Inst 1994;16:139–147.

56. Anderson TJ. Effects on breast tissue of exogenous oestrogens and proestrogens. Acta Obstet Gynecol Scand 1986;134(S):9–13.

57. Lippman ME, Huff KK, Jakesz R, et al. Estrogens regulate production of specific growth factors in hormone-dependent human breast cancer. In: Angeli A, Bradlow HL, Dogliotti L, eds. Endocrinology of the Breast: Basic and Clinical Aspects. Ann NY Acad Sci 1986;464:11–16.

58. Brugarolas J, Jacks T. Double indemnity: p53: p53, BRCA and cancer. Nature Med 1997;3:721–722.

59. Kelsey JL, Whittemore AS. Epidemiology and primary prevention of cancers of the breast, endometrium, and ovary. A brief overview. Ann Epidemiol 1994;4:89–95.

60. Brinton LA, Schairer C, Hoover RN, Fraumeni JF Jr. Menstrual factors and risk of breast cancer. Cancer Invest 1988;6:245–254.

61. Jordan VC, Piette M, Cisneros A. Metabolism of antiestrogens. In: Lindsay R,

Dempster DW, Jordon VC, eds. Estrogens and Antiestrogens. Philadelphia: Lippincott-Raven, 1997, pp. 29–41.

62. Committee on the Relationship Between Oral Contraceptives and Breast Cancer. Oral Contraceptives and Breast Cancer. Institute of Medicine, Division of Health Promotion and Disease Prevention. Washington, DC: National Academy Press, 1991.

63. Frisch RE. Body fat, menarche, fitness and fertility. In: Frisch RE, ed. Adipose Tissue and Reproduction. Prog Reprod Med 1990;14:1–26.

64. Baird DT. Amenorrhoea. Lancet 1997;350:275–279.

65. Bernstein L, Henderson BE, Hanisch R, Sullivan-Halley J, Ross RK. Physical exercise and reduced risk of breast cancer in young women. J Natl Cancer Inst 1994;86:1403–1408.

66. Dorgan JF, Brown C, Barrett M, et al. Physical activity and risk of breast cancer in the Framingham Heart Study. Am J Epidemiol 1994;139:662–669.

67. Bernstein L, Ross RK, Lobo RA. The effects of moderate physical activity on menstrual cycle patterns in adolescence: Implications for breast cancer prevention. Br J Cancer 1987;55:681–685.

68. Huang Z, Hankinson SE, Colditz GA, et al. Dual effects of weight and weight gain on breast cancer risk. JAMA 1997;278:1407–1411.

69. Azziz R. Reproductive endocrinologic alterations in female asymptomatic obesity. Fertil Steril 1989;52:703–725.

70. Ekin R. The free hormone concept. In: Hennemann G, ed. Thyroid Hormone Metabolism. New York: Marcel Dekker, 1986:77–106.

71. Hartz AJ, Rupley DC, Rimm AA. The association of girth measurements with disease in 32,856 women. Am J Epidemiol 1984;119:71–80.

72. LaVecchia C, Decarli A, DePietro S, Franceschi S, Parazzini F. Menstrual cycle patterns and the risk of breast disease. Eur J Cancer Clin Oncol 1985;21:417–422.

73. Going JJ, Anderson TJ, Battersby S, Macintyre CCA. Proliferative and secretory activity in human breast during natural and artificial menstrual cycles. Am J Pathol 1988;130:193–204.

74. Cauley JA, Gutai JP, Kuller LH, Scott J, Nevitt MC. Black–white differences in serum sex hormones and bone mineral density. Am J Epidemiol 1994;139:1035–1046.

75. Public Health Service Centers for Disease Control and Prevention, National Center for Health Statistics, Division of Health Examination Statistics, National Health and Nutrition Examination Survey II, 1976–80, and Hispanic Health and Nutrition Examination Survey, 1982–84. Washington DC: NCHS.

76. Newcomb PA, Storer BE, Longnecker MP, et al. Lactation and a reduced risk of premenopausal breast cancer. N Engl J Med 1994;330:81–87.

77. Hankinson SE, Manson JE, London SJ, Willett WC, Speizer FE. Laboratory reproducibility of endogenous hormone levels in postmenopausal women. Cancer Epidemiol Biomarkers Prev 1994;3:51–56.

78. Gail MH, Fears TR, Hoover RN, et al. Reproducibility studies and interlaboratory concordance for assays of serum hormone levels: Estrone, estradiol, estrone sulfate, and progesterone. Cancer Epidemiol Biomarkers Prev 1996;5:835–844.

79. Toniolo P, Koenig KL, Pasternack BS. Reliability of measurements of total, protein-bound, and unbound estradiol in serum. Cancer Epidemiol Biomarkers 1994; 3:47–50.

80. Reed MJ, Purohit A. Breast cancer and the role of cytokines in regulating estrogen synthesis: An emerging hypothesis. Endocrine Rev 1997;18:701–715.

81. Nandi S, Guzman RC, Yang J. Hormones and mammary carcinogenesis in mice, rats, and humans: A unifying hypothesis. Proc Natl Acad Sci USA 1995;92: 3650–3657.

82. Fabian CJ, Zalles C, Kamel S , McKittrick R, Moore WP, Zeiger S, Simon C, Kimler B, Cramer A, Garcia F, Jewell W. Biomarker and cytologic abnormalities in women at high and low risk for breast cancer. J Cell Biochem 1993;17G:153–160.

83. Longcope C, Franz C, Morello C, Baker R, Johnston CC Jr. Steroid and gonadotropin levels in women during the peri-menopausal years. Maturitas 1986;8: 189–196.

84. Wing RR, Mattews KA, Kuller LH, et al. Weight gain at the time of the menopause. Arch Intern Med 1991;151:97–102.

85. Wing RR, Matthews KA, Kuller LH, et al. Waist to hip ratio in middle-aged women. Arterioscler Thromb 1991;11:1250–1257.

86. Kleerekoper M, Nelson DA, Peterson EL, Wilson PS, Jacobsen G, Longcope C . Body composition and gonadal steroids in older white and black women. J Clin Endocrinol Metab 1994;79:775–779.

87. Kuller LH, Gutai JP, Meilahn E, Matthews KA, Plantinga P. Relationship of endogenous sex steroid hormones to lipids and apoproteins in postmenopausal women. Arteriosclerosis 1990;10:1058–1066.

88. Cauley JA, Gutai JP, Kuller LH, LeDonne D, Powell JG. The epidemiology of serum sex hormones in postmenopausal women. Am J Epidemiol 1989;129:1120–1131.

89. Jaffe RB. The menopause and perimenopausal period. In: Yen SSC, Jaffee RB, eds. Reproductive Endocrinology. Physiology, Pathophysiology and Clinical Management. Philadelphia: W.B. Saunders, 1986, pp. 406–423.

90. Schapira DV, Kumar NB, Lyman GH, Cavanagh D, Roberts WS, LaPolla J. Upper-body fat distribution and endometrial cancer risk. JAMA 1991;266:1808–1811.

91. Refubbe'-Scrive M, Eldh J, Hafström L-O, Björntorp P. Metabolism of mammary, abdominal, and femoral adipocytes in women before and after menopause. Metabolism 1986;35:792–797.

92. Hilf R. The actions of insulin as a hormonal factor in breast cancer. In: Pike MC, Sisiteri PK, Welsch CW, eds. Banbury Report 8: Hormones and Breast Cancer. Cold Spring Harbor, NY: Cold Spring Harbor Laboratory, 1981, pp. 317–337.

93. Goodwin PJ, Boyd NF. Body size and breast cancer prognosis: A critical review of the evidence. Breast Cancer Res Treat 1990;16:205–214.

94. Toniolo PG, Levitz M, Zeleniuch-Jacquotte A, et al. A prospective study of endogenous estrogens and breast cancer in postmenopausal women. J Natl Cancer Inst 1995;87:190–197.

95. Dorgan JF, Longcope C, Stephenson HE Jr, et al. Relation of prediagnostic serum estrogen and androgen levels to breast cancer risk. Cancer Epidemiol Biomarkers Prev 1996;5:533–539.

96. Cauley JA, Lucas FL, Kuller LH, Stone K, Browner W, Cummings SR. Endogenous sex steroid hormone concentrations and bone mass predict breast cancer in older women. Proceedings from the Department of Defense Breast Cancer Research Program Meeting, "Era of Hope", October 31–November 4, 1997, Vol. I. Washington, DC: U.S. Government Printing Office, 1997, pp. 506–586.

97. Dorgan JF, Stanczyk FZ, Longcope C, Stephenson HE Jr, et al. Relationship of serum dehydroepiandrosterone (DHEA), DHEA sulfate, and 5-androstene-3β, 17β-diol to risk of breast cancer in postmenopausal women. Cancer Epidemiol Biomarkers Prev 1997;6:177–182.

98. Zeleniuch-Jacquotte A, Bruning PF, Bonfrer JMG, et al. Relation of serum levels of testosterone and dehydroepiandrosterone sulfate to risk of breast cancer in postmenopausal women. Am J Epidemiol 1997;145:1030–1038.

99. Parker LN, ed. Adrenal Androgens in Clinical Medicine. San Diego: Academic Press, 1989.

100. Simpson ER, Waterman MR. Steroid hormone biosynthesis in the adrenal cortex and its regulation by adrenocorticotropin. In: DeGroot LJ, ed. Endocrinology. Philadelphia: W.B. Saunders, 1994, pp. 1630–1641.

101. Parker LN. Adrenal androgens. In: DeGroot LJ, ed. Endocrinology. 1994, pp. 1836–1852.

102. Dempster DW, Lindsay R. Pathogenesis of osteoporosis. Lancet 1993;341: 797–801.

103. Cauley JA, Lucas FL, Kuller LH, Vogt MT, Browner WS, Cummings SR. Bone mineral density and risk of breast cancer in older women. JAMA 1996;276: 1404–1408.

104. Zhang Y, Kiel DP, Kreger BE, et al. Bone mass and the risk of breast cancer among postmenopausal women. N Engl J Med 1997;336:611–617.

105. Boyd NF, Greenberg C, Lockwood G, et al. Effects at two years of a low-fat, high-carbohydrate diet on radiologic features of the breast: Results from a randomized trial. J Natl Cancer Inst 1997;89:488–496.

106. Byrne C, Schairer C, Wolfe J, Parekh N, Salane M, Brinton LA, Hoover R, Haile R. Mammographic features and breast cancer risk: Effects with time, age, and menopause status. J Natl Cancer Inst 1995;87:1622–1629.

107. Saftlas AF, Hoover RN, Brinton LA, et al. Mammographic densities and risk of breast cancer. Cancer 1991;67:2833–2838.

108. Kato I, Beinart C, Bleich A, Su S, Kim M, Toniolo PG. A nested case–control study of mammographic patterns, breast volume, and breast cancer (New York City, NY, United States). Cancer Causes Control 1995;5:431–438.

109. Telang NT, Katdare M, Bradlow HL, Osborne MP. Estradiol metabolism: An endocrine biomarker for modulation of human mammary carcinogenesis. Environ Health Perspect 1997;105:559–564.

110. Kabat GC, Chang CJ, Sparano JA, et al. Urinary estrogen metabolites and breast cancer: A case–control study. Cancer Epidemiol Biomarkers Prev 1997;6: 505–509.

111. King MC, Rowell S, Love SM. Inherited breast and ovarian cancer. What are the risks? What are the choices? JAMA 1993;269:1975–1980.

112. Ford D, Easton DF. The genetics of breast and ovarian cancer. Br J Cancer 1995;72:805–812.

113. Ahlbom A, Lichtenstein P, Malmström H, Feychting M, Hemminki K, Pedersen NL. Cancer in twins: Genetic and nongenetic familial risk factors. J Natl Cancer Inst 1997;89:287–293.

114. Peters J. Breast cancer genetics: Relevance to oncology practice. Cancer Control 1995;May/June:195–208.

115. Weber B. Breast cancer susceptibility genes: Current challenges and future promises. Ann Intern Med 1996;124:1088–1090.

116. Shattuck-Eidens D, Oliphant A, McClure M, et al. BRCA1 sequence analysis in women at high risk for susceptibility mutations. Risk factor analysis and implications for genetic testing. JAMA 1997;278:142–1250.

117. Prentice RL, Kakar F, Hursting S, Sheppard L, Klein R, Kushi LH. Aspects of the rationale for the Women's Health Trial. J Natl Cancer Inst 1988;80:802–814.

118. Gray GE, Pike MC, Henderson BE. Breast-cancer incidence and mortality rates in different countries in relation to known risk factors and dietary practices. Br J Cancer 1979;39:1–7.

119. Freedman LS, Clifford C, Messina M. Analysis of dietary fat, calories, body weight, and the development of mammary tumors in rats and mice: A review. Cancer Res 1990;50:5710–5719.

120. Wynder EL, Cohen LA, Rose DP, Stellman SD. Dietary fat and breast cancer: Where do we stand on the evidence? J Clin Epidemiol 1994;47:217–222.

121. Howe GR. High-fat diets and breast cancer risk. The epidemiologic evidence. JAMA 1992;268:2080–2081.

122. Hunter DJ, Spiegelman D, Adami H-O, et al. Non-dietary factors as risk factors for breast cancer, and as effect modifiers of the association of fat intake and risk of breast cancer. Cancer Causes Control 1997;8:49–56.

123. Liu K. Consideration of and compensation for intra-individual variability in nutrient intakes. In: Kohlmeyer L, Helsin E, eds. Epidemiology, Nutrition and Health. Proceedings of the 1st Berlin Meeting on Nutritional Epidemiology. London: Smith-Gordon, 1989, pp. 87–97.

124. Ashley JM. Lipid biomarkers of adherence to low fat diets. In: Heber D, Kritchevsky D, eds. Dietary Fats, Lipids, Hormones, and Tumorigenesis. New York: Plenum Press, 1996, pp. 115–129.

125. Kuller LH. Dietary fat and chronic diseases: Epidemiologic overview. J Am Diet Assoc 1997;97:S9-S15.

126. Rose DP, Boyar AP, Cohen C, Strong LE. Effect of a low-fat diet on hormone levels in women with cystic breast disease. I. Serum steroids and gonadotropins. J Natl Cancer Inst 1987;78:624–626.

127. Ingram DM, Bennett FC, Willcox D, deKlerk N. Effect of low-fat diet on female sex hormone levels. J Natl Cancer Inst 1987;79:1225–1229.

128. Kuller LH. Eating fat or being fat and risk of cardiovascular disease and cancer among women. Ann Epidemiol 1994;4:119–127.

129. Stoll BA. Diet and exercise regimens to improve breast carcinoma prognosis. Cancer 1996;78:2465–2470.

130. Adlercreutz H. Western diet and Western diseases: Some hormonal and biochemical mechanisms and associations. Scand J Clin Lab Invest 1990;50(S201):3–23.

131. Ingram D, Sanders K, Kolybaba M, Lopez D. Case–control study of phyto-oestrogens and breast cancer. Lancet 1997;350:990–994.

132. Messina M, Barnes S, Setchell KD. Phyto-oestrogens and breast cancer [Commentary]. Lancet 1997;350:971–972.

133. Baird DD, Umbach DM, Lansdell L, et al. Dietary intervention study to assess estrogenicity of dietary soy among post-menopausal women. J Clin Endocrinol Metab 1995;80:1685–1690.

134. Phillips RL, Kuzma JW, Lotz TM. Cancer mortality among comparable members versus nonmembers of the Seventh-day Adventist Church. In: Cairns J, Lyon JL, Skolnick M, eds. Banbury Report 4, Cancer Incidence in Defined Populations. Cold Spring Harbor, NY: Cold Spring Harbor Laboratory, 1981, pp. 93–108.

135. Ames BN, Shigenaga MK, Hagen TM. Oxidants, antioxidants, and the degenerative diseases of aging. Proc Natl Acad Sci USA 1993;90:7915–7922.

136. Dorgan JE, Schatzkin A. Antioxidant micronutrients in cancer prevention. Hematol Oncol Clin North Am 1991;5:43–68.

137. Garland M, Willett WC, Manson JE, Hunter DJ. Antioxidant micronutrients and breast cancer. J Am Coll Nutr 1993;12:400–411.

138. Powles TJ, Hardy JR, Ashley SE, et al. Chemoprevention of breast cancer. Breast Cancer Res Treat 1989;14:23–31.

10

EPIDEMIOLOGY OF POLYCYSTIC OVARY SYNDROME

Evelyn O. Talbott, Robert A. Wild,
Karen E. Remsberg, LuAnn B. Gibson,
and Annette Casoglos

It is difficult to relate any specific sex hormone to cardiovascular disease in epidemiological studies because of the complex interrelationship between gonadotropin and sex steroid hormones. A single blood measurement may not reflect production, metabolism, and excretion of these hormones, and in women it does not capture hormonal variation across the menstrual cycle. Much of the epidemiological research linking hormonal variation to cardiovascular outcomes has depended on natural experiments or clinical trials. The key observations in studies making this link have been increased atherosclerosis among women with artificial menopause; differences in coronary heart disease (CHD) rates and atherosclerosis between men and women, especially premenopausal women; changes in risk factors at puberty and menopause; and the protective effects of exogenous hormones.

The polycystic ovary syndrome (PCOS) affords another natural experiment linking hormonal changes to cardiovascular risk. This syndrome is a heterogeneous group of disorders involving altered ovarian function. The disorders have been estimated to affect 5%–10% of all women,[1] but the true prevalence of PCOS is unknown. It is characterized by chronic anovulation, hirsutism, hyperandrogenism, and obesity or a subset of these features. Over the past decade, it has been reported that women with PCOS have elevations in coronary heart disease risk factors, especially lipids, blood pressure, clotting factors, and insulin resistance.[2-14] The study of cardiovascular risk among women with polycystic ovaries is particularly interesting because PCOS provides a natural experiment of the effects of hormone alterations (androgen excess and gonadotropin abnormalities) and insulin resistance on cardiovascular risk factors and disease.[15]

This chapter presents a general characterization of PCOS and its pathophysiology, and the epidemiology of PCOS, including genetic and environmental determinants of the disease. Finally, the most recent evidence linking this disorder with other disease outcomes, particularly CHD in women, is presented.

WHAT IS POLYCYSTIC OVARY SYNDROME?

This syndrome comprises a group of endocrine disorders among women that commonly results in infertility. First termed the Stein-Leventhal syndrome by Irving Stein and Michael Leventhal in 1935,[16] the syndrome was initially described as consisting of polycystic ovaries, amenorrhea, and in some patients, increased body hair and coarse skin. The polycystic ovary is a sign that is readily discernible by ultrasound (Fig. 10–1).[17] Multiple small cysts are seen beneath the ovarian capsule, and there is a hyperechogenic dense stroma. There has been much debate about every aspect of this syndrome, including its definition, pathophysiology, and etiology, as well as optimum management and treatment strategies. Through the observations of numerous clinicians and researchers, it became apparent that the original definition of the Stein-Leventhal syndrome was restrictive. Many women presented with polycystic ovaries but

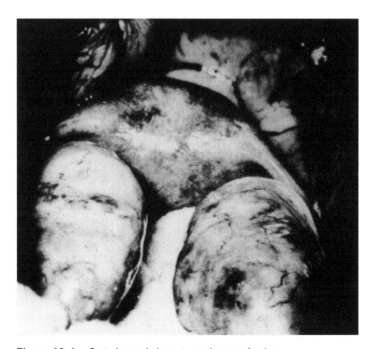

Figure 10–1. Stein-Leventhal ovaries as large as fundus

were not necessarily hirsute or oligomenorrheic. These women benefited from ovarian wedge resection, the treatment of choice for normalizing the menstrual cycle among women with Stein-Leventhal syndrome.[17] It became clear that the Stein-Leventhal syndrome was actually a heterogeneous group of disorders consisting of several criteria and symptoms. The term polycystic ovary syndrome emerged as a new identifier, most likely because of the characteristic ovarian morphology.

The diagnosis of PCOS most commonly entails the presence of polycystic ovaries in addition to abnormal biochemical measures and clinical symptoms. Women with PCOS are often obese and hirsute (with abnormal amounts of male-like hair growth on the face, chest, stomach, or inner thighs).[8,16–21] Adult acne and acanthosis nigricans (discoloration of the skin at the crural fold areas of the body) may also be present.[19,20] Biochemically, elevated levels of circulating free or total testosterone, luteinizing hormone (LH), LH to follicle-stimulating hormone (FSH) ratio (2 to 1 or greater), androstenedione, and dehydroepiandrosterone sulfate (DHEAS) are commonly found.[16,17,20–24] Oligomenorrhea or amenorrhea are also important symptoms. Normally, the menstrual cycle is perpetuated by a complex interaction of numerous hormonal interrelationships (see Chapter 6), and irregular periods occur when this balance is disrupted. Although menstrual irregularity often prompts evaluation for PCOS, there may be a substantial delay between the onset of amenorrhea or oligomenorrhea and its recognition. Menstrual patterns typically may not become regular until months to years after menarche. The pathophysiological aspects of PCOS are thought to start at the time of puberty,[25] but a diagnosis may not be made until several years later.

The prevalence of PCOS among women with menstrual abnormalities and hirsutism of unknown cause was studied in 1986 by Adams et al.[18] Their study included 173 patients referred to the gynecological endocrinology clinic in London. Twenty-five women presented with hirsutism, 75 women presented with oligomenorrhea (irregular menses), and 73 women presented with amenorrhea (no menses). They also studied 21 control women with regular menstrual cycles and normal ovaries by ultrasound examination. All of the hirsute women had regular menstrual cycles. Polycystic ovaries were defined when 10 or more cysts 2–8 mm in diameter with a widened stroma were observed. Of the 73 women with amenorrhea, 19 (26%) had polycystic ovaries by ultrasound examination. The remaining 54 had amenorrhea possibly related to other diagnoses, such as primary ovarian failure, hyperprolactinemia, or weight loss. The most common diagnosis for women with oligomenorrhea was polycystic ovaries (87%). Hyperprolactinemia (elevated prolactin level), obesity, or weight loss were associated with oligomenorrhea in the remaining 13%. Of women with idiopathic hirsutism, 92% were found to have polycystic ovaries by ultrasound. In this same study, the researchers also examined LH, FSH, LH/FSH ratios, testosterone, and androstenedione levels. They found that LH and testosterone levels were significantly higher in the women with polycystic ovaries and idiopathic hirsutism compared with controls.

Polycystic ovaries detected by ultrasound also occur in menstruating, fertile, nonhirsute women. In a study of 257 normal volunteers from the clinical and secretarial staff at St. Mary's Hospital in London, Polson et al.[26] reported that 20% of women using oral contraceptives and 23% of women not on oral contraceptives had polycystic ovaries by ultrasound examination. For those women not on oral contraceptives, menstrual pattern was a strong indicator of polycystic ovaries: 86% of irregular cycling women had PCOS compared with 7% of normally cycling women. The presence of polycystic ovaries did not invariably indicate the presence of PCOS.

PATHOPHYSIOLOGY OF PCOS

There is considerable controversy about the primary pathophysiologic defect in PCOS.[27] A broad consensus is evolving, however, that women with this condition are characterized by androgen excess, hyperinsulinemia, and abnormal gonadotropin (LH and FSH) secretion.[27,28] There is a strong relationship between insulin and androgen levels in women with PCOS; the correlation between insulin and ovarian vein androgens is in the range of 0.88 to 0.99.[29] There is also evidence that high insulin levels or insulin resistance causes elevated androgens rather than the reverse. When androgen levels are reduced by a gonadotropin-releasing hormone (GnRH) analogue (which reduces the secretion of gonadotropins and, in turn, reduces the secretion of androgens), insulin resistance remains in women with PCOS.[30] In contrast, pharmacologic reduction of insulin levels leads to a reduction in androgen levels.[31] It is currently unknown whether hyperinsulinemia increases androgen levels by increasing the production of androgen or decreasing the catabolism (breakdown) of androgens.

Examination of the metabolism of insulin and glucose in PCOS has revealed that women with PCOS have a unique defect in the early stages of insulin receptor signaling[32] even though the insulin receptor may be expressed normally.[33] In addition, a history of non-insulin-dependent diabetes mellitus (NIDDM) in a first-degree relative appears to define a subset of PCOS subjects with a greater prevalence of insulin secretory defects.[34] According to one study of 75 women with PCOS from the United States, Italy, and Japan, the prevalence of adrenal androgen excess and insulin resistance is similar across these ethnic groups.[35] Clearly, more research is needed concerning the relationships among glucose intolerance, insulin sensitivity, and PCOS. Nestler et al.[20] proposed that obesity plays an important role in the phenotypic expression of PCOS, not only by increasing the peripheral conversion of androgens to estrogens but by creating a more insulin-resistant, or hyperinsulinemic, state. They base their claims on the high incidence of insulin resistance in women with PCOS and the high positive correlation between fasting insulin values and serum androstenedione and testosterone levels. Their hypothesis is also based on the data (summarized above) indicating that hyperandrogenism is a result of hyperinsulinemia.

GENETIC BASIS AND HERITABILITY OF PCOS

The genetics of PCOS are not well understood, but several avenues have been explored regarding potential modes of inheritance. Candidate genes and biomarkers that may represent or regulate symptoms of PCOS are being examined. Because of the multietiologic nature of PCOS, many candidate genes from differing aspects of the condition are being studied. A variety of techniques, including molecular scanning and hormone assays, are currently being employed in pursuit of a genetic basis for PCOS.

Family studies have indicated a genetic predisposition to the development of PCOS.[36–38] Early research noted the disease to be sex linked, whereas more recent studies have supported an autosomal dominant mode of inheritance,[37,39] which was suggested as the most plausible pattern of inheritance in a review by Legro.[36] It is unlikely that PCOS is caused by a single gene defect. Although the predominant belief concerning PCOS is that it is inherited in an autosomal dominant pattern, there is no consensus on whether penetrance is complete—that is, whether all individuals with the dominant trait exhibit the syndrome. Gene expression in males is reportedly marked by hirsutism and male-pattern baldness.[40] Lunde et al.[40] reported a significant increase in prevalence of baldness and/or hirsutism in male relatives of women with PCOS (19.7%) compared to a referent group (6.5%). Polycystic ovaries and premature male-pattern baldness are associated with one allele of the steroid metabolism gene, CYP17.[41]

In a classic segregation analysis, Carey et al.[37] studied the first degree relatives of 10 women with PCOS who were diagnosed both clinically and by ultrasound. Data were collected on history of PCOS and premature balding, defined as loss of fronto-parietal hair before the age of 30 years. The investigators found that 31% of the males in this study presented with premature balding. A segregation ratio of 51.4% was calculated, suggesting autosomal dominant inheritance. In calculating the segregation ratio, probands were eliminated to avoid ascertainment bias and male-pattern baldness was considered to be the male phenotype.

Because PCOS is a disorder associated with a moderate level of insulin resistance or glucose intolerance, some genetic research has focused on genes responsible for insulin, the glucose transport mechanism, and general metabolism. These genes include the glycogen synthetase gene and the insulin receptor gene. Although 90 PCOS cases and 62 controls were examined for polymorphisms in the glycogen synthetase gene, no significantly different genotypes were found among cases.[42] Despite the normal gene, insulin levels were elevated in obese PCOS cases compared to controls.

Results concerning the insulin receptor gene are mixed. Among 22 unrelated women with type A extreme insulin resistance, several mutations were revealed,[43] but type A resistance is rare among women with PCOS. Conway et al.[44] amplified the tyrosine kinase domain of the insulin receptor gene and found no mutations that have been previously associated with insulin resistance. Nor were mutations found when the entire coding region of the insulin receptor gene was scanned[45] or in a separate study of three insulin-resistant women.[33] A few studies suggest that the insulin resistance in PCOS may not be due to the insulin receptor itself but instead to defective insulin secretion,[34] post-receptor miscommunication,[46–48] or defective insulin binding.[49]

These are just some of the genes that have been considered candidates for the control and/or regulation of PCOS. Future genetic studies may include molecular scanning of the human genome in regions thought to regulate symptoms of associated conditions.

CHD RISK FACTORS AND PCOS

A growing number of investigators have noted that women with chronic anovulation, hyperandrogenism, hyperinsulinemia, and obesity have an increase in cardiovascular disease (CVD) risk factors.[2–14] Most investigations have included patients seen in outpatient clinics for infertility, irregular periods, or hirsutism, and have applied varying definitions of PCOS. However, the literature describing CHD risk factors and PCOS has more recently expanded from case reports and clinical research involving specific patient populations[2–6] to larger epidemiological studies.[7–14]

Women with PCOS appear to develop NIDDM in their 30's and 40's; the age of onset in the general population is usually over 60 years of age.[50] Very few epidemiological studies have examined this relationship thoroughly, however, an increased prevalence of NIDDM has been linked with PCOS in a retrospective study ($n = 47$).[11] Rosenfield estimated that fully 40% of women with PCOS by age 26 met World Health Organization criteria for NIDDM.[51] True population-based estimates of PCOS and glucose intolerance/NIDDM comorbidities have not been obtained, since previous studies have examined PCOS cases alone or with controls in small, clinic-based studies.

In 1985, Wild and colleagues[3] found that women with PCOS had lower high-density lipoprotein (HDL) levels, higher LDL/HDL (low-density lipoprotein) ratios, and higher triglyceride levels than regularly menstruating women. More recently, Slowinska-Srzednicka et al.[52] compared 27 women with PCOS and 22 eumenorrheic controls, stratified by weight (obese, non-obese). Women

with PCOS had significantly lower levels of HDL2, higher levels of apolipoprotein B, and higher triglyceride levels—classically an adverse CVD risk profile.

Wild et al.[53] also studied 102 women referred for cardiac catheterization. A
total of 52 women had confirmed coronary artery disease and 50 women were
without coronary artery disease. A questionnaire was given to the study group
concerning the distribution of body hair and prevalence of acne earlier in life.
Twice as many cases with coronary artery disease reported excess body hair (facial hair, upper lip hair) and bad acne than controls. In another study of PCOS
and coronary artery disease, Birdsall et al.[54] evaluated 143 women less than 60
years of age who had undergone coronary angiography for investigation of
chest pain or valvular disease. When the ovaries of these women were examined
by transvaginal ultrasound, 42% were found to be polycystic. Women with
polycystic ovaries had more advanced coronary artery disease than women with
normal ovaries ($p = .01$).

Finally, Talbott et al. conducted a large-scale epidemiologic study of CHD
risk factors in women with a diagnosis of PCOS. This is the largest population-
based epidemiologic study to date and is described in detail below.[14]

Subject Recruitment

A total of 549 women with clinically diagnosed PCOS were identified (Fig.
10–2). The original cohort of women (seen at the Reproductive Endocrinology
Department at Magee–Womens Hospital between 1972 and 1986) consisted of
2,777 records. After careful medical review, 274 women (10%) met the criteria
for PCOS: chronic anovulation associated with (a) clinical symptoms consistent
with androgen excess (amenorrhea, increased body hair, acne, and male-pattern
baldness), or (b) if serum hormone levels were obtained, total testosterone >2
nmol/L or LH:FSH ratio >2. A second group consisted of 204 women meeting the criteria for PCOS who were identified from current office records
(1987–1992) of the Division of Reproductive Endocrinology at Magee–Womens
Hospital. The remaining 71 (12.9%) of the PCOS case population were non-
white women who were recruited as part of a supplemental grant aimed at increasing minority participation. This third group was identified by newspaper
advertisements, direct mailings, posters, and a medical record review of 1,500
largely non-white women who were seen at the Magee–Womens Hospital Obstetrics and Gynecology Clinic in 1989–1993 for fertility-related problems. Details of the methodology for control selection have been published elsewhere.[14]

Data Collection Procedures

All participants completed a telephone questionnaire conducted by a trained in-
terviewer. Demographic information, reproductive and gynecological history,

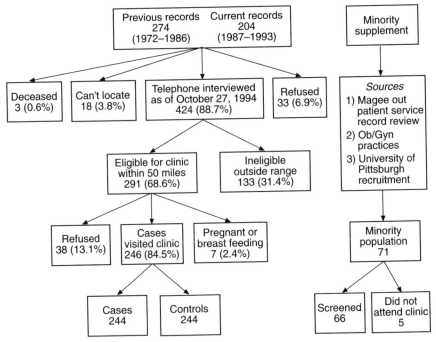

Figure 10–2. Case population in epidemiological study of coronary heart disease in women with polycystic ovary syndrome (PCOS). Age (±5 years) and race-matched neighborhood controls were selected using a combination of voter's registration tapes for 1992 for the greater Pittsburgh area and household directories.

use of oral contraceptives or hormone replacement therapy, and medical history were obtained.

Upon completion of the telephone questionnaire, women residing within the greater Pittsburgh area were asked to participate in a clinical examination after a 12-hour fast. Height, weight, waist and hip circumferences, and blood pressure were measured. A fasting blood sample was obtained for lipid and hormone assays.

Serum concentrations of total cholesterol, HDL cholesterol, subfractions HDL-2 and HDL-3, triglycerides, LDL, and very low density lipoprotein (VLDL) cholesterol were analyzed. LH and FSH, total testosterone (TT), androstenedione (A), and estradiol (E2) levels were determined using radioimmunometric assay.

Descriptive Results

A total of 244 cases and 244 age-matched controls were interviewed and examined. The mean age of the study group was 35–36 years old and the great majority were premenopausal. Women with PCOS had fewer live births on average than controls (P <.05). Body mass index (BMI) and waist/hip ratio were significantly higher among PCOS cases (P <.001) (Table 10–1).

Presence of hirsutism and reporting of ever having unwanted hair removed from face or body was reported in 43% of cases and 12% of controls, (P < .001). Presence of irregular menstrual periods was also reported more frequently by cases (94%) than by controls (36%). A pelvic transvaginal ultrasound was conducted on a subset of 75 PCOS cases and 75 controls. The presence of multiple, small subcapsular cysts with a hyperechogenic stroma on ultrasound was considered indicative of polycystic ovaries. This was found in 35.9% of cases and 9.8% of controls (P < .01).

A logistic regression model with PCOS status as the outcome was used to determine which of the risk factors were independent predictors of PCOS. Insulin (P = .016) and waist/hip ratio (P = .027) were significant predictors (Table 10–2). It must be noted that these three factors are collinear (highly intercorrelated).

Analysis of Cardiovascular Risk Factors in Relation to PCOS Status

The cardiovascular risk profile was worse among PCOS cases than controls (Table 10–3). HDL cholesterol was lower total cholesterol, and LDL cholesterol

Table 10–1. Sociodemographic and Reproductive
Factors in PCOS Cases and Controls

VARIABLE	CASES (N = 244)	CONTROLS (N = 244)
Age	35.3 ± 7.4	36.7 ± 7.7
Average Years of Education	14.2 ± 2.2	14.4 ± 2.0
Currently Married	179 (73.4%)	150 (61.5%)
Currently smoking	57 (23.4%)	63 (26%)
Currently on OCP/hormone replacement	39 (16%)	48 (20%)
Hysterectomy with bilateral oophorectomy	8 (3.0%)	3 (1.2%)
Natural menopause	3 (1.2%)	3 (1.2%)
Number of pregnancies	1.51 ± 1.7	2.03 ± 1.8*
Mean number of live births	.90 ± 1.4	1.6 ± 1.5*

*P <.01.

Table 10–2. Results of Conditional Logistic Regression

VARIABLE	COEFFICIENT ESTIMATE	S.E.	ODDS RATIO[a]	P VALUE
Insulin	.0460	.0190	1.05	.016
Waist/hip ratio	.061	.0274	1.06	.027
BMI	−.022	.0317	.978	.483

[a]One S.D. of the independent variable was used as the unit of risk.

Table 10–3. Distribution of Salient Risk Factors
(PCOS Case and Age-Matched Controls)

	CASES (N = 244) MEAN ± S.D.	CONTROLS (N = 244) MEAN ± S.D.	T	DF	P-VALUE
BMI	29.9 ± 7.95	26.6 ± 6.77	4.93	226	<.001
Total cholesterol	195.8 ± 32.95	185.7 ± 36.34	3.45	226	.001
HDL cholesterol	51.2 ± 14.74	56.1 ± 14.43	−3.39	226	.001
HDL$_2$ cholesterol	8.4 ± 6.5	11.4 ± 7.78	−4.25	215	<.001
LDL cholesterol	119.9 ± 31.8	112 ± 32.6	2.81	225	.005
Insulin	23.3 ± 17.8	13.6 ± 8.7	4.74	96	<.001
Triglycerides	123.6 ± 88.7	87.3 ± 63.1	4.95	226	<.001
Systolic blood pressure	113.5 ± 14.7	110.3 ± 13.1	2.64	215	.009
Diastolic blood pressure	72.7 ± 10.5	70.8 ± 8.3	2.09	215	.04
Waist/hip ratio	.83 ± .13	.76 ± .07	6.2	224	<.001

were higher among cases than controls (P = .001, P < .01, P = .005, respectively). Fasting insulin and triglyceride levels among cases were also greater than controls (P < .001). Likewise, mean systolic and diastolic blood pressures were greater in PCOS cases than controls (P = .009, P = .04). Diastolic blood pressure ≥ 90 mmHg occurred in 6.1% of cases and 2.6% of controls (P = .03).

By using multiple regression analysis, we determined whether lipid levels and blood pressure were higher among PCOS cases than controls after adjusting for other risk factors, including BMI, fasting insulin, age, smoking, and use of exogenous hormones and/or oral contraceptives (Table 10–4). Women with PCOS had significantly higher lipid levels than controls after adjusting for potentially confounding variables. PCOS status was not an independent predictor of systolic or diastolic blood pressure. The distribution of CHD risk factors (triglycerides, total cholesterol, HDL$_T$, LDL, triglycerides, insulin) as well as testosterone levels in cases with and without cysts was similar.

INSULIN, STEROID HORMONES, AND ENDOTHELIAL FUNCTION

Endothelial dysfunction is an important component of early atherosclerosis.[55,56] There is a progressive loss of endothelial vasodilation from normal arteries to a partial loss with hypercholesterolemia; a complete loss of this function occurs in severe atherosclerosis.[57] Endothelial vasodilation is impaired in both insulin-dependent[58,59] and non-insulin-dependent diabetes.[60] The loss of flow-mediated endothelial vasodilation occurs earlier in men than women.[55] Several studies have reported that estrogen improves endothelial-dependent, flow-mediated vasodilation in postmenopausal women. Estrogen receptors have been identified

Table 10–4. Estimated Parameters from Multiple Linear Regression: Predictors of CHD Risk Factors

INDEPENDENT VARIABLE	HDL_T	HDL_2	TOTAL CHOLESTEROL	LDL	SYSTOLIC BLOOD PRESSURE	DIASTOLIC BLOOD PRESSURE	TRIGLYCERIDES[a]
PCOS[b]	−2.512	−2.158*	9.121*	6.980*	.763	.520	.197*
Age	−.025	.031	.857*	.539*	.394*	.174*	.011*
Hormone status	.050	1.029	−3.687	−2.82	−1.041	−.468	−.046
Insulin	−.159*	−.054*	.094	−.02	.143*	.103*	.010*
BMI	−.437*	−.238*	.653*	.761*	.799*	.514*	.016*
Smoking	−.474	−.523	−1.833	−1.867	1.650*	.952*	.037

*$P < .05$. [a]log transformed. [b]Case = 1, control = 0.

on the endothelial cells.[61-67] Gilligan et al.[68] recently reported that acute intra-arterial infusions of estradiol substantially increased blood estradiol levels and potentiated forearm vasodilation induced by the endothelial-dependent vasodilator, acetylcholine. However, after 3 weeks of transdermal estradiol administration, resulting in estradiol blood levels of about 120 ± 57 pg/ml, the vasodilator responses to acetylcholine were unchanged from initial measurements. The authors suggest that acute administration of 17-β-estradiol potentiates endothelial-dependent vasodilation in the forearms of postmenopausal women, but this effect is not maintained with systemic estradiol administration within the physiological–pharmacological range. Most of these studies of the effects of estrogen administration on artery vasodilation are relatively small and of short duration, and they often include (primarily) patients with CHD.

Progression of atherosclerosis to clinical disease depends on changes in plaque morphology and rupture of plaque. A fibrous plaque is an accumulation of smooth muscle cells in the arterial wall. These cells lay down collagen and other matrix proteins that cause fibrosis and vascular rigidity. The endothelium overlying fibrous plaques have abnormal metabolism and action of vasodilatory factors such as nitric oxide. Advanced atherosclerotic plaques are characterized by extracellular oily collections of cholesterol, scarring, and calcification as well as by smooth muscle cell proliferation and foam cells.[69] Inflammation and activation of cytokines may lead to increased risk of thrombosis and clinical disease by further activation of clotting factors and increased platelet aggregation.[70] Recently, Hoffman et al.[71] reported a positive correlation between plasma levels of all four of the vitamin K–dependent clotting factors,[2,7,9,10] but not fibrinogen, with both cholesterol and triglyceride levels among healthy young adults. Interestingly enough, this relationship was less consistent for women than men. Links between the coagulation factor VII, and lipoprotein levels have also been demonstrated in a number of cross-sectional epidemiological studies,[72] as have associations between dietary fat intake and coagulation factor VII coagulation activity.[73] These relationships show that a cluster of CHD risk factors, including lipids and clotting factors, may change together and that estrogen affects all of them positively. The effects of disturbed insulin resistance, estrogen, androgen, and progesterone secretion on endothelial dysfunction as in the PCOS paradigm remains to be determined.

THE PHYSIOLOGIC LINK BETWEEN PCOS AND CHD RISK

What is the biology that links PCOS to increased risk of CHD? Two possibilities (or their combination) are most likely: increased testosterone and insulin resistance. The relationship between blood testosterone levels and CHD is controversial. Lesko et al. have noted that male-pattern baldness,[74] characterized by high levels of dihydrotestosterone, was associated with enhanced risk of CHD in men. Male-pattern baldness and android obesity have been considered by some to be the male counterpart of PCOS in women.[74] Abuse of androgenic steroids in young men is anecdotally associated with increased risk of CHD. Elevated blood testosterone in men and women, however, has not been associated with an increased risk of CHD,[75] and levels of total and free testosterone in the blood have been associated with elevated, rather than decreased, HDL cholesterol (HDLc) levels[76,77] as well as triglyceride. These studies, however, are relatively limited and most have been done in men. The higher HDLc level in women than men is primarily a function of a decline in HDLc in men at puberty, rather than a specific increase in women.[78] There is also little evidence for a substantial increase in HDLc in women at the time of the menopause.[79,80]

A recent study in primates noted that administration of testosterone to female menstruating monkeys was associated with increased atherosclerosis of the coronary arteries at postmortem examination.[81] The testosterone, however, resulted in an increase rather than a decrease in coronary artery vasodilation in the short term, this finding being inconsistent with elevated CHD risk. The testosterone-treated animals had a greater body weight and BMI, and increased triceps and subscapular skin folds. The increase in adiposity, however, was generalized rather than being limited to abdominal obesity or android obesity. Testosterone also effectively suppressed ovulation. Monkeys given a combination of androstenedione (a weak androgen) and estrone to mimic PCOS had no increase in atherosclerosis or any specific effect on their lipoprotein levels.[82]

Although there is significant evidence that diabetics have a higher incidence of cardiovascular disease, the relationship between insulin levels and CHD remains controversial. Some studies report a direct relationship between blood insulin levels and CHD risk, while others have found no such relationship, at least within the nondiabetic population.[83–87] This association has recently been reviewed by Ferrara et al.[88] In nondiabetic subjects, however, a relationship has been reported between insulin levels and degree of atherosclerosis as measured by carotid artery wall thickness and distention of the aorta.[89–91]

Within PCOS cases, fasting insulin was associated with total triglycerides and apolipoprotein A-1 after adjustment for age, BMI, and sex steroids. These results suggest that hyperinsulinemia may play a role in the lipid disturbances of PCOS.[53] These results support a 1992 study by Wild et al.[8] and a subsequent study by Wild, Alaupovic, and Parker[9] in which women with evidence of androgen excess were treated with a gonadotropin-releasing hormone agonist for 3 months, which suppressed ovarian production of estradiol and testosterone. Lipid profiles remained aberrant despite sex steroid suppression and remained correlated with insulin resistance. The authors concluded[9] that lipoprotein abnormalities appear to be associated more with insulin resistance than with endogenous androgens or estrogens.

In addition, there is evidence that high blood insulin levels suppress sex hormone binding–globulin (SHBG) production; more SHBG will reduce free sex-hormone levels. Furthermore, the reduced level of SHBG may lead to greater levels of free testosterone than free estradiol because SHBG has a greater affinity for testosterone than estradiol.

A fundamental unanswered question is whether at least some of the CHD risk that has been attributed to obesity or body fat distribution among pre-menopausal women is primarily due to polycystic ovary syndrome. Body fat appears to exert different influences on lipoprotein metabolism and CHD risk, depending on its location in the body. Intra-abdominal fat is a stronger CHD risk factor than thigh fat. Women have less intra-abdominal fat than men and testosterone may be an important factor in the development of intra-abdominal fat. The release of fatty acids from intra-abdominal fat to the liver may result in increased gluconeogenesis, increasing VLDL synthesis, depressing glucose up-take by muscle, and producing insulin resistance.

In the past, these relationships have been evaluated by quantifying upper versus lower body fat, waist-to-hip ratio (WHR), or skin folds. There is growing evidence that these measures, although useful, may not provide a completely accurate estimate of intra-abdominal versus subcutaneous fat.[92–94] Although the WHR has been the traditional method of quantifying visceral abdominal fat, WHR may not adequately predict visceral abdominal fat because of the variable amount of subcutaneous adipose tissue that constitutes a given waist circumfer-ence.[95] Seidell et al. found that the correlation between WHR and visceral ab-dominal fat as measured by computer tomography (CT) in women was only 0.55.[82] Improved methods such as CT scans and magnetic resonance imaging (MRI) of measuring intra-abdominal and subcutaneous fat as well as regional body fat provide an opportunity to test whether an increase in intra-abdominal fat is a critical determinant of atherosclerosis among women with PCOS. Ongo-ing studies are aimed at evaluating these relationships.

POLYCYSTIC OVARIAN SYNDROME AND RISK OF ENDOMETRIAL CANCER

The use of estrogens without progesterone in postmenopausal women has been clearly linked with an increased risk of endometrial carcinoma.[96] Women with PCOS have a similar unopposed endogenous hormonal milieu. That is, because they do not ovulate, they also circulate estrogen without progesterone. Endome-trial cancer has been diagnosed in young, (25–40 years) premenopausal women with PCOS.[97–102] In a cohort study of 1,270 PCOS women identified between 1935 and 1980 and followed for 14,499 person-years, a 3.1-fold increased risk (1.1–7.3) of endometrial cancer was noted. Endometrial cancer was the only cancer risk found to be elevated in these premenopausal women.[96] In fact, many of the cases of chronic anovulation were diagnosed because of symptoms of endometrial carcinoma. There are several hypothesized mechanisms by which these hormones increase the risk for endometrial cancer among women with PCOS. High levels of LH without FSH cause an increase in estrogen without progesterone opposition. This may cause an excess proliferation of endometrial cells, which has been associated with endometrial cancer.[98] Androgens, which are typically elevated in women with PCOS, lower levels of SHBG, as does insulin, which increases available estradiol in the endometrium, again causing proliferation of the endometrium. Insulin resistance is common among PCOS; hyperinsulinemia may also be a risk factor for endometrial cancer by suppressing endometrial production of insulin-like growth factor binding protein-I. Reduced binding protein enhances the stimulatory action of insulin growth factor-I, which may cause endometrial proliferation.[103]

POLYCYSTIC OVARIAN SYNDROME AND RISK OF OVARIAN CANCER

Epithelial ovarian cancer risk is highest among nulliparous women who are infertile (Odds ratio [OR] = 27.0; 2.3–315.6), as reported in a study in which fertility-enhancing drugs were used. Pregnancy, breast feeding, and oral contraceptive use seem to protect women against ovarian epithelial malignancies.[104] Whittemore et al.[104,105] reported that women with ovarian cancer were more likely to have had a diagnosis of infertility, particularly infertility related to abnormal ovarian function. Women with PCOS are likely to be nulliparous and infertile. The question remains, is PCOS an independent risk factor for ovarian cancer? Ongoing epidemiologic studies are likely to contribute the first data to address this question.

POLYCYSTIC OVARIAN SYNDROME AND RISK OF BREAST CANCER

It has been hypothesized that among women with chronic anovulation and hyperandrogenism, there is an increased risk of developing breast cancer.[106] High ovarian-produced testosterone levels and chronic anovulation are typically seen among women with PCOS and among women with abdominal obesity. Postmenopausal breast cancer has been linked to both PCOS and abdominal adiposity.[107] Current epidemiologic evidence, however, is not unequivocally supportive of this hypothesis. A historical cohort study of 1,270 women with chronic anovulation reported PCOS to be a major risk factor (relative risk [RR] = 3.6) for postmenopausal breast cancer, but not for premenopausal breast cancer.[96] However, in a retrospective study of 4,730 PCOS cases and 4,688 normal controls, a significant inverse association (OR = 0.52; 95% confidence interval [CI]

= 0.32, 0.87) for breast cancer was found.[108] Toniolo and Whittemore[109] challenged this later finding, noting that the observed protective association between PCOS and breast cancer may be a spurious one because of self-reported diagnosis and effects of treatment of PCOS that were attributed to PCOS itself.

Other studies have indirectly examined the association between PCOS and breast cancer by comparing menstrual or fertility status among cases and controls. These studies have been conflicting. A cohort of 428,653 women was asked about menstrual regularity in a 1959 questionnaire and then followed prospectively for 12 years to determine risk of breast cancer.[110] Women reporting irregular menstruation at age 20 were 0.84 times as likely to develop breast cancer (95% CI = 0.74–0.96) as women with regular menstrual patterns. A similar protective association was found for infertility and breast cancer in a case-control study.[111] Among 4,730 breast cancer cases, infertility was nonsignificantly protective, OR = 0.75. However, a slightly increased, but nonsignificant, risk of observed versus expected breast cancer cases (1.8) was found in a cohort study of 2,632 women.[106]

CONCLUSION

Polycystic ovary syndrome, a relatively common condition among women, is associated with a set of hormonal alterations, including hyperinsulinemia, increased circulating androgens, and sometimes obesity. These aberrations may put women with PCOS at increased risk of CHD and diabetes. In addition, women with PCOS may be at risk for cancers of the endometrium, ovary, and breast. Current data support a causal pathway whereby insulin (rather than testosterone) is the primary mediator of PCOS and is the primary link between PCOS and CHD. The role of adiposity in the pathophysiology of PCOS is yet to be completely understood. Cohort studies using standard definitions and measures that fully capture body fat distribution and hormonal fluctuations will help to further clarify the physiologic link between PCOS and CHD and thereby more generally elucidate the pathophysiology of CHD.

REFERENCES

    1. Yen SSC. Chronic anovulation caused by peripheral endocrine disorders. In: Yen S, Jaffe R, eds. Reproductive Endocrinology. Physiology, Pathophysiology and Clinical Management, 2nd ed. Philadelphia: W.B. Saunders, 1986, pp. 576–630.

    2. Mattson L, Culberg G, Hamberger L, Samsioe G, Silfverstolpe G. Lipid metabolism in women with polycystic ovary syndrome: Possible implications for an increased risk of coronary heart disease. Fertil Steril 1984;42(4):579–584.

    3. Wild R, Painter P, Coulson P, Carruth K, Ranney G. lipoprotein lipid concentrations and cardiovascular risk in women with polycystic ovary syndrome. J Clin Endocrinol Metab 1985;61:946–951.

4. Chang RJ, Nakamura R, Judd H, Kaplan S. Insulin resistance in nonobese patients with polycystic ovarian disease. J Clin Endocrinol Metab 1983;51:356–359.

5. Gibson M, Schiff I, Tulchindky D, Ryan KJ. Characterization of hyperandrogenism with insulin-resistance diabetes type A. Fertil Steril 1980;33:501–505.

6. Pasquali R, Venturoli S, Paradis R, Capelli M, Parenti M, Melchionda N. Insulin and C-peptide levels in obese patients with polycystic ovaries. Horm Metab Res 1982;14:284–292.

7. Slowinska-Szrednicka J, Zgliczynski S, Wierzbicki M, et al. The role of hyperinsulinemia in the development of lipid disturbances in non-obese and obese women with polycystic ovary syndrome. J Endocrinol Invest 1991;14:569–575.

8. Wild R, Alaupovic P, Givens J, Parker I. Lipoprotein abnormalities in hirsute women. Am J Obstet Gynecol 1992;167:1813–1818.

9. Wild R, Alaupovic P, Parker I. Lipid and apolipoprotein abnormalities in hirsute women. Am J Obstet Gynecol 1992;167:1191–1197.

10. Conway G, Argawal D, Betteridge, Jacobs H. Risk factors for coronary artery disease in lean and obese women with polycystic ovary syndrome. Clin Endocrinol 1992;37:119–125.

11. Dahlgren E, Janson P, Johansson S, et al. Women with polycystic ovary syndrome wedge resected in 1956–1965: A long-term follow-up focusing on natural history and circulating hormones. Fertil Steril 1992;57(3):505–513.

12. Dahlgren E, Janson P, Johansson S, Lapidus L, Oden A. Polycystic ovary syndrome and risk for myocardial infarction. Evaluated from a risk factor model based on a prospective population study of women. Acta Obstet Gynecol Scand 1992;71:599–604.

13. Cooper H, Spellacy W, Prem K, Cohen W. Heredity factors in the Stein-Leventhal syndrome. Am J Obstet Gynecol 1968;2:371–387.

14. Talbott E, Guzick D, Clerici A, et al. Coronary heart disease risk factors in women with polycystic ovary syndrome. Arterioscler Thromb Vasc Biol 1995;(15)7: 821–827.

15. Franks S. Polycystic ovary syndrome. N Engl J Med 1995:333(13):83–86.

16. Stein I, Leventhal M. Amenorrhea associated with bilateral polycystic ovaries. Am J Obstet Gynecol 1935;29:181–191.

17. Epidemiology of polycystic ovary syndrome. Figure 20–13A, 20–13B. In: Novak E, Woodruf JD, eds. Novak's Gynecologica and Obstetric Pathology with Clinical and Endocrine Relatives. Philadelphia: W.B. Saunders, 1979, pp. 392–393.

18. Adams J, Polson, Franks S. Prevalence of polycystic ovaries in women with anovulation and idiopathic hirsutism. Br Med J 1986;293:355–359.

19. Franks S, White D. Prevalence of and etiologic factors in polycystic ovarian syndrome. Ann NY Acad Sci 1993;687:112–114.

20. Nestler J, Clore J, Blackard W. The central role of obesity in the pathogenesis of the polycystic ovary syndrome. Am J Obstet Gynecol 1989;161(5):1095–1097.

21. Shelly D, Dunaif A. Polycystic ovary syndrome. Compr Ther 1990;16(11): 26–34.

22. Barbieri R. Hyperandrogenic disorders. Clin Obstet Gynecol 1990;33(3): 640–654.

23. Wild R, Applebaum-Bowden D, Demers L, et al. Lipoprotein lipids in women with androgen excess: Independent associations with increased insulin and androgen. Clin Chem 1990;36(2):283–289.

24. Wild R. Lipid metabolism and hyperandrogenism. Clin Obstet Gynecol 1991; 34(4):864–871.

25. Brook C. Polycystic ovaries in childhood. Br Med J 1988;296;878.

26. Polson D, Wadsworth J, Adams J, Franks S. Polycystic ovaries—a common finding in normal women. Lancet 1988;1(8590):870–872.

27. Barnes R, Rosenfield R. The polycystic ovary syndrome: Pathogenesis and treatment. Ann Intern Med 1989;110:386–397.

28. Barbieri RL, Smith S, Ryan KJ. The role of hyperinsulinemia in the pathogenesis of ovarian hyperandrogenism. Fertil Steril 1988;50:197–212.

29. Nagamani M, Dinh TV, Kelver ME. Hyperinsulinemia in hyperthecosis of the ovaries. Am J Obstet Gynecol 1986;154:384–389.

30. Geffner ME, Kaplan SA, Bersch N, Golde DW, Landaw EM, Chang RJ. Persistence of insulin resistance in polycystic ovarian disease after inhibition of ovarian steroid secretion. Fertil Steril 1986;45:327–333.

31. Nestler JE, Barlascini CO, Matt DW, et al. Suppression of serum insulin by diazoxide reduces serum testosterone levels in obese women with polycystic ovary syndrome. J Clin Endocrinol Metab 1989;68:1027–1032.

32. Dunaif A, Segal KR, Futterweit W, Dobrjansky A. Profound peripheral insulin resistance, independent of obesity, in the polycystic ovary syndrome. Diabetes 1989;38: 1165–1174.

33. Sorbara LR, Tang Z, Cama A, et al. Absence of insulin receptor gene mutations in three insulin-resistant women with the polycystic ovary syndrome. Metabolism 1995; 43(12):1568–1574.

34. Ehrmann DA, Sturis MM, Karrison T, Rosenfield RL, Polonsky KS. Insulin secretory defects in polycystic ovary. Relationship to insulin sensitivity and family history of non-insulin-dependent diabetes mellitus. J Clin Invest 1995;96(1):520–527.

35. Carmina E, Koyama T, Chang L, Stanczyk FZ, Lobo RA. Does ethnicity influence the prevalence of adrenal hyperandrogenism and insulin resistance in polycystic ovary syndrome? Am J Obstet Gynecol 1992;167:1807–1812.

36. Legro RS. The genetics of polycystic ovary syndrome. Am J Med 1995; 98(suppl1A):9S–16S.

37. Carey A, Chan K, Short F, White D, Williamson R, Franks S. Evidence for a single gene effect causing polycystic ovaries and male pattern baldness. Clin Endocrinol 1993;38:653–658.

38. Hague WM, Adams J, Reeders ST, Peto TE, Jacobs HS. Familial polycystic ovaries: A genetic disease? Clin Endocrinol 1988;29:593–605.

39. Cooper H, Spellacy W, Prem K, Cohen W. Hereditary factors in the Stein-Leventhal syndrome. Am J Obstet Gynecol 1968;100:371–387.

40. Lunde O, Magnus P, Sandivic L, Hoglo S. Familial clustering in the polycystic ovarian syndrome. Gynecol Obstet Invest 1989;28:23–30.

41. Carey AH, Waterworth D, Patel K, et al. Polycystic ovaries and premature male pattern baldness are associated with one allele of the steroid metabolism gene CYP17. Hum Mol Genet 1994;3(10):873–876.

42. Rajkhowa M, Talbot JA, Jones PW, Clayton RN. Polymorphism of glycogen synthetase gene in polycystic ovary syndrome. Clin Endocrinol 1996;44(1):85–90.

43. Moller DE, Cohen O, Yamaguchi Y, Assiz R, Girgorescu F, Eberle A, Morrow LA, Moses AC, Flier JS. Prevalence of mutations in the insulin receptor gene in subjects with features of the type A syndrome of insulin resistance. Diabetes 1994;43(2): 247–255.

44. Conway GS, Avey C, Rumsby G. The tyrosine kinase domain of the insulin receptor gene is normal in women with hyperinsulinemia and polycystic ovary syndrome. Hum Reprod 1994;9(9):1681–1683.

45. Talbot JA, Bicknell EJ, Tajkhowa M, Krook A, O'Rahilly S, Clayton RN. Molecular scanning of the insulin receptor gene in women with polycystic ovarian syndrome. J Clin Endocrinol Metab 1996;81(5):1979–1983.

46. Lanzone A, Caruso A, DiSimone N, DeCarolis S, Fulghesu AM, Mancuso S. Polycystic ovary disease. A risk factor for gestational diabetes? J Reprod Med 1995;40 (4):312–316.

47. Ciaraldi TP, El-Roeiy A, Madar Z, Reichart D, Olefsky JM, Yen SSC. Cellular mechanisms of insulin resistance in polycystic ovarian syndrome. J Clin Endocrinol Metab 1992;75:577–583.

48. Dunaif A, Segal KR, Shelley DR, Green G, Dobrjansky A, Licholai R. Evidence for a distinctive and intrinsic defect in insulin action in the polycystic ovary syndrome. Diabetes 1992;41:1257–1266.

49. Marsden PJ, Murdoch A, Taylor R. Severe impairment of insulin action in adipocytes from amenorrheic subjects with polycystic ovary syndrome. Metab Clin Exper 1994;43(12):1536–1542.

50. Dunaif A. Hyperandrogenic anovulation (PCOS): A unique disorder of insulin action associated with an increased risk of non-insulin-dependent diabetes mellitus. Am J Med 1995;98(1A):33S–39S.

51. Rosenfield RL. Polycystic ovary syndrome for pediatricians. The 22nd Annual Frederick M. Kenny Memorial Lecture, April 3, 1995, delivered at McClosky Auditorium, Children's Hospital of Pittsburgh, University of Pittsburgh Medical Center.

52. Slowinska-Srzednicka J, Zgliczynski S, Wierzbicki M, et al. The role of hyperinsulinemia in the development of lipid disturbances in non-obese and obese women with the polycystic ovary syndrome. J Endocrinol Invest 1991;14:569–575.

53. Wild RA, Grubb B, Hartz A, Van Nort JJ, Bachman W, Bartholomew M. Clinical signs of androgen excess as risk factors for coronary artery disease. Fertil Steril 1990;54(2):255–259.

54. Birdsall MA, Farquhar CM, White HD. Association between polycystic ovaries and extent of coronary artery disease in women having cardiac catheterization. Ann Intern Med 1997;126:32–35.

55. Celermajer DS, Sorensen KE, Spiegelhalter DJ, Georgakopoulos D, Robinsin J, Deanfield JE. Aging is associated with endothelial dysfunction in healthy men years before the age-related decline in women. J Am Coll Cardiol 1994;24:461–476.

56. Meredith IT, Anderson TJ, Uehata A, Yeung AC, Selwyn AP, Ganz P. Role of endothelium in ischemic coronary syndromes. Am J Cardiol 1993;72:27C–31C.

57. McLenachan JM, Williams JK, Fish RD, Ganz P, Selwyn AP. Loss of flow-mediated endothelium-dependent dilation occurs early in the development of atherosclerosis. Circulation 1991;84:1273–1278.

58. Johnstone MT, Creager SJ, Scales KM, Cusco JA, Lee BK, Creager MA. Impaired endothelium-dependent vasodilation in patients with insulin-dependent diabetes mellitus. Circulation 1993;88:2510–2516.

59. Calver A, Collier J, Vallance P. Inhibition and stimulation of nitric oxide synthesis in the human forearm arterial bed of patients with insulin-dependent diabetes. J Clin Invest 1992;90:2548–2554.

60. McVeigh GE, Brennan GM, Johnston GD, et al. Impaired endothelium-dependent and independent vasodilation in patients with type 2 (non-insulin-dependent) diabetes mellitus. Diabetologia 1992;35:771–776.

61. Gilligan DM, Badar DM, Panza JA, Quyyumi AA, Canon RO III. Acute vascular effects of estrogen in postmenopausal women. Circulation 1994;90:786–791.

62. Gerhard MD, Roddy M-A, Knab ST, Creager SJ, Creager MA. Acute estrogen administration improves endothelium-dependent vasodilation in postmenopausal women [Abstract]. Circulation 1994;90:1–86.

63. Lieberman EH, Gerhard MD, Uehata A, et al. Estrogen improves endothelium-dependent, flow-mediated vasodilation in postmenopausal women. Ann Intern Med 1994;121:936–941.

64. Rosselli M, Imthurn B, Keller PJ, Jackson EK, Dubey RK. Circulating nitric oxide (nitrite/nitrate) levels in postmenopausal women substituted with 17β-estradiol and norethisterone acetate: A two-year follow-up study. Hypertension 1995;25(4):848–853.

65. Keaney JF, Shwaery GT, Xu A, et al. 17β-estradiol preserves endothelial vasodilator function and limits low-density lipoprotein oxidation in hypercholesterolemic swine. Circulation 1994;89(5):2251–2259.

66. Gilligan DM, Quyyumi AA, Cannon RO III. Effects of physiological levels of estrogen on coronary vasomotor function in postmenopausal women. Circulation 1994;89(6):2545–2551.

67. Herrington DM, Braden GA, Williams JK, Morgan TM. Endothelial-dependent coronary vasomotor responsiveness in postmenopausal women with and without estrogen replacement therapy. Am J Cardiol 1994;73:591–592.

68. Gilligan DM, Badar DM, Panza JA, Quyyumi AA, Cannon RO III. Effects of estrogen replacement therapy on peripheral vasomotor function in postmenopausal women. Am J Cardiol 1995;75:264–268.

69. Biochemistry. A Case-Oriented Approach, 6th ed. Montgomery R, Conway TW, Spector AA, Chappell D, eds. St. Louis: Mosby, 1996.

70. DeFronzo RA, Ferrannini E. Insulin resistance: A multifaceted syndrome responsible for NIDDM, hypertension dyslipidemia, and atherosclerotic cardiovascular disease. Diabetes Care 1991;14:173–194.

71. Hoffman CJ, Lawson WE, Miller RH, Hultin MB. Correlation of vitamin K-dependent clotting factors with cholesterol and triglycerides in healthy young adults. Arterioscler Thromb 1994;14:1737–1740.

72. Moor E, Silveira A, Hooft F, et al. Coagulation factor VII mass and activity in young men with myocardial infarction at a young age. Arterioscler Thromb Vasc Biol 1995;15(5):655–664.

73. Nordoy A, Goodnight SH. Dietary lipids and thrombosis: Relationships to atherosclerosis. Arteriosclerosis 1990;10(2):149–163.

74. Lesko SM, Rosenberg L, Shapiro MB. A case–control study of baldness in relation to myocardial infarction in men. JAMA 1993;269(8):998–1003.

75. Cauley JA, Gutai JP, Kuller LH, Dai WS for the MRFIT Research Group. Usefulness of sex steroid hormone levels in predicting coronary artery disease in men. Am J Cardiol 1987;60:771–777.

76. Dai WS, Gutai JP, Kuller LH, LaPorte RE, Falvo-Gerard L, Caggiula A. Relation between plasma high-density lipoprotein cholesterol and sex hormone concentrations in men. Am J Cardiol 1984;53:1259–1263.

77. Pratico D, FitzGerald G. Testosterone and thromboxane: Of muscles, mice and men. Circulation 1995;91(11):2694–2698.

78. Jiang X, Srinivasan SR, Webber LS, Wattigney WA, Berenson GS. Association of fasting insulin level with serum lipid and lipoprotein levels in children, adolescents, and young adults: The Bogalusa heart study. Arch Intern Med 1995;155:190–196.

79. Kuller LH, Meilahn EN, Gutai JP, Cauley JA, et al. Lipoproteins, estrogens and the menopause. In: Korenman SG, ed. The menopause—biological and clinical con-

sequences of ovarian failure: Evolution and management. Norwell: Serono Symposia, USA, 1990, pp. 179–197.

80. Matthews KA, Meilahn EN, Kuller LH, et al. Menopause and coronary heart disease risk factors. N Engl J Med 1989;321:641–646.

81. Adams MR, Williams JK, Kaplan JR. Effects of androgens on coronary artery atherosclerosis and atherosclerosis-related impairment of vascular responsiveness. Arterioscler Thromb Vasc Biol 1995;15(5):562–570.

82. Seidell JC, Oosterlee A, Thijssen JAO, et al. Assessment of intra-abdominal and subcutaneous abdominal fat: Relation between anthropometry and computed tomography. Am J Clin Nutr 1987;45:7–13.

83. Ley CJ, Swan J, Godsland IF, Walton C, Crook D, Stevenson JC. Insulin resistance, lipoproteins, body fat and hemostasis in nonobese men with angina and a normal or abnormal coronary angiogram. J Am Coll Cardiol 1994;23:377–383.

84. Wright RA, Flapan AD, Stenhouse F, et al. Hyperinsulinemia in ischaemic heart disease: The importance of myocardial infarction and left ventricular function. Q J Med 1994;87:131–138.

85. Knight TM, Smith Z, Whittles A, et al. Insulin resistance, diabetes, and risk markers for ischaemic heart disease in asian men and non-Asian men in Bradford. Br Heart J 1992;67:343–350.

86. Welin L, Eriksson H, Larsson B, Ohison LO, Svardsudd K, Tibblin G. Hyperinsulinaemia is not a major coronary risk factor in elderly men—the study of men born in 1913. Diabetologia 1992;35:766–770.

87. Hargreaves AD, Logan RL, Elton RA, Buchanan KD, Oliver MF, Riemersma RA. Glucose tolerance, plasma insulin, HDL cholesterol and obesity—12-year follow-up and development of coronary heart disease in Edinburgh men. Atherosclerosis 1992;94:61–69.

88. Ferrara A, Barrett-Connor EL, Edelstein SL. Hyperinsulinemia does not increase the risk of fatal cardiovascular disease in elderly men or women without diabetes: The Rancho Bernardo Study, 1984–1991. Am J Epidemiol 1994;140:857–869.

89. Folsom AR, Eckfeldt JH, Weitzman S, et al. Relation of carotid artery wall thickness to diabetes mellitus, fasting glucose and insulin, body size, and physical activity. Stroke 1994;25:66–73.

90. Laakso M, Sarlund H, Salonen R, et al. Asymptomatic atherosclerosis and insulin resistance. Arterioscler Thromb 1991;11:1068–1076.

91. Kupari M, Hekali P, Keto P, Poutanen VP, Tikkanen MJ, Standerstkjold-Nordenstam CG. Relation of aortic stiffness to factors modifying the risk of atherosclerosis in healthy people. Arterioscler Thromb 1994;14:386–394.

92. Kvist H, Sjostrom L, Tylen U. Adipose tissue volume determinations in women by computer tomography: Technical considerations. Int J Obesity 1986;10:53–67.

93. Kvist H, Chowdhury B, Grangard U, Tylen U, Sjostrom L. Total and visceral adipose tissue volumes derived from measurements with computer tomography in adult men and women: Predictive equations. Am J Clin Nutr 1988;48:1351–1361.

94. Borkan GA, Gerzof SG, Robbins AH, et al. Assessment of abdominal fat content by computed tomography. Am J Clin Nutr 1982;36:172–177.

95. Pouliot MC, Despress JP, Lemieux S, et al. Waist circumference and abdominal visceral adipose tissue accumulation and related cardiovascular risk in men and women. Am J Cardiol 1994;73:460–468.

96. Coulam CB, Annegers JF, Kranz JS. Chronic anovulation syndrome and associated neoplasia. Obstet Gynecol 1983;61(4):403–407.

97. Wood GP, Boronow RC. Endometrial adenocarcinoma and the polycystic ovary syndrome. Am J Obstet Gynecol 1976;124(2):140–142.

98. Jafari K, Javaheri G, Ruiz G. Endometrial adenocarcinoma and the Stein-Leventhal syndrome. Obstet Gynecol 1978;51(1):97–100.

99. Tsoutsoplides GC. Endometrial adenocarcinoma and the Stein-Leventhal syndrome. Am J Obstet Gynecol 1983;147:844–845.

100. Farhi DC, Nosanchuk J, Silverberg SG. Endometrial adenocarcinoma in women under 25 years of age. Obstet Gynecol 1986;68:741–745.

101. Jackson RL, Dockerty MB, Minn R. The Stein-Leventhal syndrome. Am J Obstet Gynecol 1957;73:161–173.

102. Dockerty MB, Lovelady SB, Faust GT. Carcinoma of the corpus uteri in young women. Am J Obstet Gynecol 1991;61:966–981.

103. Gibson M. Reproductive health and PCOS. Am J Med 1995;98:67S–75S.

104. Whittemore AS, Harris R, Itnyre J. Characteristics relating ovarian cancer risk: Collaborative analysis of 12 US case control studies. Am J Epidemiol 1992;136:1184–1203.

105. Harris R, Whittemore AS, Itnyre J. Characteristics relating to ovarian cancer risk: Collaborative analysis of 12 U.S. case control studies. Am J Epidemiol 1992;136:1204–1211.

106. Ron E, Lunenfeld B, Menczer J, et al. Cancer incidence in a cohort of infertile women. Am J Epidemiol 1987;125:780–790.

107. Secreto G, Zumoff B. Abnormal production of androgens in women with breast cancer. Anticancer Res 1994;14(5B):2113–2117.

108. Gammon MD, Thompson WD. Polycystic ovaries and the risk of breast cancer. Am J Epidemiol 1991;134:818–824.

109. Toniolo P, Whittemore AS. Letter—Re: Polycystic ovaries and the risk of breast cancer. Am J Epidemiol 1992;136:372–373.

110. Michels-Blanck H, Byers T, Mokdad AH, Will JC, Calle EE. Menstrual patterns and breast cancer mortality in a large U.S. cohort. Epidemiology 1996;7:543–546.

111. Gammon MD, Thompson WD. Infertility and breast cancer: A population-based case–control study. Am J Epidemiol 1990;132:708–716.

III

ANATOMY OF THE GENITAL TRACT AND IMMUNOLOGY

11

ANATOMY OF THE FEMALE AND MALE GENITAL TRACTS

Giuliana Trucco

The female and male genital systems share basic similarities in morphology and function. Both exist in order to allow for reproduction. Both produce germ cells and transport these cells to the site of fertilization. There are also more subtle similarities that may appear to be differences. For example, it may seem that only a single ovum is produced once a month, while millions of spermatozoa are simultaneously ejaculated. In reality, many ova start the "challenge" of maturation each month, but only one reaches ovulation. Similarly, only one sperm "wins" the race for fertilization.

At the same time, male and female systems are profoundly different. Cyclic variation of sexual hormone levels occurs in women but not in men and these fluctuations are responsible for mood swings, fluid retention, and other changes. The clearest example of morphological difference in organs with similar capability is that between penis and uterus. The penis is composed mainly of erectile tissue with empty vascular spaces that under sexual stimulation become filled with blood, allowing for erection and intercourse by which the semen is deposited in the female vagina. The uterus is mainly composed of coiled muscular fibers that become elongated and stronger during pregnancy to permit the growth and delivery of the fetus.

The main function of the female genital organs is to allow the fertilization and development of the fetus. For this reason, the most important female genital organs are internally located. By contrast, the testes are externally located in men because the maturation of the spermatozoa requires a lower temperature. Along the ducts through which semen passes, there are several glandular structures that produce the fluid component of semen and promote sperm motility.

The following description of the anatomy of female and male genital systems is intended to underline such similarities and differences.

EMBRYOLOGY

The fetal genital system consists of primitive sex glands, or gonads, genital ducts, and externa genitalia that from an initial undifferentiated stage develop into either a male or female genital system.[1] Genetically, gender is determined at the moment of fertilization, but the Y chromosome influences sexual development.[2] In fact, at 7 weeks testis-determining factor (TDF), encoded by the gender-determining region of the Y chromosome, induces cells to differentiate into pre-Sertoli cells, which are the cells that support developing spermatogonia the precursor of spermatozoa.[3-6] The pre-Sertoli cells produce Müllerian-inhibiting substance (MIS),[7,8] which induces the regression of the paramesonephric ducts (part of the female genitalia). MIS probably also induces the differentiation of Leydig cells, which are capable of secreting androgens in the male testis. Testosterone is responsible for the male differentiation of the mesonephric ducts, which become the epididymis and vas deferens. Between the 10th and 12th weeks, seminal vesicles and prostate originate from the mesonephric ducts and the urethra, respectively. A testosterone derivative, dehydrotestosterone, induces male differentiation of the external genitalia, scrotum, and penis.

In the absence of a Y chromosome, female development takes place. In the forming ovaries the first meiotic division of the female ova is interrupted at prophase. Each of the resulting primary oocytes, surrounded by a layer of follicle cells, becomes a primordial follicle. In the absence of MIS, the mesonephric ducts degenerate, while the paramesonephric ducts develop into the Fallopian tubes, uterus, and upper portion of the vagina. The externa genitalia derive from the genital tubercle.

ANATOMY OF THE FEMALE GENITAL SYSTEM

External Genital Organs

The external genital organs, also known as vulva, consist of the mons pubis, labia majora and minora, clitoris, vulvar vestibule, vestibulo-vaginal bulbs, vaginal introitus, urethral meatus, Bartholin's glands, and Skene's glands[9-11] (Figs. 11–1, 11–2).

The *mons pubis* is the area next to the pubic symphysis. The skin is covered with coarse hair at the time of puberty. *Labia majora* are two prominent foldings of hair-bearing skin that run longitudinally from the mons pubis (anterior commissure) to the perineum (posterior commissure). In each labium there is an external pigmented and hair-bearing surface and an internal smooth surface. Mi-

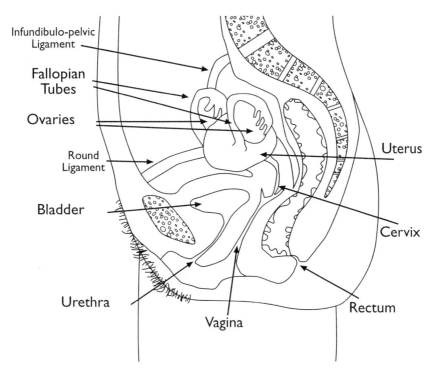

Figure 11-1. Schematic sagittal section of the pelvis of an adult woman. Reproductive organs are shown relative to the urinary bladder and rectum.

croscopically, it is possible to identify squamous epithelium with hair follicles and various types of glands.[12] Underlying the labia majora are fat tissue and smooth muscle corresponding to the dartos muscle of the scrotum in the male.

Labia minora are located inside the labia majora. They are delicate folds of squamous epithelium that outline the vaginal introitus. They join each other above the clitoris, forming the prepuce, which covers the glans clitoridis. The lower portions form the frenulum clitoridis underneath the clitoris. The *vestibule* is the area between the labia minora in which the urethral and vaginal orifices are located. Numerous glands empty into the vestibule.

The *clitoris* is the erectile female organ that corresponds to the male penis. It is partially contained within the labia minora. Like the penis, it contains two corpora cavernosa composed of erectile tissue that is limited by bands of fibrous tissue and anchored to a bone called the ischiopubic ramus. The *glans clitoridis* is a small tubercle at the apex of the clitoris consisting of erectile tissue and is covered by highly sensitive skin. The *urethral meatus* is located between the glans clitoris and the vaginal introitus, or opening. It has raised borders and is located 2.5 cm from the clitoris. The shape of the orifice can be round, crescent, or stellate.

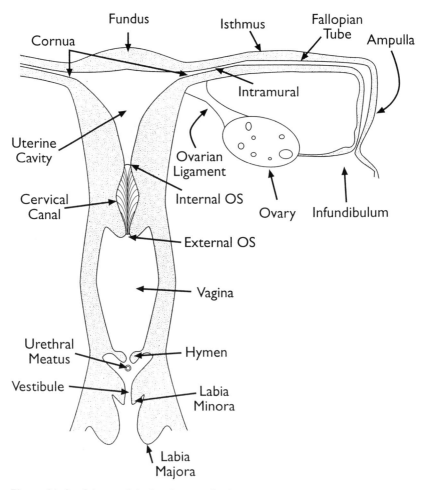

Figure 11-2. Schema of the female reproductive organs

The *vaginal introitus* is the opening of the vagina into the vestibule and varies in shape and size in relation to the *hymen*, which is a thin membrane that partially occludes it. The hymen has no known function; it can be absent or complete. When complete, it is known as an imperforate hymen. When ruptured, its small remnants constitute the carunculae hymenales.

Vestibulovaginal bulbs consist of two masses of erectile tissue located laterally to the vaginal introitus; at their largest they are 3.0 cm and they correspond to the bulb and corpora spongiosa of the penis. The two bulbs fuse above and below the introitus, ending in the greater vestibular glands. Superficially, they are covered by the bulbospongiosus muscle and underneath them is the urogenital diaphragm. They increase in size during sexual stimulation.

The *greater vestibular glands* are two round to oval mucus-secreting glands known as Bartholin's glands. They are located near the vaginal introitus at the end of the vestibular bulb.[13] They correspond to the male bulbourethal glands. Each of their ducts opens in the groove between the hymen and the labia minora. Histologically, they are tubuloacinar glands with columnar epithelium producing a clear mucus during sexual excitement. Whenever the ducts of these glands are occluded, they give rise to cyst formation or infection. Neoplasia can occasionally develop in these glands.

Skene's glands are small glands around the urethra and are analogous to the male prostate gland. They are lined by mucus-secreting, columnar epithelium, which becomes squamous epithelium in the vestibule.

Vagina

The vagina is a tubular structure that connects the vulva with the uterus.[9–11] It lies between the bladder and urethra above (anteriorly) and the rectum below (posteriorly); the vagina has an S shape and is oriented at a 90°angle in relation to the uterine axis. The posterior wall is longer than the anterior wall (9.0 cm vs. 7.5 cm). Normally, the vaginal cavity is collapsed and the inner surfaces are in contact with each other and present longitudinal mucosal ridges. A recess is present where the vagina meets the external portion of the cervix. This recess is divided into anterior, posterior, and two lateral fornices (Fig. 11–1).

The wall of the vagina comprises two main layers: mucosa and muscle (muscularis).[14] The mucosa consists of squamous epithelium. There are no glands in the vagina. It is possible to evaluate a woman's hormonal status by examining the epithelial cells that are shed (exfoliated) from the walls of the vagina. There is, in fact, a variation in the cellular pattern at different phases of the menstrual cycle. After puberty and especially after ovulation, the epithelial cells become rich in glycogen, a storage form of glucose for which the cell maturation can be evaluated.[15,16]

The vagina is not sterile and contains bacterial flora of which Doderlein's bacillus is an important component. In fact, this bacillus has a fermentative effect on glycogen-rich cells, which lowers the vaginal pH, reducing the growth of the other vaginal bacteria. Since the percentage of glycogen is lower before puberty and after menopause, women are more prone to develop vaginal infections during those times.

Uterus

Gross Anatomy. The uterus is a pear-shaped organ located in the lesser pelvis between the bladder and the rectum. At the upper portion, or fundus, the two lateral sides, or cornua, connect the uterine cavity with the fallopian tubes. At the lower end, the uterus continues through the cervix and connects with the vagina. In the adult nonpregnant woman, the size of the uterus is about 7.5 $\times 5.0 \times 2.5$ cm and the weight ranges from 30 to 40 g. The axis of the uterus is at 90° in relation to the vaginal axis but its position varies with the status of fullness of bladder and rectum[9,10,17,18] (Fig. 11–1).

The uterus can be divided anatomically and functionally into two regions: *corpus uteri*, which corresponds to the upper two-third of the organ, and *cervix uteri*, the lower third (Fig. 11–2). The corpus uteri and its cavity have a triangular shape with the lower portion being the *internal os* of the cervix and the upper portion being the fundus. The length of the uterine cavity is approximately 6.0 cm. The anterior surface is flat and adjacent to the urinary bladder. It is covered by the peritoneum, which folds between the uterus and bladder to form the uterovescical fold. The posterior surface of the uterus is slightly convex and is entirely lined by the peritoneum, which extends to cover the upper portion of the vagina. The peritoneum folds the rectum, forming the rectouterine pouch of Douglas, and to each of the convex lateral sides of the uterine body to form the broad ligaments, which extend to the pelvic wall (see below).

The cervix has a cylindrical configuration that is 2.5–3.0 cm long. The cervix is less mobile than the corpus uteri. The angle between the uterus and the vagina is 90° and is known as antiversion. When this angle is approximately 180°, the uterus lies posteriorly toward the rectum; this position is called retroversion. The flexure between corpus uteri and cervix determines its antiflexion or retroflexion, respectively. The combination of retroversion and retroflexion of the uterus may cause painful menstruation (dysmenorrhea) and infertility.

Anatomically, the cervix is divided into supravaginal and vaginal portions. The vaginal portion (or *portio vaginalis*) is a convex disc surrounded by a fold forming the vaginal fornices. The *external os,* which is round and small in nulliparous women, is centrally located and becomes flat and irregular in multiparous women. The internal and external os are connected through the cervical canal, which is a flattened cavity.

The upper third of the cervix is narrower and forms the *isthmus,* which becomes the lower uterine segment (LUS). During pregnancy, fetal membranes are not attached to the LUS, but they are to the remainder of the uterine cavity. During the menstrual cycle, the mucosa of this area undergoes less pronounced hormonal changes than that found in the rest of the uterus.

Histology

The wall of the uterus consists of three layers: the mucosa, or endometrium; the muscular layer, or myometrium; and the thin, shiny outer lining, or the serosa. The endometrial mucosa, which consists of glands, stroma, and arterioles, is functionally divided into two layers: the *stratum basalis,* or the deeper layer from which the new endometrium matures and which is not influenced by progesterone; and the *stratum functionale,* or the superficial layer, which can be subdivided into the *compactum* (the most superficial layer) and *spongiosum.*

This part of the endometrium is sensitive to estrogen and progesterone stimulation. Therefore, its appearance varies during the different phases of the menstrual cycle. Upon examining a small endometrial sample, one can evaluate the hormonal status, possible causes of infertility, and possible causes of dysfunctional or postmenopausal bleeding[19-21] (Fig. 11–3).

The first half of the menstrual cycle is termed the *proliferative phase*. The proliferative endometrium is characterized by stroma, arterioles, and glands

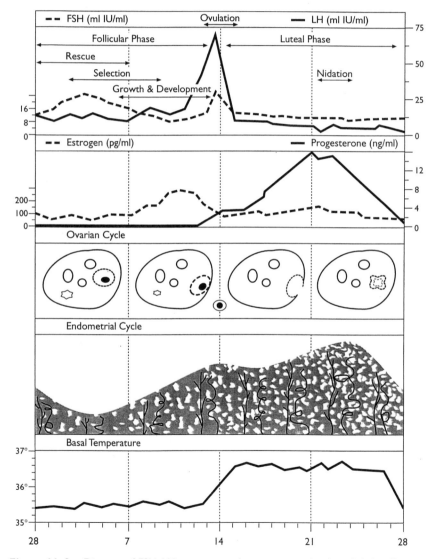

Figure 11–3. Diagram of FSH, LH, estrogen, and progesterone levels and their effects on the ovary and endometrium

that regenerate from the stratum basalis after each episode of menstrual bleeding. The glands are tubular and straight. Mitoses, signifying active cell turnover, are easily seen in the glands and in the stroma. Ovulation, which occurs at the middle of the cycle, heralds the second half, or *secretory phase,* of the menstrual cycle during which secretory changes in the endometrium occur that become obvious by day 17 with the appearance of subnuclear vacuoles in the columnar epithelium of the endometrial glands. Progesterone production, which is sustained by the newly formed corpus luteum, makes the stroma edematous (day 22) and the spiral arterioles prominent and surrounded by predecidual cells (day 23). The glands become increasingly tortuous, assuming a saw-toothed aspect. By day 26, the predecidual changes appear as a solid sheet occupying the entire endometrium. At this time, the presence of polynuclear cell infiltration is the first sign of the incumbent necrosis and hemorrhage of the endometrium, which results in menstruation. Menstrual shedding occurs on average every 28 days.[22,23] The late secretory phase is the best time to perform an endometrial biopsy to evaluate hormonal function.[24,25] If stromal edema and glandular secretion in combination with decidual changes occur, then fertilization and implantation have likely taken place.

The basalis of the endometrium continues directly down into the muscular layer, or myometrium, which constitutes most of the uterine wall. In the corpus uteri, the 1.3- to 1.5-cm thick myometrium is divided into four layers. The *stratum submucosum* which consists mostly of longitudinal muscular fibers, extends into the Fallopian tubes to form a sphincter-like structure. The *stratum vasculare*, which is rich in blood vessels, consists of longitudinal smooth muscle. The *stratum supravasculare* is composed of circular fibers and the thin *stratum subserosum* of longitudinal fibers. The last two muscular layers extend laterally into the fallopian tubes and ovarian and round ligaments. During pregnancy, the muscular layer becomes enlarged and the myocytes acquire more gap junctions so that they can contract more efficiently at the time of labor.

The cervical canal is lined by columnar, mucus-secreting cells resting on a layer of small reserve cells, which are important in the process of repair and proliferation. The columnar epithelium folds into the stroma, forming pseudoglandular structures that normally are 0.5 cm deep. When the lumens of these structures are dilated by mucous secretion, they form cysts known as Nabothian cysts.

A very delicate area is represented by the transformation zone, or *squamous columnar junction,* in which the columnar epithelium of the cervical canal continues into the squamous epithelium of the ectocervix. However, the squamous columnar junction only rarely coincides with the external os. Normally, the functional squamous columnar junction is located on the ectocervix. *Ectropion* occurs when the squamous columnar junction is more fully covered by columnar epithelium.[26] Ectropion is associated with young age and oral contraceptive use and may enhance susceptibility to sexually transmitted infections (see Chapter 17). The transformation zone is a particularly vulnerable site of origin for precancerous lesions. Cytological examination of exfoliated cells by the Papanicolaou method (i.e., Pap smear; Fig. 11–4) provides an excellent screening for early detection of premalignant lesions of the cervix.[27-32]

The muscular layer in the cervix forms a funnel-shaped array of smooth muscles enriched with elastic fibers and connective tissue. At the level of the external os, those layers become more compact and function like a valve, keeping the cervical os closed and separated from the nonsterile vaginal environment.

Uterine Ligaments

The uterine ligaments connect the uterus with neighboring organs (bladder and rectum); some of them are just peritoneal folding (uterovescical and rectovaginal) without any supportive function.[9,17] The broad ligament is a peritoneal folding that extends from each side of the uterus to the pelvic wall. It divides the pelvic cavity into two areas: the anterior containing the bladder, and the posterior containing part of the sigmoid colon and rectum. Its free margin contains the fallopian tube on both sides. The uterine arteries pass through the broad ligament.

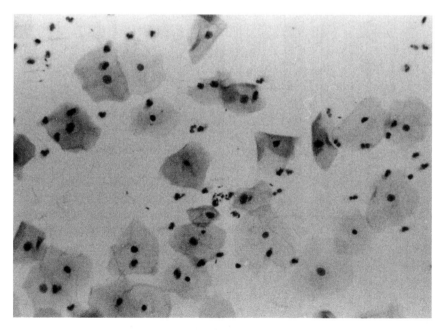

Figure 11–4. Normal cervical smear showing a population of superficial and intermediate cells. The superficial cells are large, with pycnotic hyperchromatic nucleus and abundant cytoplasm. The intermediate cells have a larger nucleus and a more blue-green cytoplasm, with evidence of active metabolism. Papanicolaou stain, ×600

The round ligaments of the uterus are two narrow, slightly flattened tubular structures 10–12 cm long that connect the upper portion of the uterus to the pelvic floor. The ovarian ligament is visible in the lower portion of the broad ligament. The round ligament corresponds to the male spermatic cord and, with the ovarian ligament, is the female counterpart to the gubernaculum testis (see below).

The cervix is held at the pelvic floor by ligaments with a very important mechanical, supportive function. The *cardinal ligaments,* or *transverse cervical ligaments of Mackenrodt,* hold tight the lateral side of the cervix, the vaginal vault, and the lateral fornices to the pelvic wall. Along with the *pubocervical* and *uterosacral ligaments,* they are responsible for supporting the uterus. The muscular structures of the urogenital diaphragm are also important in prevention of prolapse of the uterus and urinary stress incontinence—both of which are common problems in multiparous women.

Fallopian Tubes

Gross Anatomy. The fallopian tubes are paired tubular structures 8–10 cm long that extend laterally from each side of the uterus to reach the ovaries. Each tube has a uterine and an abdominal opening, or os, and can be divided into four portions (Fig. 11–2). The infundibulum, or fimbriated end, is the most lateral and largest part, characterized by the formation of finger-like projections, or fimbiriae, that float in the peritoneal cavity and extend to the ovarian surface. The function of the fimbriae is to convey the unfertilized ovum to the ampulla, which is the second portion of the fallopian tube. The lumen of the tube is larger here (up to 1.0 cm) and contains several ridges, or plicae, in which normally fertilization occurs.[33] The third portion of the fallopian tube, the isthmus, has a narrow lumen (0.2–0.5 cm) and a thicker wall that is rich in muscular fibers. The isthmus continues into the fourth portion of the tube, located within the uterine wall.

Histology. Microscopically, the fallopian tube consists of three layers:[34] mucosa; the muscular layer, with its external longitudinal and internal circular components; and serosa, which is covered by mesothelial cells.

Ovary

The ovaries are the female gonads, which are located lateral to the uterus behind the broad ligament. The anterior portion, or *hilus,* is attached to the posterior aspect of the broad ligament. The blood supply and the nerves enter the ovary at the hilus. The blood supply of the ovary and fallopian tubes originates from the ovarian artery, a branch of the abdominal aorta, and is drained through the ovarian vein. The lymphatics drain to the pelvic and aortic lymph nodes. The ovary receives innervation by sympathetic, parasympathetic, and autonomic fibers from the ovarian plexus.[35]

The ovaries are connected by the ovarian ligament to the sides of the uterus (Fig. 11–2). They are suspended to the lateral pelvic wall by the suspensory (or infundibulopelvic) ligament. In an adult, the ovaries are oval, measure about 3.5–5 ×2.0–3.0 ×1.0–1.8 cm, and weigh about 5–8 g each. The external surface is pink and smooth in young women but becomes increasingly convoluted with age. In child-bearing women, the cut surface of the ovary shows multiple cystic cavities of various sizes, representing different stages of maturation of follicles. It is also possible to recognize a yellow, occasionally hemorrhagic, partially cystic structure that is well circumscribed and corresponds to a recent corpus luteum. Remnants of old corpora lutea, or corpora albicantia, are firm white nodules. All of these structures, representing the physiologically active gonad, are located in both the external (cortex) and in part the inner (medulla) portion of the ovary. The surface of the ovary is covered by a single layer of cuboidal epithelium which is in turn covered by the tunica albuginea, a layer of fibrous tissue.[36] The vast majority of benign and malignant ovarian tumors originate from this epithelium.

The stroma of the ovary consists of dense collagenous fibers with a whorl pattern and fibroblast-like or mesenchymal cells. The medulla of the ovary is highly vascular and contains spiral arteries in loose connective tissue rich in elastic and smooth muscle fibers. Aggregates of interstitial cells, which are similar to the Leydig cells of the testis, are present and may produce androgens.

The cortex of the ovary contains most of the follicles, which at birth are represented by primordial follicles. Approximately 400,000 primordial follicles contain primary oocytes, which are large (25-μm) cells surrounded by a single layer of flat follicular, or granulosa, cells (Fig. 11–5). During childhood many of these primordial follicles degenerate and become atretic follicles, while only some of them reach complete maturation during childbearing life. After puberty, under the influence of follicle-stimulating hormone (FSH), the complete maturation of only one follicle results in ovulation every cycle.[37]

It is possible to distinguish follicles microscopically as primary, secondary, and tertiary. Primary follicles are characterized by the proliferation of follicular, or granulosa, cells around the oocyte into 3–5 concentric layers. The oocyte increases in size and acquires an extracellular membrane, the *zona pellucida* (Fig. 11–6). The granulosa is divided by a thick membrane, the *membrana limitans externa*, from the surrounding stroma cells, which differentiate into an internal theca and a thicker external theca.

The secondary, or antral, follicle is characterized by a cavity filled with clear fluid, *liquor folliculi*, which contains growth factors and hormones (mainly estradiol) secreted by granulosa cells.[38,39] The granulosa cells around the oocyte become more compact and form the *cumulus oophorus,* which pro-

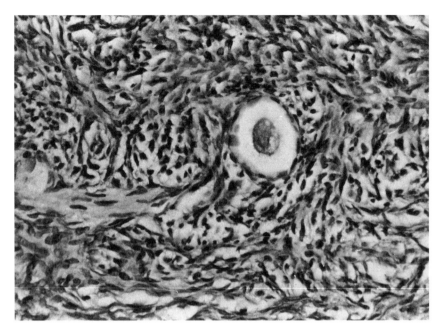

Figure 11–5. Primordial ovum. In the ovarian stroma, a large cell, the primary oocyte, is surrounded by a single layer of cuboidal follicular cells. Hematoxylin eosin, × 400

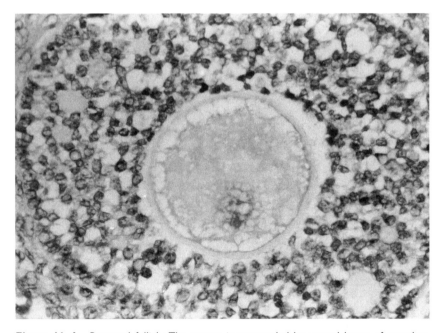

Figure 11–6. Preantral follicle. The oocyte is surrounded by several layers of granulosa cells and is characterized by a hyperchromatic nucleus and pale, indistinct cytoplasm. Small cavities "Call-Exner bodies" begin to form among the granulosa cell. Hematoxylin eosin, × 400

jects into the newly formed follicular cavity, or *antrum*.[40,41] Although more than one follicle in each cycle can reach the stage of secondary follicle, normally only one of them progresses to that of tertiaty follicle; the others become atretic.

The *Graafian follicle* is a mature follicle (Fig. 11–7) containing an oocyte surrounded by a ring of granulosa cells, the *corona radiata* (Fig. 11–8), which detaches from the wall of the antrum and floats in the follicular fluid. At this stage, the first meiotic division of the oocyte is concluded, accompanied by a reduction in the number of chromosomes and the expulsion of the first polar body. The oocyte, now called the secondary oocyte, starts the second meiotic division which stops at the metaphase. The second meiotic division will be completed only in the event of fertilization when, after the penetration of the sperm head, the two pronuclei fuse and the second polar body is expelled.

During the final stage of maturation, the follicle (about 1.5–2.5 cm in diameter) moves toward the ovarian surface and bulges through the epithelium. When the follicle ruptures (the stigma), the epithelium and stroma degenerate, probably as a result of proteolytic enzyme and prostaglandin action. The oocyte, along with its corona radiata and part of the follicular fluid, is released in the peritoneal cavity and drawn into the fallopian tube. After ovulation, the stigma, which is occluded by a coagulum composed of fibrin, follicular fluid, and blood, becomes a scar.

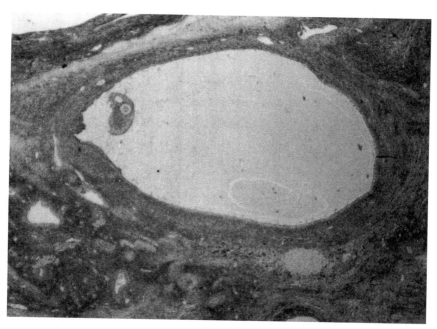

Figure 11–7. Graafian follicle. The mature follicle is characterized by a follicular cavity filled by clear fluid into which the cumulus oophorus protrudes. The wall of the follicle is composed of granulosa cells, theca interna, and theca externa. Hematoxylin eosin, ×20

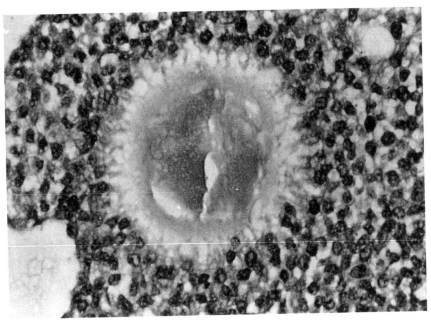

Figure 11–8. The cumulus oophorus is composed of the secondary oocyte surrounded by zona pellucida and a layer of granulosa cells radially oriented (the corona radiata).This cluster of cells protrudes into the follicular cavity and before ovulation, is detached from the follicular wall. Hematoxylin eosin, × 400

The collapsed wall of the follicle becomes the corpus luteum, and the granulosa cells are transformed into granulosa-lutein cells. These cells, which contain cytoplasm rich in carotenoid pigment, are responsible for the bright yellow color of the corpus luteum. The cells of the theca interna also become luteinized and through a breakdown of the basal lamina of the follicle, capillaries and connective tissue invade the central cavity.[42]

If fertilization does not occur, on days 8–9 postovulation the corpus luteum becomes involuted, i.e., it disintegrates. The granulosa-lutein cells become smaller and are characterized by pyknotic nuclei and a reduction in steroid biosynthesis. Following degeneration of the functional cells that are progressively replaced by fibrous tissue, the corpus luteum becomes the physiologically quiescent corpus albicans. If pregnancy occurs, the corpus luteum does not regress but increases in size. At 8–9 weeks gestation, the granulosa-lutein cells reach a maximum diameter of 50–60 μm and have major synthetic capabilities, particularly for progesterone. Progesterone production by the corpus luteum starts to decline by the end of the second month of pregnancy when steroid synthesis occurs in the placenta.

ANATOMY OF THE MALE GENITAL SYSTEM

The anatomy of the female genital system is best understood in comparison with the male genital system. That is, there are structures common to both and structures unique in each. Anatomic differences may explain some differences in disease frequency (see Chapter 14).

Testes and Epididymes

The testes are the male gonads, or sperm-producing organs. They are ovoid, paired, about $4.5 \times 2.5 \times 3.0$ cm in size, weigh 15–20 g, and are located in the scrotum where they are attached in the back to the spermatic cord.[9] Each testis is covered by a capsule composed of three layers. The outer serosa, or *tunica vaginalis* (with a flat mesothelial epithelium), divides the organ from the scrotum. The intermediate layer, known as *tunica albuginea*, consists of a network of collagen bundles that cover the organ. At the posterior surface, the tunica albuginea continues into a thick, incomplete septum containing vascular and nerve structures. Septations termed the septula testis divide the tissue into small, cone-shaped lobules that have bases toward the surface. There are approximately 250 lobules and each contains up to four seminiferous tubules (Fig. 11–9). These range in diameter between 0.12 and 0.3 mm and have basement membranes that become thicker with age. The tubules are lined by tall, columnar, ciliated and short, nonciliated cells. (Fig. 11–9). The third layer, the *tunica vasculosa,* is the innermost layer and contains a delicate vascular plexus interposed by loose connective tissue. Through a testicular biopsy in which three to five lobules are examined microscopically spermatogenesis can be assessed.[43–45]

Interspersed among the seminiferous tubules there are two other types of cell populations:[46] Leydig cells and Sertoli cells. Leydig cells are large polyhedral cells found singly or in clusters and are often associated with nerves. They resemble the interstitial cells of the ovary or the luteal cells of the corpus luteum. Leydig cells secrete androgens under the stimulus of luteinizing hormone (LH) and possibly FSH. These cells induce sperm production or spermatogenesis through the secretion of testosterone, which influences the Sertoli cells and peritubular structures to create the ideal environment for spermatogenesis. Sertoli cells are columnar cells connected to the basement membrane of tubules with cytoplasmic projections. They surround and support the germinal cells.

When the seminiferous tubules reach the apex of the lobules, they become less coiled, assume an almost straight configuration, and join to form 20–30 tubules of 0.5 mm in diameter—the *tubuli recti*. At the hilum of the testis they form the *rete testis*, which is divided into three components: septal, mediastinal,

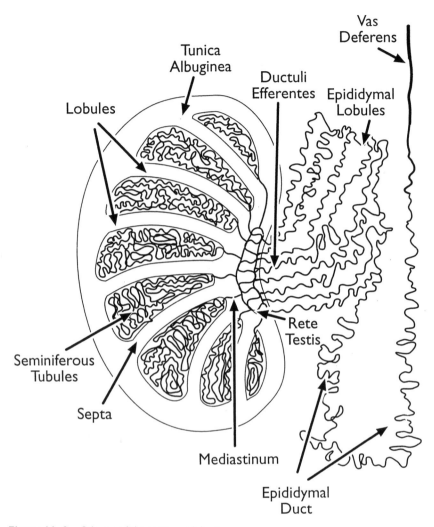

Figure 11–9. Schema of the testis epididymis

and tunical. These structures continue into the *ductuli efferentes,* which perforate the tunica albuginea, leave the testis, and reach the epididymis. The tubules in the head of the epididymis are convoluted and enlarged and constitute the epididymal lobules. These 15- to 20-cm long tubules merge into each other and become a single duct in the body and the tail of the organ. The coil is held together by fibrous tissue and continues into the deferens duct.

The epididymal epithelium is composed of three types of cells. Tall columnar, or *principal* cells have prominent cilia at the luminal end. Their function is to absorb water and secrete glycoproteins necessary for sperm maturation. The basal cells are reserve cells located between the principal cells and the basement membrane. Occasionally, columnar cells with clear cytoplasm rich in lipid droplets called the clear cells are interspersed among the other two types.

The epididymal wall is composed of a thick muscular layer that receives adrenergic innervation. This innervation is more prominent in the body and the tail, which explains why the ductules and the proximal portion of the epididymus contract slowly compared with the rapid reflex contraction of its distal portion and the vas deferens.

Spermatogenesis

The development and growth of the testes occur in three major phases. The first is static, from birth to 4 years. During this phase, seminiferous tubules filled with undifferentiated cells remain the major figures whereas the interstitial Leydig cells become hard to recognize. The second phase occurs from age 4 to 10 years and is characterized by progressive, slow growth of the seminiferous tubules, which become more tortuous and start to form a lumen. The third phase is characterized by progressive maturation of the tubules and interstitium under the influence of gonadotropins and 17-ketosteroids. Between 11 and 12 years of age mitotic activity increases and spermatid and fully developed spermatozoa appear.

The maturation of each spermatozoa takes place over a period of 70 days. It is characterized by development of the *spermatogonium,* which becomes the primary spermatocyte progressing through stages of meiotic division, including pre-leptotene, leptotene, zygotene, pachytene, and diplotene; then secondary spermatocyte and spermatid; and finally, mature sprematozoum[47] (Fig. 11–10). This maturation occurs along the seminiferous tubule in a sort of helical progression, so upon examination of a cross section of the tubule, all stages may not be present[48] (Fig. 11–11).

Deferent and Ejaculatory Ducts

The paired tubular structures that connect the epididymis with the prostate are called *vas deferens.* They ascend from the tail of the epididymis to the posterior portion of the spermatic cord and enter the abdominal cavity and the pelvis where they join the excretory duct of the seminal vesicles to form the ejaculatory duct. The vas deferens is lined by nonciliated columnar epithelium with secretory functions. This mucosa is surrounded by a thick muscular layer.[45]

Prostate

The prostate is a pear-shaped glandular organ about $4.0 \times 2.0 \times 3.0$ cm in size and weighs 20 g. It is located in the pelvis, between the bony pubic symphysis

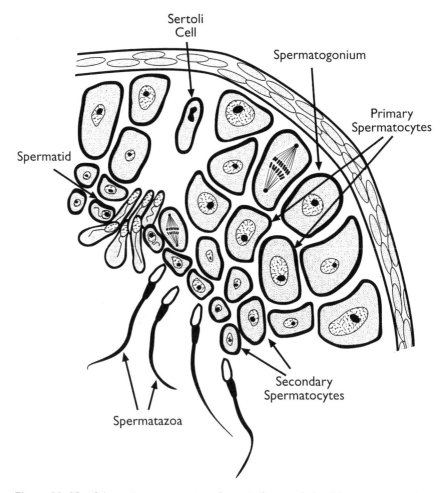

Figure 11–10. Schematic representation of a seminiferous tubule with spermatogenesis

and the rectum.[9] Its development and growth are under the influence of androgenic hormones. The function of the prostate is to expel glandular secretions into the urethra and to expand the content of the seminal fluid (3–5 ml) during sexual excitement and before ejaculation.

The base of the prostate is in direct contact with the neck of the bladder, and it is here that the urethra enters the prostate. At the top, the prostate is penetrated by two ejaculatory ducts. The prostate is anchored anteriorly to the pubis by the pub-prostatic ligament and is surrounded by a fibrous muscular layer referred to as the *capsule*. Strands of fibrous tissue divide the glandular component into different parts. Traditionally, it has been divided into anterior, middle, posterior, and two lateral lobes. More recently, this organ has been subdivided into an inner (periuretheral) region, where nodular hyperplasia or benign pro-

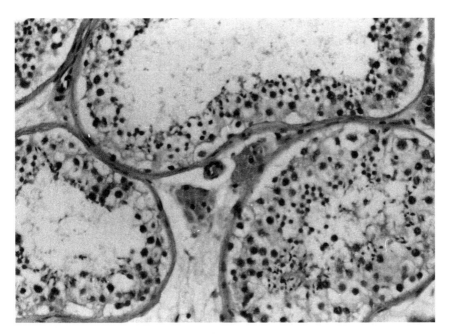

Figure 11–11. Seminiferous tubules. Cross section of seminiferous tubules with different stages of spermatogenesis interposed among clusters of Leydig cells. These large cells are characterized by abundant eosinophilic cytoplasm. Hematoxylin eosin, × 20

static hypertrophy (BPH) develops, and an outer (cortical) region, the site of origin for prostatic cancers.

The blood supply of the prostate comes from branches of the internal pudendal, inferior vescical, and middle rectal arteries. Blood from the prostate drains into the internal iliac vein. The lymphatic system drains into the pelvic lymph nodes and from there into the retroperitoneal chain. The prostate receives innervation by the prostatic nerve, a branch of the hypogastric plexus.[49]

Histologically, the prostate consists of glandular tissue that is supported by a fibrous vascular network derived from the capsule. The prostatic stroma is mainly composed of smooth muscles.[50] The glands consist of convoluted acini characterized by frequent papillary projections and large ducts. The lumens contain dense protein secretions called *amyloid bodies.*[51]

Secretory, basal, and rare neuroendocrine cells are present in both acini and ducts. The acini are lined by columnar secretory cells that produce glycoproteins called Prostatic-specific antigen (PSA) and acid phosphatase (PAP). These two products are useful as diagnostic tools because of their organ-related specificity. In addition, the lining cells have androgen receptors.[52–54] The secretory cells are separated from the basement membrane by a thin, continuous layer of cuboidal cells called basal cells. They are equivalent to the myoepithelial cells of the lobules of the breast and are considered reserve cells. The third group of cells present in the prostate are neuroendocrine cells, which can express neurotransmitters such as chromogranin A and B, serotonin, somostatin, calcitonin, and bombesin.[55]

The larger prostatic ducts open into the prostatic sinuses in the floor of the prostatic urethra; the epithelium is bistratified and continues indistinctly into transitional epithelium of the prostatic urethra. This configuration is similar to that of the bladder epithelium except that umbrella cells are present only in the latter. Areas of squamous metaplasia can be seen, particularly after estrogen therapy for prostatic carcinoma.[56]

Seminal Vesicles

The two seminal vesicles are pyramidal, 5-cm long organs located between the bladder and the rectum above the prostate. They consist of two coiled tubular structures of 3–4 mm in diameter. They connect with the vas deferens and with it they form the ejaculatory duct.[57]

The wall of the seminal vesicles is composed of three layers: the external layer is composed of connective tissue, the middle consists of two layers of muscular fibers, and the final layer is the internal mucosa. The mucosa is formed by columnar epithelium and goblet cells responsible for the secretion of important components of the seminal fluid (i.e., water, fructose, potassium ions, prostaglandin). Secretory function is controlled by the level of testosterone and its activity is controlled by nerves of the pelvic plexus.

The function of the seminal vesicle is not the storage of spermatozoa but rather the control of maturation (capacitation) and motility of the sperm. During puberty, the seminal vesicles form a functional unit with the vas deferens and ejaculatory ducts that produces 70% of the seminal fluid. This fluid, derived from the seminal vesicles, also has an immunosuppressive function in the female genital tract, which favors the survival of semen.

Penis

The penis is the male copulatory organ and consists of a root *(radix)* and a shaft *(corpus)* and is covered by the *glans* and foreskin *(prepuce)*. The radix and the corpus are composed of erectile tissue, the *crura* and *bulb;* these continue into the *corpora cavernosa* and *corpus spongiosum,* respectively.[9,58] The erection of the penis results from the rapid inflow of blood that fills the cavernous spaces and increases the pressure of the veins draining the spongy tissue.

The crura penis is attached to the ischiopubic ramus of the pubis, while the bulb is firmly attached to the perineal membrane. The bulb has an oval shape and is traversed by the urethra.The corpus of the penis has a cylindrical shape when flaccid but becomes triangular in section during erection. The erectile tissue of the corpora cavernosa and corpus spongiosum are surrounded by the tunica albuginea, which is composed of fibrous tissue.

All of these erectile structures are covered by a smooth, discontinuous muscle, the *dartos,* and an elastic sheath, known as Buck's fascia, which divides the penis into ventral and dorsal sections. The glans penis is an extension of the corpus spongiosum, which reflects posteriorly over the corpora cavernosa. The glans and the corpus forms the *balanopreputial sulcus*, which contains modified sebaceous glands and ends in the *frenulus*.[59]

In men, the urethra is divided into three segments: the prostatic urethra (traversing the prostate gland), the membranous or bulbomembranous segment (from the apex of the prostate to the bulb), and the penile segment, which runs through the corpus cavernosum. The distal portion enlarges to form the *fossa navicularis*. The epithelium of the prostatic urethra is transitional then is ciliated columnar and becomes stratified squamous at the fossa navicularis. The penile urethra appears to secrete IgA and is thus active in the immune response. The presence of many IgA-positive plasma cells has been demonstrated.[60]

Scrotum and Spermatic Cord

The scrotum is a fibromuscular sac containing the testes, adnexa, and distal spermatic cord and is suspended from the bony pubic symphysis. The wall of the scrotum consists of seven layers: the epidermis and dermis (pigmented, hair-bearing, and containing sebaceous and sweat glands), the dartos muscle (composed of smooth muscle), the Colles' fascia, which consists of three layers, and the outer lining of the tunica vaginalis. The scrotum receives its blood supply from the external and internal pudendal arteries. The venous system parallels the arteries. The scrotal lymphatics drain into the ipsilateral superficial inguinal lymph nodes. The innervation of the scrotum comes from branches of the genitofemoral, perineal, and posterior femoral cutaneous nerves.

The spermatic cord extends from the internal abdominal ring to the posterior surface of the testis, passing through the inguinal canal. The left spermatic cord is longer than the right one, which is why the left testis is lower than the right. The spermatic cord contains loose connective tissue (which surrounds the vas deferens), arteries, the convoluted venous pampiniform plexus, lymphatics, and the spermatic nervous plexus.

REFERENCES

1. O'Rahilly R. The timing and sequence of events in the development of the human reproductive system during the embryonic period proper. Acta Embryol 1983;166: 247–261.

2. Jost A, Magre S. Control mechanism of testicular differentiation. Philos Trans R Soc Lond [Biol] 1988;322:55–61.

3. McLaren A. What makes a man a man? Nature 1990;346:216–217.

4. McLaren A. The making of male mice. Nature 1991;351:96.

5. Gubbay J, Collingnon J, Koopman P, et al. A gene mapping to the sex determining region of the mouse Y chromosome is a member of a novel family of embryologically expressed genes. Nature 1990;346:245–250.

6. Koopman P, Gubbay J, Vivian N, et al. Male development of chromosomally female mice transgenic for Sry. Nature 1991;351:117–121.

7. Burgoyne PS, Buehr M, Koopman P, Rossant J. Cell autonomous action of the testis-determining gene: Sertoli cells are exclusively YX in XX-XY chimeric mouse testes. Development 1988;102:443–450.

8. Cate RL, Mattaliano RJ, Hession C, et al. Isolation of bovine and human Müllerian inhibiting substance and expression of the human gene in animal cells. Cell 1986; 45:685–698.

9. Williams PL. Gray's Textbook of Anatomy, 38th ed. New York: Churchill Livingstone, 1995.

10. Blaustein's Pathology of the Female Genital Tract, 4th ed. New York: Springer-Verlag, 1994.

11. Wendell-Smith CP, Wilson PM. The vulva, vagina and urethra and the musculature of the pelvic floor. In: Philipp E, Setchell M, Ginsburg J, eds. Scientific Foundations of Obstetrics and Gynecology. Oxford: Butterworth-Heinemann, 1991.

12. Van der Putte SCJ. Anogenital sweat glands. Histology and pathology of a gland that can mimic mammary glands. Am J Dermopathol 1991;13:557–567.

13. Rorat E, Ferenczy A, Richert RM. Human Bartholin gland, duct and duct cyst. Arch Pathol 1975;99:367–374.

14. Robboy SJ, Prade M, Cunha G. Vagina. Histology for Pathologists. New York: Raven Press, 1992.

15. Koss LG. Diagnostic Cytology and its Histopathologic Bases, 4th ed. Philadelphia: J.B. Lippincott, 1992, p. 1.

16. Rakoff AE. Hormonal cytology in gynecology. Clin Obstet Gynecol 1961; 4:1045.

17. Cunningham FG. Williams Obstetrics, 20th ed. Stamford, CT: Appleton & Lange, 1997.

18. Linde T. Operative Gynecology, 8th ed. Philadelphia: Lippincott-Raven, 1997.

19. Campbell BF, Phipps WR, Nagel TC. Endometrial biopsies during treatment with subcutaneous pulsatile gonadothropin realising hormone and luteal phase human chorionic gonadotropins. Int J Fertil 1988;33:329–333.

20. Mazur MT, Kurman RJ. Diagnosis of Endometrial Biopsies and Curettings. A Practical Approach. New York: Springer-Verlag, 1994.

21. Israel R, Mishell DR Jr, Labudovich M. Mechanisms of normal and dysfuncional uterine bleeding. Clin Obstet Gynecol 1970;13:386–399.

22. Poropatich C, Rojas M, Silverberg SG. Polymorphonuclear leukocytes in the endometrium during the normal menstrual cycle. Int J Gynecol Pathol 1987;6:230–234.

23. Bulmer JN, Lunny DP, Hagin SV. Immunohistochemical characterization of stromal leukocytes in non-pregnant human endometrium. Am J Reprod Immunol Microb 1988;17:83–90.

24. Ehrmann RL. Histologic dating of the endometrium. J Reprod Med 1969;3: 179–200.

25. Chambers JT, Chambers SK. Endometrial sampling. When? Where? Why? With what? Clin Obstet Gynecol 1992;35:28–39.

26. Malecha MJ, Miettinen M. Patterns of keratin subsets in normal and abnormal uterine cervical tissues. An immunohistochemical study. Int J Gynaecol Pathol 1992;11:24–29.

27. Koss LG. The Papanicolaou test for cervical cancer detection. A triumph and a tragedy. JAMA 1989;261:737–743.

28. Koss LG. Cervical (Pap) smear. New directions. Cancer 1993;71:1406–1412.

29. Kurman RJ, Malkasian GD Jr, Sedlis A. From Papanicolou to Bethesda. The rationale for a new cervical cytologic classification. Obstet Gynecol 1991;77:779–782.

30. Luff RD. The Bethesda System for reporting cervical-vaginal cytologic diagnoses. Report of the 1991 Bethesda Workshop. The Bethesda System Editorial Committee. Hum Pathol 1992;23:719–721.

31. The Bethesda System for reporting cervical-vaginal cytologic diagnoses. Acta Cytol 1993;37:115–124.

32. Wilbur DH, Cibas ES, Meritt S, et al. Thin Prep™ Processor. Clinical trials demonstrate an increased detection rate of abnormal cervical cytologic specimen. Am J Clin Pathol 1994;10:209–214.

33. Settlege DSF, Motoshima M, Tredway DR. Sperm transport from the external cervical os to the fallopian tube in women. A time and quantitation study. Fertil Steril 1973;24:655–661.

34. Coutinho EM, Maia H Jr, Mattos CER. Contractility of the fallopian tube. Gynecol Obstet Invest 1975;6:146–161.

35. Jacobowitz D, Wallach EE. Histochemical and chemical studies of the anatomic innervation of the ovary. Endocrinology 1967;81:1132–1139.

36. Clement PB. Histology of the ovary. Am J Surg Pathol 1987;11:277–303.

37. Fetissof F, Dubois MP, Heitz PU, et al. Endocrine cells in the female genital tract. Int J Gynaecol Pathol 1986;5:75–87.

38. Feinberg R, Cohen RB. A comparative histochemical study of the ovarian stromal lipid band, stromal theca cell, and normal ovarian follicular apparatus. Am J Obstet Gynecol 1965;92:958.

39. Erickson GF. Normal ovarian function. Clinc Obstet Gynecol 1978;21:31.

40. Balboni GC. Structural changes: Ovulation and luteal phase. In: Serra GB, ed. The Ovary. New York: Raven Press, 1983, pp. 123–141.

41. McNatty KP, Smith DM, Makris A, et al. The microenvironment of the human antral fluid, the population of granulosa cells, and the status of the oocyte in vivo and in vitro. J Clin Endocrinol Metab 1979;49:851–860.

42. Visfeldt J, Starup J. Dating of the human corpus luteum of menstruation using histological parameters. Acta Pathol 1974;82:137–144.

43. Johnson L, Petty CS, Neaves WB. The relationship of biopsy evaluations and testicular measurements to overall daily sperm production in human testes. Fertil Steril 1980;34:36–40.

44. Silber SJ, Rodriguez-Rigau LJ. Quantitative analysis of testicular biopsy. Determination of partial obstruction and prediction of sperm count after surgery for obstruction. Fertil Steril 1981;36:480–485.

45. Trainer TD. Testis and excretory duct system. In: Sternberg SS, ed. Histology for Pathologists. New York: Raven Press, 1992, pp. 731–747.

46. Schulze C. Sertoli and Leydig cells in man. Adv Anat Embryol Cell Biol 1984;88:1–104.

47. Dym M. Spermatogonial stem cells in the testis [commentary]. Proc Natl Acad Sci USA 1994;91:11287–11289.

48. Schulze W, Reimer M, Rehder U, et al. Computer-aided three-dimentional re-constructions of the arrangement of primary spertmatocytes in human seminiferous tubules. Cell Tissue Res 1986;244:1–7.

49. Benoit G, Merlaud L, Meduri G, et al. Anatomy of the prostatic nerves. Surg Radiol Anat 1994;16:23–29.

50. Cunha GR. Role of mesenchimal-epithelial interaction in normal and abnormal development of the mammary gland and prostate. Cancer 1994;74:1030–1044.

51. McNeal JE. Normal histology of the prostate. Am J Surg Pathol 1988;12: 619–633.

52. Bonkhoff H, Remberger K. Androgen receptor status in endocrine-paracrine cell type of the normal, hyperplastic, and neoplastic human prostate. Virchows Arch 1993;423(4):291–294.

53. Bonkhoff H, Stein U, Remberger K. Multidirectional differentiation in the nor-mal, hyperplastic and neoplastic human prostate: A simultaneous determination of cell-specific epithelial markers. Hum Pathol 1994;25:42–46.

54. Allsbrook WC Jr, Simms WW. Histochemistry of the prostate. Hum Pathol 1992;23:297–305.

55. Schmis KW, Helpap B, Totschn M, et al. Immunohistochemical localization of chromogranin A and B and secretogranin II in normal, hyperplastic and neoplastic pros-tate. Histopathology 1994;24:233–239.

56. Lager DJ, Goeken JA, Kemp JD, et al. Squamous metaplasia of the prostate. An immunohistochemical study. Am J Clin Pathol 1988;90:597–601.

57. Aumuller G, Riva A. Morphology and functions of the human seminal vesicle. Andrologia 1992;24:183–196.

58. Hricak H, Marotti M, Gilbert TJ, et al. Normal penile anatomy and abnormal penile conditions. Evaluation with MR imaging. Radiology 1988;169:683–690.

59. Barretto J, Caballero C, Cubilla A. Penis. In: Sternberg SS, ed. Histology for Pathologists. New York: Raven Press, 1992, pp. 721–730.

60. Pudney J, Anderson DJ. Immunobiology of the human penile urethra. Am J Pathol 1995;147:155–165.

12

BASIC PRINCIPLES OF IMMUNOLOGY AND GENITAL TRACT IMMUNITY

Peggy A. Crowley-Nowick

This chapter provides an introduction to the basic concepts of immunology and immunity in the reproductive tract of women. Immunology is a complex field, and our understanding of the intricate mechanisms used by the immune system to protect individuals from the massive onslaught of pathogens in our environment expands each day. Therefore, it is impossible to cover all aspects of immunity in a single chapter. This chapter is meant only to be an overview of a field that is reviewed in more detail elsewhere.[1,2] To simplify the immunologic concepts, it is divided into four sections: *(1)* antigens; *(2)* the humoral and cellular aspects of innate immunity; *(3)* the humoral and cellular factors of adaptive immunity; and *(4)* immunology of the female genital tract.

ANTIGENS

In order to initiate an immune response, the immune system must recognize a foreign substance called an antigen. An *antigen* is any substance that may be specifically bound by an antibody molecule. It can be any type of protein or biologic molecule including sugars, lipids, hormones, as well as macromolecules such as complex carbohydrates, phospholipids, and nucleic acids. However, a large molecule is usually required to initiate the immune response. After the immune response has started, small pieces of the macromolecule can be recognized and bound by an antibody. An antibody binds to a specific portion of the macromolecule called the determinant (or epitope). Antigens come in all shapes and sizes. Viruses and bacteria express many proteins and DNA molecules that are recognized as antigens by the immune system.

In addition to foreign antigens, every human cell has specific antigens expressed on the cell surface called human leukocyte antigens (HLA) or major histocompatibility complex (MHC) in the mouse. These antigens are unique to each individual person yet are the same in identical twins. Although they are called antigens, the individual's immune cells do not recognize them as foreign. The immune system has developed a mechanism to teach immune cells the difference between self and non-self. This is a mechanism of learning that is critical to prevent autoimmunity. However, if a virus infects human cells, those cells become altered and the normal HLA molecules on the cell surface are then recognized as foreign.

It is possible to transplant a liver from one mouse into another mouse of the same strain and the immune system will not recognize that as foreign because all the MHC antigens are the same among animals of a single strain of inbred mice. Humans are not inbred, so each individual has a unique set of proteins expressed on the surface of their cells. A transplant of a liver from one person to the next cannot occur unless the HLA antigens are matched from the donor to the recipient to prevent the immune system from recognizing that liver as foreign. This is the concept of transplantation immunology. If a transplantation occurs from one individual to the next without matching surface antigens, an adaptive immune response occurs. The immune system will recognize that liver as foreign and attack, destroying the liver, and in the process, possibly killing the individual.

ADAPTIVE VERSUS INNATE IMMUNITY

A summary of the most important players in innate and acquired immunity is found in Figure 12–1. This figure separates the humoral and cellular aspects of acquired and innate immunity into their respective components. Although the individual components interact extensively to prevent an infection, there are several basic concepts that make innate immunity unique from acquired immunity.

Innate immunity is the first line of defense designed to stop pathogens before infection is established. The characteristic feature of innate immunity is the lack of memory for an antigen upon second exposure. This type of immunity is primarily represented as a barrier form of protection. In comparison, acquired immunity is specific immunity developed against particular antigens. The main feature of adaptive immunity is the memory response that allows for a rapid and intense immune response when an antigen is encountered a second time. The most important fact about the adaptive immune system is the ability of this system to recognize self versus non-self.

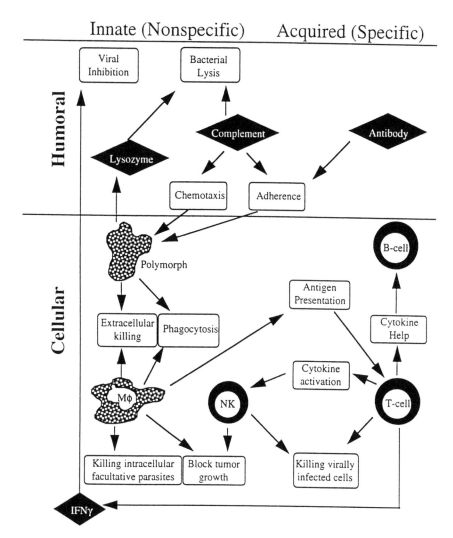

Figure 12–1. Summary of the humoral and cellular components of innate and acquired immunity and how the two types of immunity interact with each other [adapted from Roitt, 1994[1]].

Humoral Systems of Innate Immunity

The innate system is a barrier form of protection comprised of enzymes, acids, and mechanical mechanisms to prevent infection. The primary sites of pathogen invasion are all protected by components of the innate immune system. The most significant barrier is skin. The multilayers of epithelial cells that form skin act as an impressive barrier to invasion. A break in the skin such as an abrasion or burn compromises the innate barrier and increases the potential for infection. The mucosal surfaces are also potential sites of invasion. They are protected by multiple innate factors in the mucosal secretions. Lysozyme is an important enzyme found in most mucosal secretions whose function is to split bonds in the cell wall of many types of bacteria, therefore killing the bacteria before the adaptive immune system even recognizes an invasion has occurred. Mucins secreted at the cervix, lungs, and gut form a mechanical barrier to an invasion by capturing the pathogens. The pH of secretions in the stomach and vagina act in a bacteriostatic manner to prevent infection. These all represent examples of the humoral components of the innate immune system.

The complement system is also considered part of humoral innate immunity. Complement is a group of 20 serum proteins that work together to eliminate microorganisms. Although the proteins are part of the innate immune system, complement crosses the barrier between innate immunity and the adaptive immune system. Production of complement is spontaneously activated by the invasion of microorganisms. The three main functions of complement are to directly lyse microorganisms, induce chemotaxis (directed movement) of immune cells from both the adaptive and innate immune systems into the area where the microorganisms have invaded, and to opsonize, or coat, the microorganisms, making them more susceptible to phagocytosis by the immune cells. Although the three main functions of complement are innate in nature, they are essential for the triggering of the adaptive immune system.

Cellular Systems of Innate Immunity

Phagocytes, including macrophages and polymorphonuclear neutrophils, are cells that are involved with the ingestion and uptake of microbes that have evaded the mechanical barriers of the innate immune system. Before phagocytosis occurs, the microbe must adhere to the surface of the polymorphonuclear neutrophil, or the macrophage. This contact is enhanced by the process of opsonization, where complement binds to and coats the microbe. Complement receptors on the phagocytes then bind to the microbe, enhancing their ability to engulf the microbes and complete the process of phagocytosis. Alternatively, antibody molecules (humoral adaptive immune factors) may bind to the microbe and the contact is made by specific interactions of receptors for antibody molecules on the phagocytes and the antibody leading to uptake by phagocytes. The function of phagocytes is to engulf, internalize, and destroy the microbes. In the process of doing that, the microbe is destroyed, but pieces of the microbe are expressed on the cell surface of the macrophage. These pieces are antigens (peptides) and are presented to the adaptive immune system in order to initiate an adaptive immune response. Antigen presentation is an essential function of the cellular components of the innate immune system.

The third important cell type in innate immunity is the natural killer (NK) cell. These cells are important immune cells for the destruction of virally infected cells and tumor cells. NK cells are large granular lymphocytes. They have characteristic morphology granules within their cytoplasm that contain enzymes such as perforin and other proteases required for extracellular killing. Although they do not bind in an antigen-specific manner, they do recognize altered cells. By binding to a tumor cell, the NK cell injects its enzymes and induces target cell death. A second mechanism of killing is apoptosis, a mechanism of programmed cell death that causes the very rapid degradation and fragmentation of nuclear material in the cell.

The final innate immune cell population is the eosinophil. These cells have distinct granules that identify them. The granules in the eosinophils have specific enzymes unique from those found in NK cells that allow eosinophils to participate in the destruction of large parasites. In order for an eosinophil to bind to a parasite, complement must first opsonize the parasite, then, in a receptor-mediated fashion, the eosinophils make contact with the parasites and deliver their lethal enzymes.

The combination of physical barriers and cellular components of the innate immune system function together to form the first line of defense against invading pathogens and to initiate an adaptive immune response. Although innate immunity has developed to establish a barrier to infection, opportunistic pathogens have found multiple ways to evade innate immunity, therefore the adaptive immune response is necessary for protection.

ADAPTIVE IMMUNITY

As in the innate immune system, there is both a cellular and a humoral component to the adaptive immune response. The effectors of the humoral arm of the adaptive immune response are antibodies. These are proteins that can bind to antigen, leading to the removal and eventual destruction of the antigen. The cellular component is composed of different types of mononuclear cells. These immune cells are involved in the production of antibody, killing of virally infected cells, and production of cytokines that are responsible for stimulating other lymphocytes. In comparison to innate immunity, adaptive immunity can specifically recognize an antigen as foreign by means of receptors that are specific for individual antigens. The effector cells of adaptive immunity are found among layers of epithelial cells, in the stroma beneath the epithelium, in peripheral blood, and in organized lymphoid tissue such as the thymus, spleen, bone marrow, and lymph nodes, among other locations.

Humoral Systems of Adaptive Immunity

Peripheral blood can be separated into two components—plasma and cells. Plasma, the fluid constituent of blood, contains antibodies, complement, and clotting factors, whereas the cellular component contains all of the immune cells and red blood cells. Antibodies are a class of protein molecules produced by B lymphocytes that are found in plasma or bathing the mucosal surfaces.

Multiple functions have been defined for each specific antibody, yet each antibody molecule is specific for only one antigen. Neutralization of viruses and toxins is a major function of antibody. In addition, binding of antibody to an antigen such as a microbe enhances activity of macrophages and polymorphonuclear neutrophils. Both macrophages and polymorphonuclear neutrophils have constant fragment (Fc) receptors specific for the constant region of the antibody molecule. Antibody molecules also activate complement so that it can perform its functions of lysis, chemotaxis induction, or opsonization. The functions of antibodies demonstrate the continuing cross talk between the innate and adaptive immune systems.

Antibodies consist of amino acids with carbohydrates attached and have a structure typically depicted as a Y shape (Fig. 12–2). Structurally, the Y shape is important because it separates the antigen-binding portion of the molecule from the effector function of the molecule. An antibody is produced with two heavy molecular weight protein chains and two light protein chains held together by disulfide bonds. The amino terminal portion of the molecule, signified with an N in Figure 12–2, is the antigen binding portion of the molecule. This is an area of hypervariable amino acid composition, indicating that the antigen-binding sequence is very different from one specific antibody molecule to the next. The variability allows for significant diversity in the types of antigens that can be bound by each antibody. This structure creates two antigen-binding sites for

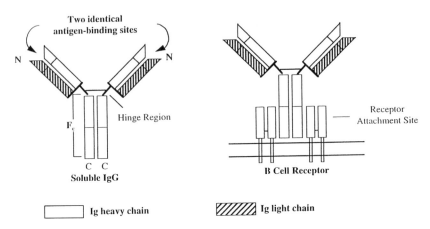

Figure 12–2. This cartoon represents the structure of a soluble IgG molecule and a membrane-bound IgG molecule with the B cell receptor. The figure is meant to represent the structural conformation of the heavy and light chain of the immunoglobulin molecule as it is held together by disulfide bonds.

each molecule and allows for cross-linking of antigens, which is critical for agglutinating antigens so that they may be taken up and removed by the innate immune system. The carboxy terminal end, designated with a *C* in Figure 12–2, is the effector end of the molecule. This is called the constant region, also known as the constant fragment (Fc). In this portion of the molecule there are very few changes in amino acids from one molecule to the next. The changes are limited and the amino acid structure can be separated into five different Fc regions that define the five isotopes of immunoglobulins. The Fc region is important because the function of each isotype is defined by this portion of the molecule. In addition to the antigen-binding site and the effector site of the molecule is a hinge region. This is the area where the light chain and heavy chain are joined together by disulfide bonds. The hinge allows for movement and bending of the molecule so that it has flexibility to bind multiple antigens.

The antibody molecule has two forms—a soluble and a membrane-bound form (Fig. 12–2). The soluble form has the Y structure and is detected in plasma or mucosal secretions. The membrane-bound form of antibody serves as a receptor on B lymphocytes and is identical to the structure of secreted antibody, except for a few additional amino acids in the Fc region. B lymphocytes are cells that have the potential to make antibody.

Only five different constant regions are produced by plasma cells even though there is an unlimited number of hypervariable regions. The five types of immunoglobulin are defined as α, γ, μ, ε, and δ; Table 12–1 summarizes the functions of these molecules. The different isotopes of immunoglobulin, IgA, IgG, IgM, IgE, can each be differentiated by function, concentration, and molecular structure.

IgM is produced and secreted during the first exposure to antigen in a primary immune response. Structurally, IgM is a pentamer structure consisting of five Y-shaped molecules attached by a protein-joining chain. The attachment of these five molecules occurs at the constant region of the molecule, therefore

Table 12–1. Properties of Immunoglobulin Isotypes

IMMUNOGLOBULIN	IgM	IgG	IgA	IgE	IgD
Primary Ag exposure	+	−	−	−	−
Secondary Ag exposure	+/1	+	+		
Concentrations mg/ml	1.2	10	2	0.03	.0005
Allergies	−	−	−	+	−
Placental transfer	−	+	−	−	−
Complement fixation	+	+	−	−	−
Molecular form	Pentamer	Monomer, dimer, polymer	Monomer	Monomer	Monomer

freeing the antigen-binding end of the molecules and resulting in ten antigen binding sites.

IgG is produced in significant concentrations after the second exposure of the immune system to antigen. In plasma, it is the most abundant immunoglobulin, and structurally it is present as a monomeric molecule (single Y-shaped molecule). IgG activates complement and therefore is a potent immunoglobulin molecule for clearance of pathogens. It is also transferred across the placenta and participates in passive immune protection of newborn infants.

IgA protects the mucosal surfaces of the gut, lungs, genital tract, and oral cavity, and it is the second most abundant immunoglobulin in serum. Unlike IgG or IgM, IgA is found in multiple molecular forms. In plasma it is predominantly a monomer, but in secretions it can exist as either a dimer (two attached molecules) or a polymer (multiple attached molecules). The constant region of IgA does not activate complement, which is important because of its function at the mucosal surfaces. These are sensitive sites where a massive immune response could induce destruction of normal healthy tissue in the process of killing the pathogen if complement were activated. The inability of IgA to activate complement is a regulatory mechanism of the immune response. However, IgA is quite capable of eliminating pathogens or antigens because of the multiple binding sites, yet in a less pathogenic manner. IgA is also passed from mother to infant in breast milk and is important for early protection of infants.

In an immune response, the humoral effector molecules, i.e., antibodies, are produced in a specific pattern depending on the timing of antigen exposure. Primary exposure to antigen usually results in a minimal immune response. IgM is the first antibody isotype produced, then the protein machinery switches within the B cell, resulting in the production of IgG. The time frame for generation of an IgG response is approximately 7 days after a primary exposure. In a secondary immune response, when the immune system is exposed to antigen the second time, IgG is produced in significant quantities within 48 hours after exposure, and IgM concentrations remain low. The secondary exposure demonstrates the memory response of the adaptive immune system. This aspect of immunity explains how protection is achieved by vaccine administration. Vaccines are designed to mimic the actual pathogen and initiate the primary antigen exposure, priming the immune system prior to exposure of the actual pathogen. The reason for the massive secondary response is called the theory of clonal selection and is related to the cellular arm of adaptive immunity (see below).

Cellular Systems of Adaptive Immunity

B lymphocytes (B cells) are immune cells that express an antigen-binding receptor on their cell surface. The receptor is the membrane-bound form of antibody molecules. After antigen combines with the B cell receptor, it induces maturation of the B cell into a plasma cell or a factory for antibody production. Upon binding and cross-linking of these surface antibody receptors and under the influence of specific cytokines or growth factors in the local environment, the cells are induced to proliferate and then differentiate into the plasma cells. Plasma cells do not make plasma, they secrete antibody molecules. Plasma cells no longer express antibody on the cell surface, but they produce and secrete large quantities of specific antibody. Although there are different types of immunoglobulin, each plasma cell secretes only one type of antibody and it is very specific for one antigen. The process of proliferation and differentiation leads to expansion of cellular clones producing specific antibody. This expansion is known as the theory of clonal selection, an essential concept of immunology, and is summarized in Figure 12–3. Essentially, each B cell is programmed to make one antibody and each B cell has a different antigen-binding receptor.

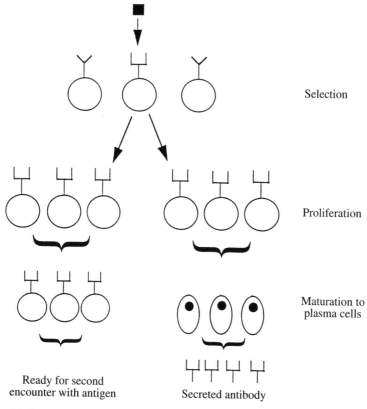

Selection

Proliferation

Maturation to plasma cells

Ready for second encounter with antigen

Secreted antibody

Figure 12–3. Summary of clonal selection. Of the multiple clones available, one antigen fits the antigen receptor on a single B cell. The binding of that antigen leads to cellular proliferation. Some of these new B cell clones will mature to become plasma cells and secrete antibody or will remain as memory B cells, in preparation for a second encounter with antigen.

When that receptor binds antigen, the cells proliferate massively. Some of those cells mature and differentiate and become plasma cells. A portion of those cells remain as memory B cells; now they are ready for a second exposure to the specific antigen. Therefore, on secondary exposure a larger number of B cells are present with the specific antigen receptor on their cell surface and are prepared for antigen encounter. When antigen is encountered again, all of those B cells can be triggered to proliferate and repeat the process.

T lymphocytes (T cell) do not have antibody on their cell surface. However, they do express their own unique antigen-binding receptor, the T cell receptor. Unlike B cells, the T cells do not mature and secrete T cell receptors. In addition to the differences in the antigen-binding receptor, there are other points that distinguish T cells from B cells. T cells do not recognize whole antigen in a soluble form. Whereas B cells recognize free antigen, a T cell is required to recognize a small piece of antigen called a peptide that must be presented in a unique form on the cell surface of antigen-presenting cells. The antigen-presenting molecules are the HLA antigens introduced earlier in this chapter. In order for a T cell to recognize the peptide, it must be expressed on the cell surface in the presence of HLA antigens.

Two types of major histocompatibility antigens, MHC class I and MHC class II, are important for adaptive immunity. MHC is the designation used for the mouse system, whereas in humans, the HLA class I and class II designation defines the same antigens on human cells. HLA class I antigens are found on all nucleated cells. HLA class II antigens are only expressed on specialized antigen-presenting cells such as macrophages, Langerhans cells, and some epithelial cells. HLA antigens actually act like a hand holding a pencil out on the surface of the cell. The peptide (the pencil) fits nicely into a cleft on the HLA antigen (hand) and is tightly bound yet exposed on the cell surface. This structure is designed to allow the T cell receptors to make contact and bind to the antigen. If HLA antigens are not holding the peptide, a T cell cannot recognize the peptide as foreign.

In addition to the two types of HLA antigens, there are two subpopulations of T cells that are restricted in their capacity to recognize antigen based on the type of HLA molecule presenting the antigen. T helper and T cytotoxic cells can be identified by their HLA restriction or function, or by surface marker expression (Fig. 12–4). T helper cells are defined by the expression of a marker on their cell surface called CD4, and T cytotoxic cells are defined by a marker on their cell surface called CD8. As the names state, CD4+ T helper cells provide help to the immune system. After binding peptide in HLA class II antigens, these cells secrete cytokines that are critical for proliferation and maturation of B cells and other cytokines that stimulate T cytotoxic cell function. Alternatively, CD8+ T cytotoxic cells kill viral infected cells and tumor cells. Their method of killing is similar to NK cells in the innate immune system, but T cy-

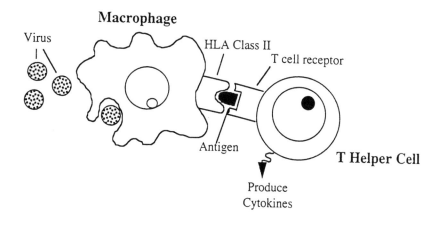

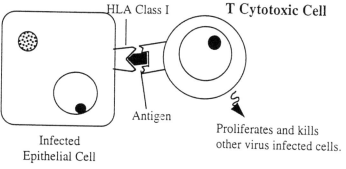

Figure 12–4. Binding of antigen by T cells. T helper cells can only recognize antigen when it is presented on class II HLA antigens, and cytotoxic cells can only recognize antigen when presented in HLA class I antigens. The binding of antigens for T helper cells leads to the production of cytokines used to help in other immunologic responses. The binding of a T cytotoxic cell leads to proliferation and killing of virus-infected cells.

totoxic cells perform their function in an antigen specific manner, triggered by binding of the T cell receptor to peptide antigens in HLA class I molecules.

The ratio of these two cell types is important in defining changes in disease states. For example, in HIV infection, the definition of AIDS is partly based on the level of CD4 cells that are still present in the individual or by the ratio of CD4 to CD8 cells. In HIV infection, the number of CD4+ cells decline as disease progresses, meaning that the number of T helper cells decreases. With their decline, the host becomes immunocompromised because the appropriate help signals are not sent to B lymphocytes or T cytotoxic cells when an antigen is encountered.

Phagocytes are antigen-presenting cells that engulf microbes or soluble antigens. Once the antigens are inside of the phagocytes, they are processed, chopped up, and cleaved into small pieces (peptides). Inside the cell, the peptides become bound to HLA class II, which is then expressed on the surface of the phagocyte and can stimulate T helper cells. Alternatively, T cytotoxic cells recognize other cells that are altered in such a way that they no longer represent self. This explanation is known as the altered self hypothesis. For example, T cytotoxic cells recognize tumor cells because these are altered cells. As normal cells go through the carcinogenic process, unique proteins are produced and expressed on the cell surface in conjunction with HLA class I. These proteins are recognized as foreign by CD8+ T cytotoxic cells (Fig. 12–4). A second example is provided by virally infected cells that express viral antigens on the cell surface in class I antigens. The self HLA antigens that are present on all nucleated cells become altered by the virus and therefore, T cytotoxic cells recognize the changes in self. T cytotoxic cells function by binding to the altered cell through the T cell receptor and then inducing cell death by apoptosis.

Both T helper and T cytotoxic cells produce growth factors or cytokines that are critical for the growth, differentiation, and regulation of immunity. At one time, it was thought that cytokines, called lymphokines, were produced only by lymphocytes. It is now known that all cell types produce some type of growth factors. These factors are small peptides that function in a way similar to hormones but act locally and are critical to the regulation of cell growth and differentiation. For a review of the different types of cytokines and their functions, see the R and D Systems Catalog.[3] At this time, there are over 20 different types of cytokines that have been characterized and designated as interleukin-1 (IL-1) through interleukin-20 (IL-20). In addition to the interleukins, there are also a number of other growth factors that have different designations. Currently, an intense area of research is the regulation of cytokine secretion and function, because the regulatory functions of these molecules make them critical for disease elimination or progression. Both T and B cells are triggered to produce certain cytokines when their receptors make contact with antigen. T cytotoxic cells can kill by contact as described, or alternatively, they may produce cytokines that mediate lysis of the altered cells. Two in particular are called tumor necrosis factor α (TNF-α) and interferon γ (IFN-γ). Both of these T cytotoxic cell products have direct killing activity. Control of the immune system appears to be regulated by production of what is known as TH1- or TH2-type cytokines, which are produced and secreted by T helper lymphocytes. TH2-type cytokines push the immune response toward production of antibody, whereas TH1-type cytokines push the immune system towards induction of a T cell–mediated immune response, including phagocytes, T cytotoxic cell, and NK cell activation. TH2-type cytokines are IL-4, IL-5, IL-10, and IL-13. TH1-type cytokines are IL-2, IFN-γ, and TNF-α (Figs. 12–5, 12–6).

TH2-type cytokines have very specific functions that enhance production of antibody. IL-5 is important for the proliferation of B cells. IL-6 and IL-10 are critical for the terminal differentiation of B cells into plasma cells for the production and secretion of antibody. IL-10 also inhibits the secretion of TH1-type cytokines, thereby participating in a feedback mechanism regulating the TH1/TH2 responses (Fig. 12–5). For activation of cellular immunity, TH1 cytokines IL-2 and IFN-γ stimulate T cytotoxic lymphocytes and NK cells, again demonstrating the integration of both the adaptive and innate immune systems (Fig. 12–6).

Cytokines are involved in the fine-tuning of the immune response. The intricate cross talk between the different cytokines and the delicate balance of concentrations are critical for maintaining proper health and the ability to mount appropriate immune responses against invading pathogens. Just as pathogens have developed mechanisms to evade the innate immune system, they have also evolved mechanisms to alter the appropriate synthesis of cytokines by the host immune response to evade the adaptive immune response. Viruses and bacteria can take advantage of the fine-tuning of the immune system with cytokine production in order to trick the system and avoid detection. If a virus infects a cell, the only way an immune system can detect the presence of the virus and eliminate it is to produce a T cytotoxic lymphocyte response that can kill that virally infected cell. Therefore, TH1-type cytokines must be produced in order to stimulate T cytotoxic cells. It would be an advantage to the virus if it could fool the immune system into producing antibody and to shut off T cytotoxic lymphocytes. IL-10 is known to shut down the T cytotoxic response. Epstein Barr virus (EBV) is an example of a virus that takes advantage

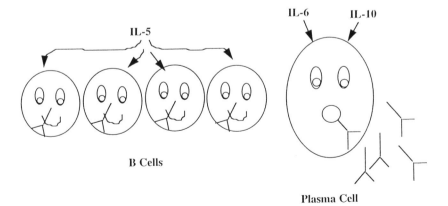

Figure 12–5. Role of cytokines in the development of plasma cells. IL-5 is critical for proliferation of B cells, whereas IL-6 and IL-10 are important for the maturation and differentiation of B cells into plasma cells secreting antibody.

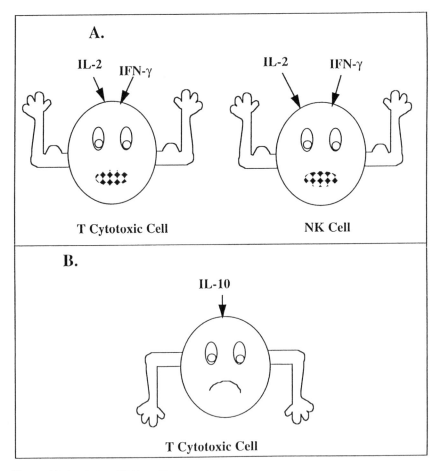

Figure 12–6. Role of TH1 and TH2 cytokines in regulation of cellular immunity. TH1-type cytokines, IL-2 and IFN-γ, activate T cytotoxic cells and NK cells, **(A)** whereas IL-10 down-regulates the cytotoxic cell response **(B)**.

of this mechanism. EBV produces a molecule very similar to IL-10 and shuts down a TH1-type response in the cytotoxic T lymphocytes that could potentially kill the virally infected cells.

PATHOGEN SURVIVAL STRATEGIES

For bacteria, a common mechanism of escape from phagocytosis is the synthesis of an outer capsule that does not adhere readily to phagocytic cells and covers carbohydrate molecules on the bacterial surface that would otherwise be recognized by phagocytic receptors. An example of this would be an encapsulated pneumococci. Genetic variation is another strategy that pathogens use to avoid detection by the adaptive immune response. By varying their surface antigen, they avoid a host antibody response. Influenza and HIV are two examples of viruses that use this mechanism to avoid detection. Some strains of bacteria, such as tubercle, leprosy bacilli, listeria, and brucella organisms, escape detection of the immune system by establishing an intracellular infection within macrophages, thus avoiding the antigen presentation phase and hiding from the immune system. The bacteria are phagocytized by macrophages, but once inside, they are not degraded through the normal mechanisms. Instead they actually continue to replicate within the macrophage and antigens from the bacteria are not presented in HLA antigens.

IMMUNE PROTECTION: INTERACTIONS OF INNATE AND ADAPTIVE IMMUNITY

Immunity to a bacteria is dependent in most cases on the cell wall components of the bacteria, and antibody is essential to prevent infection. Actual bacterial destruction requires phagocytic cells. Protection from bacteria includes synthesis of antibody to the bacterial surface antigens, such as fimbria and capsules. The innate immune system can be triggered by the outer layer of the bacteria, initiating the complement cascade. The final process of bacterial elimination is antibody-binding, providing opsonization for phagocyte uptake of bacteria. Inside the phagocytes, enzymes destroy the bacteria and eliminate it. Bacteria can produce toxins that are destructive to the host. Antibodies that neutralize these toxins are usually essential for protection from the sequelae of bacterial infections.

Several different layers of adaptive immune protection exist to prevent viral infection. Initial infection and replication in the epithelium requires protection by IgA and interferon. Interferon (IFN), a cytokine, is a direct inhibitor of viral replication while IgA antibodies can neutralize virus. If the virus becomes systemic, antibody neutralization is essential to prevent further infection. Usually, IgG is important at this stage. However, if the virus avoids the first two phases of protection, a combination of complement, cell-mediated immunity, antibody, and IFN are essential to eliminate viral infection.

A viral infection can lead to several different outcomes. The infection can initiate in an acute phase and, if the virus is cleared, lifelong immunity exists. Alternatively, the acute phase may clear leading to latent existence of the virus or possibly a subclinical infection, as occurs with hepatitis B. Latent infections can continue to recur and cause acute illness, such as that which occurs with herpes simplex virus (HSV) and varicella virus. Alternatively, latent virus can continue to cause a chronic illness, such as measles. With each recurrence of illness, the immune system is fighting to re-establish control and eliminate the viral pathogen or reduce the viral levels below the level of detection by the immune system.

LYMPHOID SYSTEM

Antigen presentation, maturation of immune cells, and the production of anti-bodies or stimulation of T cytotoxic cells all occur within a highly organized system of organs, constituting the lymphoid system. The organs of this system are composed of lymphocytes, epithelial cells, and stromal cells organized into discrete capsulated organs or as an accumulation of diffuse tissue. The lymphoid organs are separated into primary and secondary organs. The primary lymphoid organs are the thymus and bone marrow. The thymus is the site of T cell education, where self versus non-self is learned during the maturation of T cells. In the thymus, T cells are exposed to self HLA antigens. If they react with those antigens, the T cells die. This training results in the elimination of self-re-active T cells and prevents autoimmunity. Bone marrow is the site of B cell lymphopoiesis and the major production site for antibody secreted into the serum. The secondary lymphoid organs, the lymph nodes, tonsils, adenoids, spleen, and Peyer's patch, form the environment for lymphocyte interactions. In these organs, antigen presentation occurs to initiate immune responses.

The movement and homing of immune cells is an important aspect of immunity. Initial maturation and development of lymphocytes occurs in the primary lymphoid organs. The cells then migrate into the circulation and are directed to specific secondary lymphoid organs. In the lymph nodes, interactions occur with antigen and the lymphocytes then leave the lymph nodes and recirculate either to tissue sites or to the bone marrow for the production of antibody. The migration and production of antibody and stimulation of T cells in the systemic immune system is defined by this movement of cells.

MUCOSAL IMMUNITY

The mucosal surfaces of the body combined form the largest surface area in the body. These surfaces are protected by the mucosal immune response, which varies somewhat from the systemic response. Although the mucosal immune system has components and parts of the innate and adaptive immune system already described, differences exist in tissue distribution of cells, the origins of cellular precursors, and the maturation patterns for the immune cells. In addition, the immunoglobulin molecules in external secretions are predominantly polymeric, secretory IgA (s-IgA). These molecules are produced locally, transported by a receptor-mediated pathway through the epithelial cells, and deposited in the external secretions. Therefore, mucosal secretions, unlike serum, which contains predominately IgG and monomeric IgA, have a significant proportion of s-IgA.

The production of s-IgA requires protein expression by two different cell types. Plasma cells are required for production of polymeric IgA, and epithelial cells express the secretory piece. Plasma cells express both IgA and the joining chain and the product secreted by these cells is a combined polymeric IgA molecule (Fig. 12–7). After secretion, polymeric IgA is then bound by a receptor expressed on epithelial cells, called secretory piece. Secretory piece serves as a receptor for the transcytosis of IgA across the epithelial cells. When IgA is secreted out of the epithelial cells, the secretory piece remains attached and this differentiates the secretory IgA from serum IgA (Fig. 12–8).

IgA serves an important role in the protection of mucosal surfaces. The multimeric structure of the molecules has extra antigen-binding sites that lead to a high capacity for viral neutralization and inhibition of microbial adherence. IgA is also resistant to enzymatic proteolysis, which is important in areas with high enzyme content such as the mucosal secretions. In addition, IgA does not activate the complement cascade. This fact is important because the complement cascade initiates a rigorous immune response that may damage healthy bystander cells, and damage on the mucosal surfaces would result in a breakdown of the barrier mechanism required for innate protection.

Unlike the systemic immune system where antigen presentation occurs in the lymph nodes and antibody production in the bone marrow, the mucosal immune system has very specific inductive and effector sites. These inductive sites are areas of lymphoid follicles covered by specialized epithelial cells and are found in the tonsils, colon, lungs, and rectum. In the colon they are called Peyer's patches, which are domes of epithelium covered by M cells. These are specialized antigen-sampling cells that take in antigen, transcytosis the antigen, and deposit it into the lymphoid follicle just below the epithelium. Within the

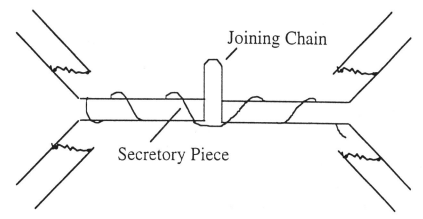

Figure 12–7. Structural representation of secretory IgA molecule demonstrating the structural components as two IgA molecules bound together by a joining chain and the additional secretory piece that is added to the molecule after transcytosis through epithelial cells

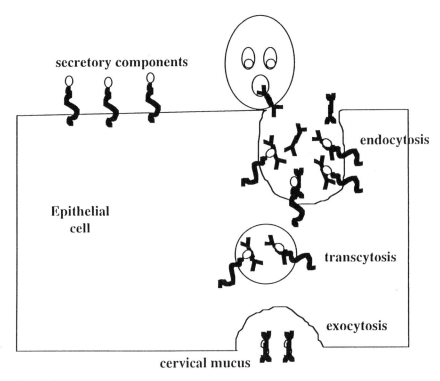

Figure 12–8. Cartoon representing the transcytosis process for secretory IgA

lymphoid follicle there are immature T cells, B cells, dendritic cells, and macrophages, so that antigen presentation can occur locally. After presentation has occurred, these T and B cells circulate to the lymph nodes where they proliferate and mature, re-enter the blood circulation, and home to effector sites, such as the lungs, breast, intestine, and genital tract. At the effector sites B cells undergo final differentiation to plasma cells under the influence of cytokines available in the local environment and begin secreting polymeric IgA. These IgA molecules are bound to the secretory piece on epithelial cells, transcytosed or moved across the epithelial cells, and deposited into the external secretions. This process leads to the protection of all mucosal surfaces. If an antigen is encountered at one inductive site, the stimulated cells will eventually home to all the effector sites, creating the common mucosal immune system.

FEMALE GENITAL TRACT IMMUNITY

The genital tract is considered to be a member of the common mucosal immune system. The components that have been described as essential to the production of secretory IgA are all found within the tissue of the female genital tract. The secretory piece is present on epithelial cells lining the endocervix. A large percentage of plasma cells are located in the stroma beneath the epithelium of the cervix, and the plasma cells consist of both IgA and IgG secreting cells. The IgA plasma cells also produce j-chain, an essential protein for the production of polymeric IgA. The final evidence is provided by the concentrations and structure of immunoglobulins in the lower genital tract. Cervical secretions contain high concentrations of polymeric secretory IgA. The mucosa of the genital tract represents a site with unique characteristics because the immune system must defend against pathogen invasion yet still allow for the deposition of sperm, a foreign antigen, in order for reproduction to occur. In addition to sperm, the system encounters many antigenic sources: both commensals and pathogenic organisms such as bacteria, fungi, and viruses. All of the components necessary for immunity are active in the genital tract.

Studying the human female genital tract is difficult because of a number of problems that are encountered. Unlike serum immunoglobulin concentrations, which remain fairly constant in individuals unless they become infected, immunoglobulin concentrations in genital tract secretions vary throughout the menstrual cycle. In addition to total immunoglobulin concentrations changing, there is also a shift in the subclass of both IgA and IgG that are produced at different phases of the menstrual cycle. These problems are compounded by the constant introduction of foreign products into the vagina and the influence of exogenous hormones. As a result of these complications, very little information is available describing immunity in the human genital tract. Many of the studies describing genital tract immunity have been carried out in rats or mice. Unfortunately, many of the processes described for rats do not correspond directly to humans. To simplify the confusion regarding human versus animal model systems, only information regarding human genital immunity will be presented here. For greater details and information, see references 4–6 for reviews of immunity in the genital tract.

There are several innate protection mechanisms in the genital tract. The squamous epithelium, which is similar to skin, protects the vagina and ectocervix. As part of the innate barriers, cervical mucus, acid pH, and high zinc concentrations function to impede bacterial infection by a mechanical trapping mechanism and an inhibition of replication, respectively. NK cells are also available in the cervical tissue. The adaptive immune system provides both specific antibodies in cervical and vaginal secretions and lymphocytes, such as T helper cells and T cytotoxic cells.

Cellular Components of Genital Tract

Unlike the Peyer's patch described in the gut, the genital tract of women does not have any organized lymphoid tissue or aggregated follicles. However, macrophages and dendritic cells are present in the cervical stroma. These cells are in close contact with T and B cells, indicating the potential for antigen presentation. The predominant lymphocyte population is B cells in a healthy cervix. However, T cells are available and the ratio of CD4+ to CD8+ is 1.0, indicating an equal proportion of T helper and T cytotoxic cells. Changes in this ratio can be seen in disease states or in viral infection of the cervix. An infiltrate of CD8+ cells occurs when women have cervical neoplasia caused by human papillomavirus infection, leading to a significant reduction in the CD4 : CD8 ratio. In addition to T and B cells, a large population of plasma cells is located in the cervix and the density of these cells changes when the cervix is infected. Although infection or disease is the major cause of change in cellular content, changes also occur throughout the menstrual cycle. It has been suggested that these changes occur in response to cycling ovarian hormones.

The Influence of Hormones on Immunity in the Genital Tract

It has been hypothesized that women are more susceptible to infection during particular phases of the menstrual cycle. Anecdotal data suggest that women are more susceptible to chlamydia (and gonococcal) infections during the time of menses and during the proliferative phase, whereas they are less likely to become infected during the secretory phase.[7] The connection between susceptibility to infection and hormonal changes indicates possible changes in immunocompetence occurring throughout the menstrual cycle. During the proliferative phase, serum estradiol concentrations rise steadily while serum progesterone levels remain low. At the time of ovulation, mid-cycle, luteinizing hormone (LH) surges, estradiol levels decline, and progesterone concentrations sharply rise. If pregnancy does not occur, then both estradiol and progesterone levels decrease in the late secretory phase, resulting in menstruation.

Three distinct phases in immunoglobulin concentrations in cervical mucus have also been demonstrated. It has been noted in several studies that a significant drop in the concentration of both IgG and IgA concentration occurs at ovulation.[8-10] However, investigators do not agree when concentrations of IgA peak. Collections during both the end of the secretory phase[11] and the proliferative phase[9] have been noted to have high IgA concentrations. These cyclical changes in IgA levels have also been noted in salivary IgA concentrations, which are highest during the proliferative phase.[12] In studies from the 1970s, women on oral contraceptives were shown to have elevated IgG and IgA concentrations, similar to women with cervical/vaginal infections.[13,14] Modern oral contraceptives have lower concentrations of estrogen and progesterone and raise IgA or IgG approximately four times higher than concentrations found in ovulating women. In addition, cyclic variation in IgA and IgG concentrations is not as great in women on oral contraceptives.

S-IgA concentrations in cervical mucus may be regulated indirectly by hormonal effects on secretory component expression and the migration of IgA+ plasma cells. Free secretory component comprises a major proportion of cervical mucus proteins, and its regulation appears also to be controlled by hormones.[15] The expression of secretory component can directly influence the concentration of IgA present in genital tract secretions.[16,17] Secretory component appears to be increased at mid- and late secretory phase in women.[16] At the same time, epithelial cells containing IgA (in the process of transcytosis) tend to increase compared with that described for the proliferative phase; this leads to the hypothesis that progesterone plays a role in this regulation. Progesterone has also been theorized to influence the migration of plasma cells to the cervix, resulting in increased numbers late in the secretory phase.[11,18] By immunohistochemistry the number of IgA+ lymphocytes present in the cervix during the proliferative phase is similar to that found in women using oral contraceptive pills and during early and late pregnancy.[11]

The mechanism of action by ovarian hormones on immunity has not been defined. Estrogen receptors are not present on B cells, therefore, a direct effect on antibody secretion is unlikely.[19,20] However, the changes in immunoglobulin concentrations and immunocompetence may be related to indirect effects of hormones on other cells involved in antigen processing and presentation, production of cytokines, or the expression of HLA antigens. Expression of estrogen receptors has been demonstrated on CD8+ T cells.[19,20] Therefore, estrogen may have a direct effect on these cells and their production of cytokines. IL-1 and IL-6 are produced by mononuclear cells under the influence of estrogen and may indirectly influence the function of B cells and CD4+ T cells.[21–23] Changes in the concentrations of these cytokines during the menstrual cycle may correlate with changes in the concentration of immunoglobulin present in cervical mucus and regulate immunoglobulin synthesis.

Immunologic Suppression Induced by Semen

A well-characterized phenomenon of genital tract immunity is the lack of immune response generated against allogeneic sperm. Although the vaginal mucosa is an area abundant in lymphatic drainage, indicating a possibility of antigen uptake, immune responses to repeated semen deposition rarely occur.[24] In mice it has been demonstrated that the weight of the draining nodes increases after semen deposition, which suggests that antigen uptake occurs.[25] However, immunosuppressive factors within the seminal plasma appear to abrogate the development of an immune response (for review, see reference 26).

In vitro, seminal plasma has been shown to inhibit T cell/B cell proliferation,[27] eliminate recognition by NK cells and cytotoxic T lymphocytes,[28] and impair phagocytic uptake by macrophages and polymor phonuclear neutrophilic leukocyes (PMNs). In addition, it inhibits the complement cascade, possibly abrogating any response induced by IgG recognition.[29] A number of studies have begun to analyze the factors involved in this specific immunosuppression. The effect of seminal plasma on NK cells appears to be mediated by prostaglandin. Fc-blocking factors are also found in seminal plasma which prevent opsonization, uptake by macrophages, and the development of reactive oxygen species.[30] Seminal plasma also contains a large number of degradative enzymes capable of cleaving immunoglobulins and possibly degrading cytokines.[31] Although semen appears to have significant effects on the immune system, most human studies to date have focused exclusively on the subject of infertility among couples rather than examining susceptibility to infection and suppression of immune status in healthy women outside the subject of fertility.

In addition to the immunosuppressive effects, factors within seminal plasma are also responsible for enhancing the migration of immune cells into the vaginal secretions. Almost immediately after the deposition of sperm, dramatic increases in the number of immune cells can be detected. Within 4 to 6 hours this increase can be measured; within 24 hours, it has already begun to decrease. Phagocytosis of immobilized sperm appears to occur between 12 and 24 hours. An additive effect occurs if sperm is redeposited into the vagina within 60 hours of the last time of intercourse.[32] On the second deposition the cell numbers increase dramatically yet decrease by 24 hours. In Rhesus monkeys the migration of immune cells to the cervix and vagina varies, depending on the phase of the menstrual cycle. There is an increase in cell number in the luteal phase 6 hours postcoitum. However, this response is suppressed at mid-cycle and does not occur in the secretory phase.[33] The majority of the cells found in human postcoital vaginal fluid are PMNs. Approximately 1% represent B and T cells.

The recruitment of T cells and macrophages to the vagina in response to semen deposition represents a potential mode of HIV infection, because mononuclear cells are present in semen. In a small study examining 17 fertile men, a median value of 4.1×10^3 CD4+ T cells/ml of semen was measured.[34] The number of lymphocytes in semen from men with sexually transmitted diseases (STDs) have not been described or quantitated. Prior to the discovery of cell-free HIV transmission, HIV+ T cells in semen were considered the primary mode of HIV transmission. The deposition of HIV-infected cells into an immunosuppressed environment containing host (female) CD4+ T cells and Mφ as potential target cells may enhance this transmission.

At this time, scientists are on the cutting edge of understanding how menstrual cycle hormones can affect the health of women. This information is critical for the development of immunological treatments or prevention strategies for sexually transmitted diseases. As the knowledge of hormone influence increases, this knowledge will be incorporated into clinical vaccine trials, in the hope of achieving the eradication of some STDs.

REFERENCES

1. Roitt I. Essential Immunology. London: Blackwell Scientific Publications, 1994.

2. Abbas AK, Lichtman AH, Pober JS. Cellular and Molecular Immunology. Philadelphia: W.B. Saunders, 1991.

3. R & D Systems Catalog. Minneapolis, MN: West End Games, Inc, 1998.

4. Kutteh WH, Hatch KD, Blackwell RE, Mestecky J. Secretory immune system of the female reproductive tract: I. Immunoglobulin and secretory component containing cells. Obstet Gynecol 1988;71:56–60.

5. Kutteh WH, Kutteh C, Blackwell RE, Carr B, Gorr H, Mestecky J. Secretory immune system of the female reproductive tract. II. Local immune system in normal and infected fallopian tube. Fertil Steril 1990;54:51–55.

6. Wira CR, Sandoe CP. Origin of IgA and IgAG antibodies in the female reproductive tract: Regulation of the genital response by estradiol. Recent advances in mucosal immunology: Part I. In: Mestecky J, ed. Cellular Interactions. New York: Plenum Press, 1986, pp. 403–423.

7. Sweet RL, Blankfort-Doyle M, Robbie MO, Schachter J. Chlamydial salpingitis tends to occur early in the menstrual cycle. JAMA 1986;255:2062–2064.

8. Davis KP, Maciulla GJ, Yannone ME, Gooch GT, Lox CD, Whetstone MR. Cervical mucus immunoglobulins as an indicator of ovulation. Obstet Gynecol 1983;62:388–392.

9. Kutteh WH, Prince SJ, Hammond KR, Kutteh CC, Mestecky J. Variations in immunoglobulins and IgA subclasses of human uterine cervical secretions around the time of ovulation. Clin Exp Immunol 1996;104:538–542.

10. Crowley-Nowick PA, Krasnow J, Kulhavy L, Wolf K, Gooding B, Edwards RP. The influence of progesterone on cervical mucus immunoglobulin and cytokine concentrations. Clinical Immunol Immunopathol 1995;76:541.

11. Murdoch AJM, Buckley CH, Fox H. Hormonal control of the secretory immune system of the human cervix. J Reprod Immunol 1982;4:23–30.

12. Gomez E, Ortiz V, Saint-Martin B, Boeck L, Diaz-Sanchez V, Bourges H. Hormonal regulation of the secretory IgA (sIgA) system: Estradiol- and progesterone-induced changes in sIgA in parotid saliva along the menstrual cycle. Am J Reprod Immunol 1993;29:219–223.

13. Chipperfield EJ, Evans BA. Effect of local infection and oral contraception on immunoglobulin levels in cervical mucus. Infect Immun 1975;11:215–221.

14. Chipperfield EJ, Evans BA. The influence of local infection on immunoglobulin formation in the human endocervix. Clin Exp Immunol 1972;11:219–223.

15. Kooij RJV, Kathmann GAM, Kramer MF. Secretory piece and plasma proteins in human cervical mucus during the cycle. J Reprod Fertil 1983;68:63–68.

16. Sullivan DA, Richardson GS, McLaughlin DT, Wira CR. Variations in the levels of secretory component in human uterine fluid during the menstrual cycle. J Steroid Biochem 1984;20:509–513.

17. Wira CR, Sullivan DA. Estradiol and progesterone regulation of immunoglobulin A and G and secretory component in cervicovaginal secretions of the rat. Biol Reprod 1985;32:90–95.

18. Vargas-Linares CERD, Burgos MH. Migration of lymphocytes in the normal human vagina. Am J Obstet Gynecol 1968;102:1094–1101.

19. Cohen JHM, Danel L, Cordier G, Saez S, Revillard J-P. Sex steroid receptors in peripheral T cells: Absence of androgen receptors and restriction of estrogen receptors to OKT8-positive cells. J Immunol 1983;131:2767–2771.

20. Stimson WH. Oestrogen and human T lymphocytes: Presence of specific receptors in the T-suppressor/cytotoxic subset. Scand J Immunol 1988;28:345–350.

21. Stanisz AM, Kataeva G, Bienenstock J. Hormones and local immunity. Int Arch Allergy Immunol 1994;103:217–222.

22. Lynch EA, Dinarello CA, Cannon JG. Gender differences in IL-1α, IL-1β, IL-1 receptor antagonist secretion from mononuclear cells and urinary excretion. J Immunol 1994;153:300–306.

23. Hu S-K, Mitcho YL, Rath NC. Effect of estradiol on interleukin 1 synthesis by macrophages. Int J Immunopharmacol 1988;10:247–252.

24. Head JR, Billingham RE. Concerning the immunology of the uterus. Am J Reprod Immunol 1986;10:76–81.

25. Beer AE, Billingham RE. Immunoregulatory aspects of pregnancy. Fed Proc 1978;37:2374–2378.

26. Alexander NJ, Anderson DJ. Immunology of semen. Fertil Steril 1987;47:192–205.

27. Haq A, Al-Tufail M, Sheth K, et al. Immunosuppression by human seminal plasma fractionated by DEAE sephadex A-50 ion exchange chromatography. Andrologia 1992;24:87–94.

28. Prakash C, Coutinho A, Moller G. Inhibition of in vitro immune responses by a fraction from seminal plasma. Scand J Immunol 1976;5:77–85.

29. Anderson DJ, Tarter TH. Immunosuppressive effects of mouse seminal plasma components in vivo and in vitro. J Immunol 1982;128:535–539.

30. Brooks GF, Lammel CJ, Petersen BH, Stites DP. Human semina plasma inhibition of antibody complement-mediated killing and opsonization of *Neisseria gonorrhoeae* and other gram-negative organisms. J Clin Invest 1981;67:1523–1531.

31. Anderson DJ, Hill JA. Cell-mediated immunity in infertility. Am J Reprod Immunol Microbiol 1988;17:22–30.

32. Pandya IJ, Cohen J. The leukocytic reaction of the human uterine cervix to spermatozoa. Fertil Steril 1985;43:417.

33. Jaszczak S. Migration of sperm in the cervix and uterus of non-human primates. In: Elstein M, Moghissi KS, Borth R, eds. Cervical Mucus in Human Reproduction. Copenhagen: Scriptor, 1973, pp. 33–44.

34. Wolff H, Anderson DJ. Immunohistologic characterization and quantitation of leukocyte subpopulations in human semen. Fertil Steril 1988;49:497–504.

13

URINARY INCONTINENCE

Kathryn L. Burgio, Patricia S. Goode,
Julie L. Locher, and Jibike Adegbile

Urinary incontinence, the accidental loss of urine from the bladder, is a prevalent condition that affects both men and women of all ages. It is so common among older adults that it is often considered a natural and even inevitable consequence of normal aging. However, while certain changes that occur normally with aging can predispose individuals to incontinence, it is neither normal nor inevitable. In fact, incontinence is also a significant problem among young and middle-aged adults and among healthy, community-dwelling people. Many people manage incontinence with relative ease, wearing absorbent products such as incontinence pads and continuing their lifestyles without significant disruption of daily life. Others, especially those with more frequent or severe forms of incontinence, experience debilitating consequences ranging from embarrassment and depression to severe social isolation and restriction of daily activities. For these individuals, incontinence is the bane of their existence and the problem around which they live their lives.

While incontinence affects both men and women, it is much more prevalent among women. The vast majority of incontinent patients are women, and most studies of the treatment of incontinence have been conducted among women. This chapter provides background information for the reader to understand incontinence as a health problem. It describes the epidemiology of incontinence with special emphasis on factors that relate to gender differences and distinguish incontinence as a women's health issue.

THE PHYSIOLOGY OF URINARY CONTINENCE AND INCONTINENCE

Normal micturition and urinary continence involve a complex set of physiological responses, described in depth by Bradley, Timm, and Scott.[1] As the bladder fills, stretch receptors in the bladder will signal the sacral spinal cord. At a critical threshold volume, a spinal cord reflex (the micturition reflex) stimulates the bladder to empty. This is accomplished by rhythmic contractions of the detrusor muscle, the smooth muscle in the bladder wall, and relaxation of the external urinary sphincter, a striated muscle that surrounds the urethra and controls the outlet. The micturition reflex stimulates bladder emptying in infants and young children as well as spinal cord–transected patients. Voluntary control over urination is accomplished through inhibition of the micturition reflex via neural circuits from the cerebral cortex. Continence requires that the individual anticipate the threshold for bladder emptying and avoid incontinence by voiding before the threshold is reached, or more commonly, by perceiving bladder distention and inhibiting reflex contractions until an appropriate setting for urination is reached. One must also be able to occlude the urethra to prevent incontinence during uninhibited bladder contraction or sudden increases in bladder pressure associated with physical activities such as coughing or sneezing. Also important to the maintenance of continence is the ability to voluntarily empty the bladder.

Failure to emit these physiological responses at the appropriate times result in the following most common types of incontinence: urge incontinence, in which bladder contractions are not inhibited; and stress incontinence, in which the outflow is not effectively prevented during transient pressure rises.

TYPES AND CAUSES OF INCONTINENCE

There are several types of incontinence and a multitude of contributory factors. Understanding of the type or types of incontinence and thus, the mechanism of urine loss is important in making rational decisions about treatment. In community-dwelling older adults, the most common types of incontinence are stress incontinence, urge incontinence, and mixed symptomology of stress and urge incontinence. Together these three types account for more than 80% of incontinence.[2]

Urge Incontinence

Urge incontinence is the accidental loss of urine associated with an uncontrollable urge to urinate. This category encompasses a group of disorders, including bladder instability, detrusor hyperreflexia, spastic bladder, neurogenic bladder, or uninhibited bladder. This type of urine loss is associated with uncontrolled contractions of the detrusor muscle that force urine out of the bladder through the urethra.

This inability to inhibit detrusor contraction can be caused by neurological disorders or injuries that impair central nervous system control, such as cerebrovascular accident, brain tumor, dementia, Parkinsonism, multiple sclerosis, or spinal cord injury. Bladder dysfunction can also be produced by local inflammation or irritation of the bladder or urethra resulting from such conditions as urinary tract infection, fecal impaction, benign prostatic hypertrophy, uterine prolapse, or bladder carcinoma.

It has also been asserted that bladder instability can result from poor bladder habits such as frequent voiding. Repeated low-volume voiding prevents the bladder from accommodating normal urine volumes and is purported to decrease bladder capacity, resulting in increased urinary frequency and urgency.[3,4]

Often, urge incontinence is characterized by large-volume urinary accidents, which can lead to embarrassment and serious restriction of activities even if such incontinence episodes are infrequent. Urge incontinence also presents as small-volume losses that are less disruptive but often more frequent.

Stress Incontinence

Stress urinary incontinence is the involuntary loss of urine that occurs following a sudden rise in intra-abdominal pressure produced by such physical activities as coughing, sneezing, jogging, or lifting. Incontinence occurs when a corresponding rise in bladder pressure exceeds urethral pressure in the absence of detrusor contraction. Stress incontinence is due to a defect of the bladder outlet (sphincter insufficiency, incompetent sphincter) such that the resistance provided by the urethra is inadequate to prevent leakage.

Stress incontinence occurs so commonly in women that mild incontinence is accepted as normal by many women, and a surprising number are not inconvenienced enough to seek or accept treatment. One study of the prevalence of stress incontinence in young, nulliparous women reported that 51% experienced stress incontinence although only 15% had daily leakage.[5] In men, stress incontinence is uncommon and is usually a result of urologic surgery, such as prostatectomy.

One commonly accepted etiologic factor in female stress incontinence is perinatal damage to the supporting tissues of the pelvic floor. The precise mechanism of urine loss is a topic of debate. Anatomical explanations emphasize the loss of the correct vesicourethral angle, the angle between the bladder and urethra, due to overstretched or damaged pelvic floor tissues. A normal angle between the bladder floor and urethra provides transmission of pressure to the urethra and bladder simultaneously during physical activities. This closes off the urethra during transient rises in intra-abdominal pressure and prevents leakage.

When the position of the urethra is altered by loss of urethral support, sudden increases in abdominal pressure are transmitted to the bladder only, leaving urethral pressure unaffected and allowing urine to escape.

Functional explanations of stress incontinence attribute urinary leakage to a lack of awareness or voluntary control of pelvic muscles and a failure of these muscles to contract during transient rises in intra-abdominal pressure.[6,7] The usual method for improving weak muscles is pelvic muscle training and exercise.

Stress incontinence is also commonly associated with atrophic vaginitis in postmenopausal women and is thought to be due to mucosal thinning in the urethra. Estrogen increases mucosal vascularity and thickness of the submucosa which theoretically increases mucosal coaptation. Estrogen also increases the sensitivity of the urethra and bladder neck to alpha-adrenergic stimulation, increasing bladder outlet resistance. Studies of estrogen therapy have reported beneficial effects on urinary control.[8–10]

Clearly, there are many factors that contribute to the development of female incontinence. Evaluation of the problem may reveal the mechanisms of urine loss but rarely distinguishes the etiological factor or factors. It is not usually essential to understand the specific causes of incontinence in order to choose or implement appropriate therapy. However, a better understanding of the many causes in general would be important for the development of programs to prevent or delay the onset of incontinence in women. Many epidemiological studies have been conducted in various populations and reveal a number of variables related to incontinence, including several possible risk factors or contributing variables.

PREVALENCE OF INCONTINENCE

Overview

Studies of the prevalence of urinary incontinence have yielded rates ranging from 2% to 83%.[2,5,11–53] The tremendous range of prevalence data reported for incontinence in these studies is probably related to the great diversity between the study populations and sampling procedures, the differences in study methodologies, and the various definitions and methods for measurement of incontinence used by the various investigators. For example, the highest rates of incontinence are found in populations of institutionalized individuals whose incontinence quite often is secondary to the physical or cognitive impairments that led to their placement. In community-dwelling populations, the prevalence of incontinence ranges from 2% to 62.7%

Of particular importance in these studies are the ways in which incontinence is defined. Examining measures of frequency or severity allows one to make a distinction between occasional incontinence and regular or severe incontinence that might be seen as a clinical problem. Thus, although urine loss occurred in approximately half of the women surveyed, a much smaller proportion of these had leakage frequently enough to be considered a problem.[5]

Another issue involved in the definition of urinary incontinence in epidemiological studies is the potential for lack of correspondence between incontinence based on the respondent's self-report and clinical or urodynamic findings. For example, in a community-based study by Sandvik and colleagues[11] comparing survey results with urodynamic findings, the survey found that 51% of incontinent women experienced stress incontinence, 39% mixed incontinence, and 10% urge incontinence. In contrast, urodynamic findings indicated that 77% of incontinent women experienced stress, 11% mixed, and 12% urge incontinence.

Longitudinal studies of the incidence of incontinence are lacking. A large study of community-dwelling older adults showed that the 1-year incidence rate was 10% for men and 20% for women.[54] Two studies that investigated the 3-year incidence rate of incontinence in women reported rates of 8% and 4.7%.[27,28] In the first of these two studies, the criterion for incontinence was based on a frequency of urine loss at least once per month. The higher incidence rate of 8% was found in a group of healthy perimenopausal women who were slightly older than the women in the study reporting the lower rate.

Gender Differences

The literature indicates consistently that women are significantly more likely to experience incontinence than are men. All community-based studies that examined gender differences in younger, middle-aged, and older adults reported higher prevalence rates for women than men.[2,17,19,26,44,45] Those for women range from 11% to 63%,[2,5,11–45] and those for men, 2% to 19%.[2,17,19,26,44,45]

In a population-based sample of 1,955 non-institutionalized older adults, Diokno and colleagues reported that 30.0% had experienced incontinence within the previous 12 months.[2] The prevalence rate was 37.7% for women compared to 18.9% for men, indicating that women are more likely to have incontinence by a ratio of approximately 2 to 1. In addition, men and women tended to have different types of incontinence. Men were more likely to have pure urge incontinence and much less likely to have pure stress incontinence. Incontinent women, on the other hand, were most likely to have a mixture of stress and urge incontinence or pure stress incontinence.

While men and women may have incontinence caused by some of the same factors, the gender differences in the overall rates of incontinence and the types of incontinence suggest that they differ in the types of predisposing or causal factors or their susceptibility to these factors. Gender differences are partially explained by anatomical differences as shown in Figures 13–1 and 13–2. Men are less susceptible to stress incontinence due to urethral insufficiency because of a significantly longer urethra through which greater pressure is required to move fluid. Also, the angulation of the male urethra as it traverses anteriorly once it passes through the prostate gland may contribute to urethral resistance. Further, the striated muscle composing the external urethral sphincter surrounds the urethra circumferentially in men. In women, the muscle separates posteriorly in the midline to accommodate the vagina. This creates a weaker area in the urogenital diaphragm which may allow bladder descent in women and contribute to stress urinary incontinence related to bladder hypermobility. Since the anterior portion of the proximal urethra is held more firmly in place by dense suspensory ligaments immediately behind the pubis, the posterior portion of the urethra tends to descend further than the anterior portion, opening the proximal

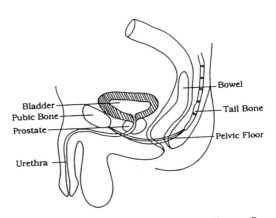

Figure 13–1. Side view of the male pelvis [Source: Burgio et al., 1989[77]]

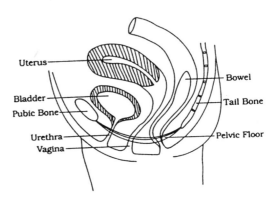

Figure 13–2. Side view of the female pelvis [Reproduced from Staying Dry: A Practical Guide to Bladder Control, Burgio, et al., page 40, February 1989.[77]]

urethra and contributing to urethral insufficiency,[55] the other major cause of stress urinary incontinence. In men, the bladder is more fully supported by the pelvic floor, thus stress incontinence is uncommon.

Another anatomic difference that may contribute to a lower incidence of incontinence in men is the testosterone-related increase in overall skeletal muscle bulk, which could have a beneficial effect on the muscles of the pelvic floor. Also, the difference in the bony structure of the pelvis in men could suspend the pelvic floor in such a manner that it is more resistant to excess pressure related to obesity or straining at stool.

It is often assumed that incontinence in women is attributable to the weakening, stretching, and nerve damage to the pelvic floor during pregnancy and childbirth. In addition, the loss of estrogen and resulting changes in tissue are thought to contribute to incontinence in women. These and other health issues related uniquely to the continence mechanism in women are explored in the following sections of this chapter.

RISK FACTORS FOR INCONTINENCE IN WOMEN

Age

Because incontinence is so common among older women, it is often regarded as a normal and inevitable part of the aging process. In fact, when an older woman reports a problem of incontinence to her health care provider, it is not unusual that she is told, "Well, you're getting older now, this is to be expected." Most studies indicate that incontinence is indeed correlated with age.[18,21,25,28,29,31,42,44] In one well-known study, a random sample of 842 women 17–64 years of age were interviewed.[42] The prevalence rates increased steadily with age. In another large survey, prevalence of incontinence in women 46–86 years old increased progressively over seven birth cohorts (1900–1940) from 12.1% to 24.6%.[18]

Incontinence is not to be considered normal with aging; however, there are changes in the bladder and the pelvic structures that occur with age and which can contribute to incontinence.[56–60] For example, it has been shown that older people have smaller bladder capacity and are more likely to have bladder spasms. It is known that striated muscle mass is reduced with aging. Therefore, it is plausible that similar changes in the musculature of the pelvic floor could occur with age and increase susceptibility to incontinence. Further, incontinence is often attributable to medical problems or diseases that can disrupt the mechanisms of continence (e.g., diabetes mellitus), many of which are more common among older adults.

Pregnancy

Incontinence in women is often assumed to be attributable to the effects of pregnancy and childbirth. Pregnancy may cause women to experience incontinence because of the increased pressure of the uterus on the bladder and pelvic floor. In addition, progesterone causes hypotonia of the detrusor which may lead to incomplete emptying with increased susceptibility to stress and urge incontinence. Progesterone also decreases sensitivity of the bladder neck and proximal urethra to alpha-adrenergic stimulation, increasing susceptibility to stress incontinence. Finally, pregnant women may experience a greater incidence of urinary tract infections which may result in symptoms of urinary incontinence.

Incontinence is a more common occurrence among pregnant women compared with other groups of women. Prevalence rates of 30.6%, 46.4%, and 59.5% have been reported in three separate studies.[23,30,61] Incontinence during pregnancy is a self-limiting condition for most women. Regaining control of continence following delivery usually occurs in the weeks or months after delivery. However, there is some speculation that women who are incontinent during pregnancy may be predisposed to experiencing incontinence at later times in their lives, such as during a subsequent pregnancy, or as they age. Indeed, older women during clinical interview will often associate the onset of their incontinence as occurring concomitantly with pregnancy.

Childbirth

The potential mechanisms of the relationship between childbirth, particularly vaginal delivery, and incontinence are somewhat more clear. The role of childbearing in predisposing women to incontinence is supported by several studies that have demonstrated a link between incontinence and parity.[16,29,35,40,41,44,61-64]

There are several explanations that may be offered. First, childbirth may result in relaxation of the pelvic floor as a consequence of weakening and stretching of the muscles and connective tissue during delivery. The connective tissue, particularly the suspensory cardinal and uterosacral ligaments which insert into the cervix, may be affected by the large amounts of collagenase that cause collagen breakdown and subsequent cervical "ripening."[65] Second, damage may occur as a result of spontaneous lacerations and episiotomies during delivery. The result of these events can be impaired support of the pelvic organs and alteration in their positions. Particularly relevant is the descent of the bladder and proximal urethra that prevents proper pressure transmission to resist urine leakage during transient rises in intra-abdominal pressure. As the bladder and urethra descend further, the anterior and posterior walls of the urethra separate because of the continued ligamentous suspension of the anterior urethra and the lack of support of the posterior urethra. This results in intrinsic sphincter deficiency.

A third hypothesis is that the stretching of the pelvic tissues during vaginal delivery may damage the pudendal and pelvic nerves, as well as the muscles and connective tissue of the pelvic floor, and can interfere with the ability of the

striated urethral sphincter to contract promptly and efficiently in response to increases in intra-abdominal pressure or detrusor contractions. Damage to the delicate sympathetic plexus during vaginal delivery most likely results in increased
detrusor and urethral instability, decreased bladder neck tone, and mixed urge
and stress incontinence, the most common type of incontinence in women.

The evidence for the relationship between childbearing and incontinence is
presented in several studies. For example, Thomas and colleagues reported that
incontinence was most likely to occur in parous rather than nulliparous women
at all ages (15–64 years).[44] Furthermore, incontinence was most common in
women who had four or more children. Holst and Wilson found that incontinence was less common in nulliparous women but found no association with
rates of incontinence and increasing parity.[37] In another study, Jolleys suggested
that the relationship between increasing rates of incontinence and increasing
parity was linear.[35] In addition, pregnant women with incontinence have been
found in one study to have a history of more pregnancies and more births than
pregnant women who were continent.[61] Vaginal delivery in particular is believed to cause pelvic neuropathy that could instigate urinary incontinence.[66,67]

Two studies of middle-aged women have found no association between
parity and incontinence. Hording and colleagues found that frequency of urinary incontinence in 45-year-old women was not associated with frequency of
births.[40] Similarly, Burgio and colleagues found that healthy perimenopausal
women with incontinence were not any more likely to have delivered more children than continent women.[27] The relationship between pregnancy and childbirth and incontinence requires further study.

Menopause

Menopause, the physiological cessation of menses, occurs as a result of decreased ovarian function and related decreases in circulating estrogen. Clinically, it has long been understood that urinary symptoms are an integral part of
the transition from the premenopausal to the postmenopausal state. Loss of estrogen causes atrophic changes not only in the vagina but in the bladder, urethra, and periurethral tissues as well. Tissues become thin and friable. Presumably, the loss affects the bulk of the periurethral tissues and the coaptation of the
urethral mucosa. In addition, the atrophic changes increase susceptibility to urinary tract infections and cause irritative symptoms such as urethritis, urinary
frequency, urgency and dysuria, vaginal dryness, and dyspareunia. Irritation in
the bladder wall and urethra is believed to cause the bladder to spasm, causing
urge incontinence. The female pelvic floor contains estrogen and progesterone
receptors. Given the evidence that atrophy of these tissues can be reversed with
estrogen,[68] and that estrogen replacement reduces incontinence in many cases,
it seems reasonable to propose that estrogen loss contributes to the problem.

The literature is inconsistent in describing the role of menopause and estrogen loss as significant contributors to incontinence. Positive findings were reported by Rekers and colleagues, who compared premenopausal women (n = 355) with postmenopausal women (n = 858) and found no significant difference in the prevalence of incontinence between the two groups (25% v. 26%).[25] However, there were significant differences in the frequency of incontinence episodes, indicating that postmenopausal women had more severe incontinence. Postmenopausal women were more likely to have incontinence on a daily basis or more frequently (7.1%), compared with the premenopausal women (3.1%). Postmenopausal women were less likely, however, to have large-volume accidents, and there were no differences in the types of incontinence. Postmenopausal women were much more likely to have irritative symptoms of urgency (P <.05) and nocturia (P <.05), but there were no differences in the symptoms of urinary frequency (>6/day) or dysuria (or cystitis).

These investigators also examined the time frame between menopause and the onset of incontinence. A significant increase in the incidence of incontinence occurred 10 years before the menopause, and an even larger increase was found at menopause. Among postmenopausal women with incontinence, 28.4% had onset before menopause, 18.0% around the time of menopause, and 53.6% after menopause. Finally, women who experienced a surgical menopause had a higher rate of incontinence (36.0%) compared with those who experienced a natural menopause (21.5%).

One study of menopause status found that among 45-year-old women, the frequency of incontinence was not higher among those who were postmenopausal compared with those who were premenopausal.[40] A second study found that postmenopausal women were actually less likely to have incontinence on a regular basis.[27] A third study showed a significantly lower prevalence rate among postmenopausal women (35%) than among premenopausal women (47%).[35] Thus, there is a clear physiological basis for a relationship between incontinence and menopause. However, epidemiological data are mixed in identifying the role played by menopause.

Hysterectomy

When asked about the onset of incontinence, many women will report that it began immediately following hysterectomy. As described above, a hysterectomy with oophorectomy that puts a woman into surgical menopause may have a hormonal mechanism as the primary cause of incontinence. Recently, with the development of electrodiagnosis technology to measure neurologic impairment of the pelvic floor, the question has been raised whether the development of posthysterectomy incontinence might be caused by nerve damage during the procedure. Milson and colleagues, in a survey of 3,896 women, reported that those who had a hysterectomy were more likely to report incontinence than those who had not (20.8% vs. 16.4%), and that this trend occurred across five birth cohorts from 1900 to 1920.[18] Further study of the relationship of hysterectomy to incontinence could yield surgical techniques that would reduce the incidence of incontinence similar to nerve-sparing procedures for prostatectomy that reduce the incidence of post-prostatectomy incontinence.

Obesity

Obesity is often viewed as a factor that can cause incontinence or contribute to the severity of the condition. It is believed that the added weight of obesity, like pregnancy, may bear down on pelvic tissues, causing chronic strain, stretching and weakening of the muscles, nerves, and other structures of the pelvic floor. Anecdotally, patients are known to report improvement in symptoms of incontinence associated with weight loss and increased severity with weight gain.

In addition, there is clear epidemiological support for the role of obesity in incontinence.[12,27,29,41,69] Incontinence in women has been associated with higher body mass index (BMI)[12,27,69] and greater weight.[29,41] In one study, a significant relationship was found between urinary incontinence and BMI such that women with regular incontinence had the highest mean BMI and those who had never been incontinent had the lowest mean BMI.[27] Dwyer and colleagues found that obesity was significantly more common among women with detrusor instability, as well as among those with stress incontinence, compared with continent women.[70] Similarly, in another study, obesity was found to be an independent risk factor for incontinence.[71] Other investigators found no differences between continent and incontinent women on BMI.[72] However, they did find that women with a positive stress test (i.e., clinically demonstrated loss of urine with physical stress [coughing]) had a higher BMI than those who had a negative stress test.

In addition to the associations found between obesity, body mass index, and incontinence, confirmatory results have been reported for intervention studies. Bariatric surgery was used in one study to drastically reduce weight in a group of morbidly obese women.[73] As a group, the women had both subjective and objective resolution of stress as well as urge incontinence.

In another study, weight reduction by bariatric surgery resulted in reduction of stress incontinence from 61.2% to 11.6% of the group.[74] Thus, there is strong evidence to support the causal role of excess weight in the development of urinary incontinence. A link between body mass and incontinence supports the concept that weight gain may increase susceptibility to incontinence and suggests that weight loss may decrease incontinence.

Race

Most epidemiological studies of incontinence have been conducted on white populations. But some comparative data exist, and they provide evidence that white women may be more susceptible to incontinence than black women. Data on middle-aged women has indicated that white women were more likely than black women to report regular incontinence at least once per month and also more likely to report even infrequent incontinence.[27] Racial differences have also been reported among pregnant women. However, the differences were evident only for stress incontinence and not for urge incontinence or other types of urine leakage.[61] In a clinical study of patients referred for evaluation of incontinence or prolapse, Bump found that a larger proportion of white women reported symptoms of stress incontinence (31% vs. 7%), and a larger proportion were diagnosed urodynamically as having genuine stress incontinence (61% vs. 27%).[75] These findings among white women may be attributable to a relative weakness of pelvic support that is perhaps due to a difference in collagen content, type, or structure. In postmenopausal women, the increased levels of circulating estrogen in obese black women due to conversion of adrenal hormones in adipose tissue may cause sufficient positive effects on the urethra, bladder, and surrounding tissues to contribute to a lower prevalence of urinary incontinence, since obesity is more common among black women.

Other Factors

Other published articles have reported correlations between incontinence and several other variables, including cystitis or urinary tract infections,[5,12] previous gynecological surgery,[16,35] use of diuretics,[29] perineal suturing,[35] cystocele,[40] uterine prolapse,[40] impaired function of the levator muscles,[40] childhood bed wetting,[15] and current and former cigarette smoking.[76]

CONCLUSION

While urinary incontinence is a prevalent condition, affecting both men and women of all ages, women are more likely to develop the condition. Knowledge of female anatomy and physiology, together with epidemiological data, has provided considerable information regarding the multitude of factors that contribute to female incontinence. Women have a shorter urethra and less skeletal muscle bulk and strength. They have a posterior opening in the urogenital diaphragm that allows the bladder to descend, interfering with the urethrovesical junction, causing intrinsic urethral insufficiency, and allowing bladder hypermobility. The higher prevalence of obesity in women, as well as the experiences of pregnancy and childbirth can largely explain the damage or compromise to pelvic structures that produces incontinence. In addition, the estrogen depletion associated with menopause can alter the urethral tissues, lowering urethral coaptation and resistance and possibly making women more susceptible to urine loss.

There are several types of incontinence and many predisposing or contributing factors. Sometimes the onset of incontinence is acute with a readily identifiable cause, such as stroke or injury. In most cases, however, the onset of incontinence is gradual, beginning with small or infrequent episodes and gradually increasing in severity to the point when the person views it as a problem. It is extremely common for women to seek treatment for incontinence only after months or typically years of living with the condition. In evaluation, the clinician is frequently unsure of when the physical changes producing incontinence actually began. For example, there may have been a gradual loss of tissue support or a gradual decrease in bladder capacity. Alternatively, there may have been an accumulation of different predisposing factors. We do not have a full understanding of why some women are more susceptible than others, nor do we understand what occurs over time that eventually leads to incontinence. Most important, we do not know if these processes might be slowed or stopped by intervening at a very early stage. However, the growing understanding of risk factors, female anatomy, and the mechanisms by which incontinence evolves is valuable in developing methods for preventing or delaying the onset of incontinence.

REFERENCES

1. Bradley W, Timm GW, Scott FB. Innervation of the detrusor muscle and urethra. In: Lapides J, ed. Symposium on Neurogenic Bladder, Philadelphia: W.B. Saunders, 1974, pp. 3–27.

2. Diokno AC, Brock BM, Brown MB, Herzog AR. Prevalence of urinary incontinence and other urological symptoms in the noninstitutionalized elderly. J Urol 1986; 136:1022–1025.

3. Frewen WK. An objective assessment of the unstable bladder of psychosomatic origin. Br J Urol 1978;50:246–249.

4. Frewen WK. The management of urgency and frequency of micturition. Br J Urol 1980;52:367–369.

5. Wolin L. Stress incontinence in young, healthy nulliparous female subjects. Urology 1969;101:545–549.

6. Kegel AH. Progressive resistance exercise in the functional restoration of the perineal muscles. Am J Obstet Gynecol 1948;56:238–248.

7. Kegel AH. Stress incontinence of urine in women: Physiologic treatment. J Int Coll Surg 1956;25:487–499.

8. Fantl JA, Cardozo L, McClish DK. Hormones and Urogenital Therapy Committee. Estrogen therapy in the management of urinary incontinence in postmenopausal women: A meta-analysis: first report of the hormones and urogenital therapy committee. Obstet Gynecol 1994;83:12–18.

9. Judge TG. The use of quinestradol in elderly incontinent women, a preliminary report. Gerontol Clin 1969;11:159–164.

10. Walter S, Walf H, Barlebo H, Jensen H. Urinary continence in postmenopausal women treated with oestrogens: a double-blind clinical trial. Urol Int 1978;33:135–143.

11. Sandvik H, Hunskaar S, Vanvik A, Seim A, Hermstad R. Diagnostic classification of female urinary incontinence: an epidemiological survey corrected for validity. J Clin Epidemiol 1995;48(3):338–343.

12. Mommsen S, Foldspang A. Body mass index and adult female urinary incontinence. World J Urol 1994;12(6):319–322.

13. Nielsen AF, Walter S. Epidemiology of infrequent voiding and association symptoms. Scand J Urol Nephrol 1994(suppl);157:49–53.

14. Mommsen S, Foldspang A, Elving L, Lam GW. Association between urinary incontinence in women and a previous history of surgery. Br J Urol 1993;72(1):30–37.

15. Foldspang A, Mommsen S. Adult female urinary incontinence and childhood bedwetting. J Urol 1994;152(1):85–88.

16. Harrison GL, Memel DS. Urinary incontinence in women: its prevalence and its management in a health promotion clinic. Br J Gen Pract 1994;44(381):149–152.

17. Lagace EA, Hansen W, Hickner JM. Prevalence and severity of urinary incontinence in ambulatory adults: an UPRNet study. J Fam Pract 1993;36(6):610–614.

18. Milsom I, Ekelund P, Molander U, Arvidsson L, Areskoug B. The influence of age, parity, oral contraception, hysterectomy and menopause on the prevalence of urinary incontinence in women. J Urol 1993;149(6):1459–1462.

19. Brocklehurst JC. Urinary incontinence in the community—analysis of a MORI poll. BMJ 1993;306(6881):832–834.

20. Foldspang A, Mommsen S, Lam GW, Elving L. Parity as a correlate of adult female urinary incontinence prevalence. J Epidemiol Community Health 1992;46(6):595–600.

21. Rekers H, Drogendijk AC, Valkenburg HA, Riphagen F. The menopause, urinary incontinence and other symptoms of the genito-urinary tract. Maturitas 1992;15(2):101–111.

22. Minaire P, Jacquetin B. The prevalence of female urinary incontinence in general practice [Abstract]. J Gynecol Obstet Biol Reprod 1992;21(7):731–738.

23. Metanyi S. Urinary incontinence in pregnancy and puerperium [Abstract]. Orv Hetil 1992;133940:2551–2553.

24. Nemir A, Middleton RP. Stress incontinence in younger nulliparous women: Statistical study. Am J Obstet Gynecol 1954;68:1166–1168.

25. Rekers H, Drogendijk AC, Valkenburg H, Riphagen F. Urinary incontinence in women from 35 to 79 years of age: Prevalence and consequences. Eur J Obstet Gynecol Reprod Biol 1992;43(3):229–234.

26. O'Brien J, Austin M, Sethi P, O'Boyle P. Urinary incontinence: Prevalence, need for treatment, and effectiveness of intervention by nurse. BMJ 1991;303(6813):1308–1312.

27. Burgio KL, Matthews KA, Engel BT. Prevalence, incidence and correlates of urinary incontinence in healthy, middle-aged women. J Urol 1991;146(5):1225–1229.

28. Krsnjavi H, Uglesic M. Urinary incontinence in female workers in the area of Zagreb [Abstract]. Archiv Za Higijenu Reda i Toksikologiju 1991;43(2):235–238.

29. Simeonova Z, Bengtsson C. Prevalence of urinary incontinence among women at a Swedish primary health care centre. Scand J Prim Health Care 1990;8(4):203–206.

30. Mellier G. Delille MA. Urinary disorders during pregnancy and post-partum [Abstract]. Rev Fr Gynecol Obstet 1990;85(10)525–528.

31. Lam GW, Foldspang A, Elving LB, Mommsen S. Urinary incontinence in women aged 30–59 years. An epidemiological study. Ugeskr Laeger 1990;152(44): 3244–3246.

32. Sommer P, Bauer T, Neilsen KK, et al. Voiding patterns and prevalence of incontinence in women. A questionnarie survey. Br J Urol 1990;66(1);12–15.

33. Elving LB, Foldspang A, Lam GW, Mommsen S. Descriptive epidemiology of urinary incontinence in 3,100 women age 30–59. Scand J Urol Nephrol Suppl 1989;125: 37–43.

34. Iosif CS, Bekassy Z, Rydhstrom H. Prevalence of urinary incontinence in middle-aged women. Int J Gynaecol Obstet 1988;26(2):255–259.

35. Jolleys JV. Reported prevalence of urinary incontinence in women in a general practice. Br Med J (Clin Res Ed) 1988;296(6632):1300–1302.

36. Hagstad A. Gynecology and sexuality in middle-aged women. Women Health 1988;13(3–4):57–80.

37. Holst K, Wilson PD. The prevalence of female urinary incontinence and reasons for not seeking treatment. New Zealand Med J 1988;101(857):756–758.

38. Mohide EA, Pringle DM, Robertson D, Chambers LW. Prevalence of urinary incontinence in patients receiving home care services. Can Med Assoc J 1988;139(10): 953–956.

39. Hagstad A, Janson PO. The epidemiology of climacteric symptoms. Acta Obstet Gynecol Scand Suppl 1986;134:59–65.

40. Hording U, Pedersen KH, Sidenius K, Hedegaard L. Urinary incontinence in 45-year-old women. An epidemiological survey. Scand J Urol Nephrol 1986;20(3): 183–186.

41. Yarnell JW, Voyle GJ, Richards CJ, Stephenson TP. Factors associated with urinary incontinence in women. J Epidemiol Community Health 1982;36(1):58–63.

42. Yarnell JW, Voyle GJ, Richards CJ, Stephenson TP. The prevalence and severity of urinary incontinence in women. J Epidemiol Community Health 1981;35(1):71–74.

43. Iosif S, Henriksson L, Ulmsten U. The frequency of disorders of the lower urinary tract, urinary incontinence in particular, as evaluated by a questionnaire survey in a gynecological health control population. Acta Obstet Gynecol Scand 1981;60(1):71–76.

44. Thomas T, Plymat K, Blannin J, et al. Prevalence of urinary incontinence. Br Med J 1980;281:1243–1245.

45. Feneley R, Shepherd A, Powell P, et al. Urinary incontinence: Prevalence and needs. Br J Urol 1979;51:493–496.

46. Harris T. Aging in the eighties, prevalence and impact of urinary problems in individuals age 65 and over. NCHS Advance Data 1986;121:1–7.

47. Herzog AR, Fultz NH. Prevalence and incidence of urinary incontinence in community-dwelling populations. J Am Geriatr Soc 1990;38:273–281.

48. Jeter KF, Wagner DB. Incontinence in the American home: A survey of 36,500 people. J Am Geriatr Soc 1990;38:379–383.

49. Somer P, Bauer T, Neilson KK, et al. Voiding patterns and prevalence of incontinence in women: A questionnaire survey. Br J Urol 1990;66:12–15.

50. Vetter NJ, Jones DA, Victor CR. Urinary incontinence in the elderly at home. Lancet 1981;2:1275–1277.

51. Ouslander JG. Urinary incontinence in nursing homes. J Am Geriatr Soc 1990; 38:289–291.

52. Ouslander, JG, Schnelle JF. Incontinence in the nursing home. Ann Intern Med 1995;122:438–449.

53. Ouslander JG, Morishita L, Blaustein J, Orzeck S, Dunn S, Syre J. Clinical, functional and psychosocial characteristics of an incontinent nursing home population. J Gerontol 1987;42:631–637.

54. Herzog, AR, Diokno, AC, Brown, MB, Normolle, DP, Brock BM. Two-year incidence, remission, and change patterns of urinary incontinence in non-institutionalized older adults. J Gerontol 1990;45:M67–M74.

55. Mostwin JL, and Burnett AL. Anatomic aspects of urinary incontinence. In: O'Donnell PD, ed. Urinary Incontinence. St. Louis: Mosby-Year Book, 1997, pp. 16–25.

56. Fantl JAA, Newman DK, Colling J, et al. Urinary incontinence in adults: Acute and Chronic Management. Clinical Practice Guideline, No. 2, 1996 Update. Rockville, MD: U.S. Department of Health and Human Services. Public Health Service, Agency for Health Care Policy and Research. AHCPR Pub. No. 96-0682. March 1996.

57. Staskin DR. Age-related physiologic and pathologic changes affecting lower urinary tract function. Clin Geriatr Med 1986;2:701–710.

58. Diokno AC, Brown MB, Brock MB, et al. Clinical and cystometric characteristics of continent and incontinent noninstitutionalized elderly. J Urol 1988;140:567–571.

59. Resnick NM. Initial evaluation of the incontinent patient. J Am Geriatr Soc 1990;39:311–316.

60. Diokno AC. Diagnostic categories of incontinence and the role of urodynamic testing. J Am Geriatr Soc 1990;38:300–305.

61. Burgio KL, Locher JL, Zyczynski H, et al. Urinary incontinence during pregnancy in a racially mixed sample: Characteristics and predisposing factors. Int Urogynecol J Pelvic Floor Disfunction 1996;7:69–73.

62. Crist T, Shingleton HM, Koch F, Koch GG. Stress incontinence and the nulliparous patient. Obstet Gynecol 1972;40:13–17.

63. Sommer P, Bauer T, Nielsen KK, et al. Voiding patterns and prevalence of incontinence in women. Br J Urol 1990;66:12–15.

64. Foldspang A, Mommsen S, Lam GW, Elving L. Parity as a correlate of adult female urinary incontinence prevalence. J Epidemiol Community Health 1992;46: 595–600.

65. Norton, PA. Pathogenesis of stress urinary incontinence: The role of connective tissue. In: Ostergard DR, Bent AE, eds. Urogynecology and Urodynamics, Theory and Practice, 4th ed. Baltimore, MD: Williams and Wilkins, 1996, pp. 283–286.

66. Smith ARB, Hosker GL, Warrell DW. The role of pudendal nerve damage in the aetiology of genuine stress incontinence in women. Br J Obstet Gynaecol 1989;96: 29–32.

67. Snooks, SJ, Swash M, Henry MM, Setchel M. Risk factors in childbirth causing damage to the pelvic floor innervation. Int J Colorectal Dis 1986;1:20–24.

68. Tapp AJS, Cardozo L. The postmenopausal bladder. Br J Hosp Med 1986;1–4.

69. Brown JS, Seeley DG, Fong J, Black DM, Ensrud KE, Grady D. Urinary incontinence in older women: Who is at risk? Obstet Gynecol 1996;87:715–721.

70. Dwyer PL, Lee ETC, Hay DM. Obesity and urinary incontinence in women. Br J Obstet Gynaecol 1988;95:91–96.

71. Wingate L, Wingate MB, Hassanein R. The relation between overweight and urinary incontinence in postmenopausal women: A case control study. J North Am Menopause Soc 1994;1:199–203.

72. Kolbl H, Riss P. Obesity and stress urinary incontinence: Significance of indices of relative weight. Urol Int 1988;43:7–10.

73. Bump RC, Sugerman HJ, Fantl FA, McClish DK. Obesity and lower urinary tract function in women: Effect of surgically induced weight loss. Am J Obstet Gynecol 1992;166:392–399.

74. Deitel M, Stone E, Kassam HA, Wilk EF, Sutherland DJA. Gynecologic-obstetric changes after loss of massive excess weight following bariatric surgery. J Am Coll Nutr 1988;7:147–153.

75. Bump RC. Racial comparisions and contrasts in urinary incontinence and pelvic organ prolapse. Obstet Gynecol 1993;81:421–425.

76. Bump RC, McClish DK. Cigarette smoking and urinary incontinence in women. Am J Obstet Gynecol 1992;167(5):1213–1218.

77. Burgio KL, Pearce KL, Lucco AJ. Staying Dry: A Practical Guide to Bladder Control. Baltimore: Johns Hopkins University Press, 1989.

14

ANATOMIC INFLUENCES ON SEXUALLY TRANSMITTED BACTERIAL DISEASES

Roberta B. Ness

It is a common belief that women suffer adverse consequences from having sexually transmitted bacterial infections whereas men do not. Sexually transmitted pathogens are endemic in both men and women. It is estimated that in the United States, there are about two million cases of *Neisseria gonorrhoeae* and four million cases of *Chlamydia trachomatis* per year.[1] These sexually transmitted pathogens primarily infect the cervices of women[2-5] and the urethras of men. In both sexes, gonorrhea and chlamydia may then ascend into the organs inside the pelvis where they infect, induce inflammation, and damage the delicate structures involved in normal fertility. In women, this upper genital tract infection is termed pelvic inflammatory disease (PID) and may involve the uterus, fallopian tubes, ovaries, and/or adjacent structures. In men, upper genital tract involvement is termed epididymo-orchitis for the typically dual involvement of epididymis and testes. Although men and women are both commonly infected with and develop cervicitis and urethritis from gonorrhea and chlamydia, women appear to be more likely to develop PID than men are likely to develop epididymo-orchitis. Women also appear to suffer more frequently than men from chronic pelvic pain and infertility after sexually transmitted infections.

This chapter summarizes and compares the actual evidence that links cervicitis, PID, and infertility in women with the evidence that links urethritis, epididymo-orchitis and infertility in men. It critically reviews the belief that women suffer more adverse reproductive sequelae from sexually transmitted infections than men. It then reviews hypotheses as to why women may experience the consequences of sexually transmitted diseases with a different frequency and/or severity than men. The theme of this chapter is that differences in risk of disease between men and women, and determinants of higher risk among certain subgroups of women, are primarily determined by biologic factors that interact with external influences. The biologic factors include sex-steroid hormone metabolism, anatomy, and immunologic function. External influences come from the sociocultural environment. The chapter explores the question whether the observed gender-specific variation in reproductive disease frequency and severity may be understood as a product of these biologic and/or social factors, that is, whether gender differences in the frequency of infertility and other adverse health outcomes from sexually transmitted infections provide clues about mediation by any of these factors.

DO WOMEN SUFFER MORE REPRODUCTIVE CONSEQUENCES FROM SEXUALLY TRANSMITTED DISEASES THAN MEN?

Epidemiologic Studies Linking Bacterial Sexually Transmitted Diseases (STDs) and Infertility Among Women

One out of nine women (11%) in the United States report having had PID at some time in their reproductive lives.[6] More direct estimates of PID incidence are difficult to obtain because it is not a reportable disease, it is treated in a broad variety of medical settings, and there are inconsistencies in diagnosis. Nevertheless, from 1979 to 1988 it was estimated that there were about 200,000 hospitalizations for PID per year and about 400,000 outpatient office visits for new cases of PID per year.[7] However, adding in Emergency Department visits (a common source of PID-related care) and women who do not seek care, it has been estimated that PID affects at least one million women per year.[8] Tubal infertility accounts for about 15%–20% of the 4.9 million cases of infertility estimated to exist among women aged 15–44 in the United States.[9]

Strong epidemiologic and biologic evidence links cervicitis and PID. First, cross-sectional studies show that from 28% to 65% of women with cervicitis have concomitant endometritis (inflammation of the endometrium in association with infection).[10–12] This high rate of concomitant lower and upper genital tract involvement is seen both in women who manifest pelvic pain, a sign of upper genital tract inflammation, as well as in women with cervicitis but without pelvic pain. Second, *C. trachomatis* and *N. gonorrhoeae* are isolated from the cervices of about two-thirds of women with PID. *N. gonorrhoeae* and *C. trachomatis* are also commonly isolated from the fallopian tubes of women with PID, although with lower rates of isolation than from cervical cultures. Smaller numbers of organisms may reach the fallopian tubes than infect the cervix and exposure to fallopian tube–neutralizing antibodies reduces the viability of organisms in culture.[13] Notably, gonorrhea and chlamydia are not the only organisms associated with PID. Bacterial vaginosis, which represents an overgrowth of "bad" over "good" normally occurring vaginal anaerobes and aerobes, is also more common in the lower genital tracts of women with PID.[14,15] There is substantial debate about whether bacterial vaginosis causes PID or whether gonorrhea or chlamydia initiate cervical and tubal infection and inflammation, thereby creating an environment ripe for the development of bacterial vaginosis and for the ascension of anaerobes or aerobes into the upper genital tract as secondary invaders.[15] Evidence reveals that, among women with untreated or partially treated cervicitis, about 30%–40% develop clinical symptoms of PID.[16,17] Finally, in a recent randomized, controlled clinical trial, aggressive chlamydial screening and treatment reduced the number of clinically verified cases of PID by over 50%.[18] These data suggest that the elimination of cervical infection with chlamydia reduces PID, strongly supporting the causal role for chlamydia in the etiology of PID. Ecologic data from Sweden have also shown that marked reductions in the incidence of gonorrhea and chlamydia were followed by declines in the occurrence of PID.[19]

Further, animal and in vitro data suggest that infection with chlamydia or gonococci may damage the normal barriers to ascending infection such as the mucus that plugs the endocervix.[20] These infections also alter the local cervical and vaginal environments by consuming nutrients and producing metabolic wastes, thereby altering pH and oxygen concentration. Ultimately, these local changes may alter the efficiency of the immune response.

Strong evidence also links PID with infertility. In the pre-antibiotic era, over 70% of women became infertile after an index episode of PID.[21] More recent studies, particularly one large, long-term prospective study from Scandinavia, showed that 16% of women with treated PID were infertile compared with 2% of controls.[22] This infertility was almost entirely the result of tubal occlusion, otherwise known as tubal infertility. The Scandinavian study was a particularly important milestone in associating PID with infertility because of the careful methodology employed. The diagnosis of PID was a specific one, consisting of visual evidence of tubal inflammation as seen during laparoscopy (see below), follow-up rates were excellent, and infertility outcomes were validated and refined by testing for type of infertility. Confirmatory retrospective studies have shown that between 36% and 91% of women with tubal infertility have serologic evidence of past chlamydial infection (Table 14–1).[23–33] In contrast, between 0% and 55% of infertile women without tubal damage or fertile control women had past evidence of chlamydial infection in these studies. In individual studies, women with tubal obstruction or damage were anywhere from two to eight times more likely to have a positive chlamydial antibody titer than control women. Infertile women *without* tubal damage were no more likely to have a positive chlamydia antibody titer than were controls.

The pathology that mediates the occurrence of infertility after endometritis and salpingitis is acute and chronic inflammation.[34] Microscopic examination of the fallopian tubes shows intraluminal exudate, microabscesses and polymorphonuclear leukocyte and mononuclear cell infiltration. The fragile cilia in the fallopian tubes that usually propel the egg toward the uterus are denuded, and this lesion alone might be sufficient to predispose to tubal infertility and ectopic pregnancy. In addition, adhesions form inside the fallopian tube and obstruct egg passage. Adhesions also form within the pelvis and distort tubal and adnexal anatomy, resulting in pelvic pain.

Epidemiologic Studies Linking Bacterial STDs and Infertility Among Men

Among men there is similar, although more limited, evidence linking gonorrhea/chlamydia to urethritis and epididymo-orchitis. However, there are conflicting results regarding the association between urethritis and male infertility. In addition, the rates of upper genital tract disease among individuals with lower genital tract infection appear to be lower in men than in women. That is, women with cervicitis are more likely to have PID than men with urethritis are to have epididymo-orchitis. Given that young men have more sexual partners than young women, it might be expected that the prevalence of epididymo-orchitis would equal or exceed the prevalence of PID, assuming equal pathogen transmission and ascension between sexes. However, estimates for the rate of epididymo-orchitis among men are about half to two-thirds the estimates for the rate of PID among women. Although data on the incidence of both diseases are limited, Walrath et al. reported that 7% of men in one work setting recalled a history of this syndrome.[35] National estimates of the rates of epididymo-orchitis have ranged from 500,000 cases/year to over 700,000 cases/year in the United States.[36–38]

Three lines of evidence link urethritis to epididymo-orchitis. First, gonorrhea and chlamydia are pathogens commonly isolated from men with urethritis and from men under the age of 35 with epididymo-orchitis.[39–42] *N. gonorrhoeae* is isolated from about 20% of men with urethritis. Among men with non-gonococcal urethritis, it has been estimated that 30%–50% are associated with *C. trachomatis*, 10%–40% are associated with *U. urealyticum* and 20%–30% are associated with none of these isolates.[43] The most common urethral pathogens isolated from men with epididymo-orchitis are also gonorrhea, chlamydia, and ureaplasma. Second, in the pre-antibiotic era, epididymo-orchitis occurred as a complication in 10% to 30% of cases of gonococcal urethritis.[44] However, among men treated for urethritis, Stamm et al. did not document any cases of

Table 14–1. Retrospective Studies Linking Past Infection with Chlamydia and Infertility

REFERENCE	NUMBER INFERTILE/CONTROLS	% OF WOMEN WITH TUBAL INFERTILITY WITH CHLAMYDIAL ANTIBODIES	% OF WOMEN WITHOUT TUBAL INFERTILITY OR CONTROLS WITH CHLAMYDIAL ANTIBODIES
Moore et al., 1982[23]	186 infertile patients	79% with abnormal HSG, ab >1:32 73% with abnormal distal occlusion on laparoscope, ab >1:32	11% with normal HSB, ab > 1:32
Conway et al., 1984[24]	123 infertile patients 40 sterilized controls 63 termination controls 72 barrier contraception controls	75% with damaged tubes on laparoscope or HSG, ab >1:32	24%–48% ab >1:32
Guderian and Trobough, 1986[25]	245 infertile patients	83% with "residues of PID" by laparoscope, ab >1:8	16% without residues, ab >1:8
Gump et al., 1983[26]	204 infertile patients	64% with old PID on laparoscope or HSG, ab >1:16	28% without PID, ab >1:16
Anestad et al., 1987[27]	105 infertile patients 90 pregnant controls	91% with tubal occlusion IgG >1:8 84% with tubal adhesions IgG >1:8 16 ≤24% with occlusion adhesions IgM >1:8	47%–55% IgG >1:8 2%–3% IgM >1:8

Kane et al., 1984[28]	164 infertile patients 162 family planning controls 38 sterilization controls	36% with tubal disease, ab ⊕titer	11% control, ab ⊕ 12% without tubal disease, ab ⊕
Jones et al., 1982[29]	172 infertile patients	60% with tubal disease, ab >1:8	17% without tubal disease, ab >1:8
Punnonen et al., 1979[30]	128 infertile patients, female contacts of males with non-gonoccal urethritis	57% infertile, ab >1:16 86% female contacts, ab >1:16	29% pregnant females, ab >1:16
Miettinen et al., 1990[31]	104 infertile patients	46% damaged tubes, ab ⊕titer	7% normal tubes, ab ⊕
Sellors et al., 1988[32]	52 tubal factor infertility patients 114 sterilized controls 99 hysterectomy controls	79% with tubal infertility IgG ab >1:400 or IgM ab >1:800	38% sterilized, ab ⊕ 38% hysterectomy, ab ⊕
WHO, 1995[33]	78 tubal factor infertility patients 155 other infertile controls 466 fertile controls	80% with tubal occlusion, ab ⊕for chlamydia or gonorrhea	60% fertile ab ⊕

HSG, hysterosalpingogram; ab, antibody titer.

gonococcal epididymo-orchitis among 150 men following urethral infection.[45] This suggests that treatment markedly reduces the upper genital tract spread from urethritis. Third, in animals, infective epididymo-orchitis has been produced by urethral inoculation of bacterial pathogens and intraluminal spread.[46] Whether this occurs in humans is unclear.

Whether genital infection with gonorrhea or chlamydia induces infertility in men is unclear. In support of this association are data from clinical series that consistently show high rates of infertility among men with histories of epididymo-orchitis. Pelouze reported that 23% of men with a history of unilateral and 42% of men with bilateral epididymo-orchitis were infertile.[44] Similarly, Campbell found that among men with bilateral epididymo-orchitis, 40% were infertile.[47] A prospective study by Osegbe followed 45 men with gonococcal urethritis and epididymo-orchitis.[48] Biopsies during the acute phase showed extensive seminiferous tubular necrosis and inflammatory cell infiltration. At 2 years of follow-up, 27% were found to have persistent azoospermia and 33% had no significant improvement in sperm density. Also of import was Osegbe's finding that many men with unilateral epididymo-orchitis had contralateral biopsies showing bilateral gonadal damage, and some of these men experienced azoospermia. This suggests that epididymo-orchitis may be clinically silent and yet pathologically devastating. However, the interpretation of these studies is limited by the fact that none involved control groups.

There is a pathologic similarity between epididymo-orchitis and PID. Both produce acute and chronic inflammation. This pathologic lesion, which can cause tubal occlusion in women, may also result in vas damage in men, including unilateral or bilateral occlusion.

Several case–control studies have shown a higher prevalence of antibodies to chlamydia among infertile men compared with fertile men (Table 14–2).[49–54] However, in none of these small studies was the difference significant. In most of these studies, infertile men were about 50% more likely than controls to have serum IgG or IgM antibodies to chlamydia. Greendale et al. reported the most strongly positive findings among 52 men from infertile couples with idiopathic infertility and 79 control first-time expectant fathers.[53] Infertile men were 3.4 times more likely than fertile men to have a higher titer (> 1:64) of IgG antichlamydial antibodies. This difference was significant even after controlling for multiple confounding factors. In addition, Helstrom et al. found that infertile men were threefold more likely than fertile men to report previous genital infections and tetracycline usage.[50] Of the two studies that examined culture results among infertile and fertile men, one found positive chlamydia cultures among 9.6% of infertile men vs. 5.7% of fertile men (a nonsignificant difference). In the other, only one subject had a positive *C. trachomatis* culture and there were no differences for ureaplasmas or mycoplasmas between fertile and infertile men.[50,54]

Although these small case–control studies have not typically shown significant associations, they consistently show a positive link between high antibody titers and male infertility. However, the strength of the association for men, a 50% increase in the rate of serologic evidence for past chlamydial infection between infertile and fertile men, is well below the two- to ninefold increase in the rate of serologic evidence for past chlamydial infection among women with tubal infertility compared with fertile women. This lesser strength of association linking chlamydia to infertility in men may be due to less precise knowledge of the specific lesion caused by sexually transmitted pathogens. In women, tubal obstruction is clearly the lesion caused by chlamydia and gonorrhea. In men, the specific marker (if any) for these infections is not known.

Indeed, a multitude of studies have shown no relationship between urethritis or previous chlamydia infection and sperm characteristics (Table 14–3).[49,55–68] The consistency of these negative studies is strengthened by their having been conducted in a wide variety of geographic locations; the multiplicity of infections tested (*M. hominis*, *U. urealyticum*, *C. trachomatis*, or nonspecific bacterial infections); the many methods for detecting infections (culture, serology, polymerase chain reaction); the different proportions of control men infected; and the numerous sperm parameters considered (volume, pH, sperm counts, motility, viability, proportion morphologically abnormal, or sperm agglutinating antibodies). However, these studies of semen parameters among infertile men suffer from a serious potential bias. Comparisons within an infertile population may yield results biased toward the null because there may be many reasons for sperm aberrations among infertile men. That is, men with sexually transmitted infections may have abnormal semen parameters, but uninfected "control" infertile men may also have abnormal parameters for other reasons. In addition, even if there were no association between sexually transmitted pathogens and sperm characteristics, this does not exclude a link between infection and infertility. Instead, it excludes the tested parameters as intermediate markers of an effect. More than anything, these data confirm that we cannot identify any specific, visually evident sperm lesion associated with bacterial infections.

Overall, then, the reproductive morbidity from sexually transmitted diseases has been more clearly and strongly demonstrated in women than in men. The reasons for this differential morbidity have received little study and are not obvious since in both sexes chlamydia and gonorrhea initially infect the lower genital tract structures (urethra and cervix) that communicate with the upper genital tract reproductive organs. Also in both sexes, these pathogens spread along intraluminal linings to the structures that transport sperm and ova (epididymis and tubes).

Table 14-2. Serology Case–Control Studies

REFERENCE	N	POPULATION	FACTORS INVESTIGATED	FINDINGS
Auroux et al., 1987[49]	143	28 infertile males with past medical history of genitourinary infection, 54 infertile males without past medical history of genitourinary infection, 61 fertile male controls (France)	Serum IgG chlamydial antibodies; semen analysis (see Table 14–3)	28% of infertile men without past history of genitourinary infection were IgG chlamydial antibody positive. 53% of infertile men with history of genitourinary infection were IgG chlamydial antibody positive. 26% of fertile controls were chlamydial IgG antibody positive.
Hellstrom et al., 1987[30]	97	52 males attending infertility clinic whose wives had no identifiable cause of infertility, 45 fertile males (San Francisco, USA)	Serum IgG and IgM chlamydial antibodies (positive titer = 1:16); semen cultured for *M. hominis* and *U. urealyticum*	71% of cases were chlamydial IgG antibody positive vs. 57% of controls. 7.6% of cases were IgM chlamydial positive vs. 6.6% of controls. Infertile men were 3 times more likely to report prior history of genital infection.
Quinn et al., 1987[51]	118	79 males attending infertility clinic, 13 partners of repeat aborters, 36 partners of "normal" pregnancies (Toronto, Canada)	Serum IgG chlamydial antibodies (positive titer = 1:32)	17% of men from idiopathic infertile couples were IgG chlamydial antibody positive. 11% of men from fertile couples were IgG chlamydial antibody positive.
Gregoriou et al., 1989[52]	240	120 infertile males from couples with idiopathic infertility, 120 fertile males (Greece)	Serum IgG chlamydial antibodies (positive titer = 1:16); semen analysis (see Table 14–3)	34% of infertile males were IgG chlamydial antibody positive vs. 26% of fertile males. No significant differences in semen parameters by chlamydial serology.

| Greendale et al., 1993[53] | 131 | 52 males attending infertility clinics, 79 males from prenatal classes (San Francisco, USA) | Serum IgG chlamydial antibodies; semen analysis (see Table 14–3) | Infertile men were 3.4 times more likely than fertile controls to have a higher titer of chlamydia (>1:64). No significant association found between reported genitourinary disease and infertility. No differences between semen characteristics of antibody-positive and antibody-negative infertile men. |
| Samra et al., 1994[54] | 223 | 135 males from infertility clinic, 88 males from prenatal care clinic (Israel) | Serum IgA, IgG, and IgM chlamydial antibodies; semen IgA and IgG chlamydial antibodies; semen and urethral cultures for genital mycoplasma and *C. trachomatis* | 13% of infertile males vs. 1% of fertile males had *M. hominis* isolated. 10% of infertile males vs. 6% of fertile males had *C. trachomatis* isolated. 9% of infertile males vs. 1% of fertile males were semen IgA chlamydial antibody positive. No significant differences between fertile and infertile males for semen IgG, serum IgA, IgG, or IgM. |

[Reprinted with permission from Fertility and Sterility, Vol. 68, No. 2, "Do Men Become Infertile After Having Sexually Transmitted Diseases," page 207, 1997, Elsevier Science Inc.[54a]]

Table 14-3. Results from Semen Studies

REFERENCE	N	POPULATION	FACTORS INVESTIGATED	FINDINGS
Witkin and Toth, 1983[55]	100	Males attending infertility clinic (New York City, USA)	Semen analysis (motility, number, volume); semen cultured for *U. urealyticum*, *C. trachomatis*; and anti-sperm antibodies (IgG, IgA, and IgM)	38% of semen samples were *U. urealyticum* culture positive, 27% were *C. trachomatis* culture positive. Semen analysis parameters did not correlate with infection status. 48% of infected men had anti-sperm antibodies. IgA was the most common antibody isotype.
Naessens et al., 1986[56]	120	Males attending infertility clinic (Belgium)	Semen analysis (number, motility, morphology, viscosity); semen cultured for *U. urealyticum*, *M. hominis*, and aerobic and anaerobic bacteria	97% of semen samples had microbial isolates. 33% were *U. urealyticum* culture positive, 9% were *M. hominis* culture positive. Oligospermia and abnormal motility were significantly associated with *U. urealyticum* positive culture.
Auroux et al., 1987[49]	143	28 infertile males with past medical history of genitourinary infection, 54 infertile males without past medical history of genitourinary infection, 61 fertile male controls (France)	Semen analysis (volume, count, motility, PMNS, sperm agglutinins); serum IgG chlamydial antibodies	No significant differences in semen parameters in relation to serology.

Reference	N	Population	Methods	Results
Close et al., 1987[57]	305	Males attending infertility clinic (Washington State, USA)	Serum IgG and IgM chlamydial antibodies (positive titer = 1:16). Anti-sperm antibodies in a subset of patients	5.9% were IgG or IgM chlamydial antibody positive. 50% of seropositive men had sperm agglutinating antibodies vs. 16% of seronegative men.
Gregoriou et al., 1989[58]	225	Infertile males (Greece)	Semen analysis (volume, motility, viability, morphology, count); semen cultured for *U. urealyticum*, *M. hominis*, *C. trachomatis*, and aerobic and anaerobic bacteria	100% of semen samples had microbial isolates. 38% were *U. urealyticum* culture positive. 12% were *C. trachomatis* culture positive. No significant differences in semen parameters between positive and negative *U. urealyticum* or *C. trachomatis* specimens.
Bornman et al., 1990[59]	100	Males attending infertility clinic (South Africa)	Semen analysis (morphology, motility, volume, forward progression, count); semen cultured for *U. urealyticum*, *M. hominis*, and aerobic bacteria	21% of semen were aerobic bacteria culture positive, 42% were *U. urealyticum* culture positive and 28% were *M. hominis* culture positive. No significant differences in semen analysis parameters by mycoplasma status (calculated from presented data).
Nagy et al., 1989[60]	184	Asymptomatic males attending infertility clinic (Hungary)	Semen analysis (motility, morphology, count); semen cultured for aerobic bacteria, *M. hominis*, *U. urealyticum*, *C. trachomatis*, and post-doxycycline treatment on semen parameters	14% of semen were *C. trachomatis* culture positive. No significant differences in semen analysis parameters by chlamydial status. 88% of repeat cultures were negative for *C. trachomatis* following 2 weeks of doxycycline therapy.

(Continued)

Table 14-3. Results from Semen Studies (*Continued*)

REFERENCE	*N*	POPULATION	FACTORS INVESTIGATED	FINDINGS
Custo et al., 1989[61]	1073	1023 males attending clinic with symptomatic genitourinary infection, 50 controls (Italy)	Semen analysis (count, motility, morphology, leukocytes); prostate secretion and urethral specimen cultured for *C. trachomatis*	9% of semen were *C. trachomatis* culture positive. No significant differences in semen analyses parameters by chlamydial status. 90% of repeat cultures were negative for *C. trachomatis* following antibiotic treatment. Also noted were improved semen analysis parameters by composite index following antibiotic treatment.
Gregoriou et al., 1989[52]	240	120 infertile males from couples with idiopathic infertility, 120 fertile males (Greece)	Semen analysis (volume, motility, count, morphology); serum IgG chlamydial antibodies (positive titer = 1:16)	34% of infertile males were IgG chlamydial antibody positive vs. 26% of fertile males. No significant differences in semen parameters by chlamydial serology.
deJong et al., 1990[62]	634	569 males attending infertility clinic, 75 fertile males (semen donors) (France)	Semen analysis (volume, count, motility morphology); semen cultured for *U. urealyticum* and other microbial pathogens, and post-doxycycline treatment on semen parameters	7% of infertile males were *U. urealyticum* culture positive vs. 5% of fertile males. Very low prevalence of other microbial pathogens. No significant differences in semen analysis parameters by *U. urealyticum* status. 78% of repeat cultures were negative for *U. urealyticum* following 10 days of doxycycline therapy. Following successful therapy, 30% demonstrated improved sperm motility, and 20% demonstrated increased sperm count.

Eggert-Kruse et al., 1990[63]	491	Asymptomatic males attending infertility clinic (Germany)	Semen analysis (count, motility, sperm-cervical mucus penetration test); semen cultured for *M. hominis, U. urealyticum*, aerobic and anaerobic bacteria; serum IgG chlamydial antibodies (positive titer ≥1:64); semen IgG and IgA anti-sperm antibodies	10% of semen samples were mycoplasma culture positive. 59% of serum were IgG chlamydial antibody positive. 7% of semen samples had anti-sperm IgG antibody positive and 5% had semen anti-sperm IgA antibody. No significant differences in semen analysis parameters by any culture or antibody status.
Micic et al., 1990[64]	386	326 infertile males, 60 fertile males without infection (Yugoslavia)	Urine and semen culture; urethral smear; seminal plasma anti-sperm antibodies	36% of urine or semen cultures or urethral smears were positive for *C. trachomatis*, gram-negative bacteria, or other microorganisms. No significant difference for positive anti-sperm antibodies by fertility or culture status.
Ruijs et al., 1990[65]	184	Males attending infertility clinic (The Netherlands)	Semen analysis (count, motility, morphology); urethral smears for *C. trachomatis*; serum IgA and IgG chlamydial antibodies; semen IgG, IgM, and IgA chlamydial antibodies	3% of urethral smears were *C. trachomatis* culture positive. Chlamydial infection significantly correlated with serum IgG (positive titer ≥1:640), and semen IgA (positive titer ≥ 1:160). Semen analysis parameters did not correlate with antibody status or chlamydial infections status. (Calculated from presented data) *(Continued)*

Table 14–3. Results from Semen Studies (*Continued*)

REFERENCE	N	POPULATION	FACTORS INVESTIGATED	FINDINGS
Soffer et al., 1990[66]	175	Males attending infertility clinic excluding those with urethritis or acute genitourinary infections (Israel)	Semen analysis (motility, count, morphology); urethral swab for *C. trachomatis*; semen cultured for *M. hominis* and *U. urealyticum*; serum and semen anti-sperm autoantibodies	7% of urethral smears were *C. trachomatis* culture positive. 33% of semen were *M. hominis* or *U. urealyticum* culture positive. Semen analysis parameters did not correlate with infection status. Semen anti-sperm autoantibodies were significantly increased among those with positive cultures. Sperm egg penetration was significantly decreased among those with positive serum or semen anti-sperm autoantibodies, but not by infection status.
Wolff et al., 1991[67]	209	Males attending infertility clinic (Germany)	Semen analysis (volume, motility); IgG (positive titer = 1:8) and IgA (positive titer = 1:4); semen chlamydial antibodies, semen *U. urealyticum* culture	15% of semen were IgG or IgA chlamydial antibody positive. 16% of semen were *U. urealyticum* culture positive. *C. trachomatis* was significantly correlated with decreased semen volume and increased semen PMN-elastase compared to microbiologically negative semen.

Study	N	Population	Methods	Results
Greendale et al., 1993[53]	131	52 males attending infertility clinics, 79 fertile males attending prenatal clinic (San Francisco, USA)	Semen analysis (volume, count, motility morphology); serum IgG chlamydial antibodies (positive titer = 1:64); past medical history	No significant difference in semen analysis parameters among infertile males by IgG chlamydia antibody status.
Witkin et al., 1993[68]	28	Infertile males who had negative semen cultures for *C. trachomatis* (New York City, USA)	Semen analysis; *C. trachomatis* testing detected by PCR; sperm anti-sperm antibodies IgA and IgG positive test, 20% binding; serum IgM chlamydial antibodies (positive titer = 1:128); semen *C. trachomatis* assay by PCR	39% of semen were positive for *C. trachomatis* by PCR. (0/15 fertile controls *C. trachomatis* PCR detected semen positive) No significant differences in semen analysis by *C. trachomatis* status. 4/11 semen PCR-chlamydia positives also positive for IgG and IgA on motile sperm.

[Reprinted with permission from Fertility and Sterility, Vol. 68, No. 2, "Do Men Become Infertile After Having Sexually Transmitted Diseases," page 208–209, 1997, Elsevier Science Inc.[54a]]

POTENTIAL MEDIATORS

Possible explanations for the differential morbidity observed between males and females after infection with sexually transmitted diseases lie in gender-specific anatomy, immunology, or care-seeking behavior. Although this chapter will propose several hypotheses to explain the epidemiologic data, much further research is required in order to verify these. There may be several points in the process of infection during which anatomic, immunologic, or care-seeking differences between men and women may influence disease manifestations. These include pathogen transmission, adherence to susceptible cells, symptomatology and thereby treatment, and ascension into the upper genital tract (see below). Another set of explanations for differential morbidity between men and women from sexually transmitted pathogens is methodologic, i.e., related to bias or confounding. This will be discussed first.

Measurement of Exposures and Outcomes: Potential Sources of Bias

The study of sexually transmitted pathenogensis has been critically affected by measurement of exposures (chlamydia, gonorrhea, and other pathogens) and outcomes (PID, epididymo-orchitis, and infertility). In the past few years, the measurement of exposures has been greatly improved by the application of the DNA amplification techniques of polymerase chain reaction (PCR) and ligase chain reaction (LCR) that, theoretically, allow a single organism to be detected. In comparison to PCR or LCR, cell culture isolation of chlamydia has been reported in only 70%–85% of endocervical specimens from women and in only 50%–75% of urethral specimens from men. The insensitivity of culture results on which much of the previous epidemiology was based may have resulted in *(1)* an underestimation of the prevalence of cervicitis and an even greater underestimation of urethritis, and *(2)* an underestimation of the association between chlamydia and upper genital tract disease. Because men are less likely to be correctly identified as being infected by culture tests, the association between infections and epididymo-orchitis may be most severely underestimated in men.

Measurement of PID, epididymo-orchitis and infertility outcomes remains a very imperfect science. PID is the name given to a clinical syndrome of pelvic pain in concert with tenderness of upper pelvic organs. The clinical diagnosis is often, but not always, associated with infection and inflammation of upper pelvic structures. PID is more definitively diagnosed by laparoscopy, a technique of direct visualization using a scope inserted into the pelvic cavity through the umbilicus. Laparoscopy reveals inflammation of the tubes (salpingitis) and/or ovaries (oophoritis). Estimates of the positive predictive value of clinical signs and symptoms, including *(1)* pelvic pain, *(2)* uterine and adnexal tenderness, and *(3)* vaginal discharge or cervical mucopus in comparison to visualized salpingitis, have ranged from 67% to 89% but typically approximate the lower end of this range.[69] This variation in estimates may result from the application of somewhat different diagnostic criteria or from different characteristics of study populations and of the pathogens involved. PID may also be diagnosed by endometrial biopsy, a safe procedure wherein a tiny piece of endometrial tissue is snipped off using a catheter inserted through the cervix. Endometritis has been shown to predict salpingitis typically anywhere from 71% to 89% of the time.[70] One study by Sellors et al. reported a lower sensitivity of only 33%, probably because in that study, a diagnosis of endometritis was made only upon the diagnostic agreement of three pathologists.[71]

The diagnosis of epididymo-orchitis is also clinically based and may be misclassified. Men with this condition present with a complaint of scrotal pain and frequently with dysuria or urinary frequency and urethral discharge. Clinical findings include scrotal pain, redness, swelling, and tenderness. Competing diagnoses include testicular torsion, tumor, and trauma, among others.[72] Because testicular biopsy is infrequently used even in a research setting, there are no data on the predictive value of clinical diagnosis versus any gold standard.

Infertility is an outcome that comprises a variety of etiologies. In women, it has clearly been shown that PID causes tubal obstruction. In turn, bilateral, and to a lesser degree, unilateral tubal obstruction is associated with irreversible infertility. In men, sperm abnormalities have typically served as a proximate measure of infertility. Controlled studies have shown no relationship between past chlamydial infection and abnormal sperm characteristics. In addition, semen analysis is not highly predictive of individual male fertility.[73-75] In studies evaluating semen parameters and fertility, there are always men who conceive with "poor" parameters (low sperm counts, low sperm densities, and poor motility) and those who fail to conceive with "normal" semen analyses. Therefore, sperm characteristics may not be the best parameter to test the association between sexually transmitted pathogens and infertility. Identification of an infection-associated lesion might increase the probability of finding an association between infertility and infection in men.

Also, infertility is a problem arising in a couple and is not always immediately attributable to the male or the female. When infertility is attributable to a specific (nontubal) factor in the female, it is less likely to be a function of infection in the male. In contrast, when the infertility is a function of female tubal factor, both partners may be more likely to have experienced a sexually transmitted infection because the infection is passed between partners. For this reason, it has been argued that the appropriate case group in studies of male infertility is men from couples with idiopathic infertility.[53]

Confounding

Sexual behavior both alters the probability of acquiring a sexually transmitted pathogen and of being infertile. Case–control studies that compare fertile with infertile couples typically do not consider the impact of this potentially important confounding factor. That is, fertile controls will almost surely differ from infertile cases with respect to number of sexual partners, use of contraception, frequency of intercourse, and perhaps other factors that may have bearing on the probability of acquiring a sexually transmitted disease. A recent study examined the possibility for bias resulting in unequal exposure opportunity among cases and controls by evaluating the reported rates of monogamy among both groups.[53]

Anatomy and Transmission

True biologic differences may also explain the differential reproductive morbidity between men and women after sexually transmitted infections. There are limited and conflicting data on transmission of gonorrhea or chlamydia from males-to-females versus females-to-males. Some studies have suggested that within couples with discordant infection status, men transmit chlamydia to their female partners slightly more frequently than females transmit chlamydia to their male partners.[76–79] In one study, transmission of chlamydia occurred 40% of the time from males to females whereas transmission occurred 32% of the time from females to males.[13] Similarly, it has been suggested that the transmission rate for gonorrhea is higher for male-to-female spread than for female-to-male passage. Support for gender differences in disease transmission also comes from the study of HIV transmission. Several studies show that males are more likely than females to transmit HIV to their opposite sex partner. In a study by Padian et al.,[80] the odds of a female becoming infected with HIV from her HIV-infected male partner were almost ninefold higher than for an HIV infection to occur in a male partner of an infected female. Differential transmission for HIV may reflect viral load, concurrent reproductive tract infections, cervical surface area, contraception, and the menstrual cycle.[81]

However, a recent large and carefully conducted study by Quinn et al. refuted the finding of differential transmission rates between sexes for chlamydia.[82] Using a cross-sectional design and enrolling 494 sexual partnerships in which one or both partners sought treatment at a sexually transmitted disease clinic, the authors first confirmed previous reports that *C. trachomatis* was isolated by culture in significantly more males than females. However, using the more sensitive technique for identification of infection, polymerase chain reaction (PCR), more infections were identified in both males and females (14%–16% infected). The PCR-based prevalence of infection was similar in both sexes. Also, the concordance of chlamydia infection within a couple was similar, regardless of whether the male partner or the female partner was infected.

These data suggest that the reason for the appearance of more efficient transmission of chlamydia from male to female than for female to male is the insensitivity of cell culture isolation, in particular for males. However, confirmatory studies will be necessary.

Anatomy and Adherence

Chlamydia and gonorrhea infect the columnar epithelial cells that line the cervix and urethra. In women, there is evidence that lower-tract infection is more likely the larger the surface area of the cervix and urethra. Thus, factors associated with extension of columnar epithelium beyond the endocervix (termed cervical ectopy), are also associated with higher rates of lower genital tract infection. These factors include young age, oral contraceptive use, and pregnancy.[83] Analogously, the fact that women have more exposed epithelium in the cervix than men have in the urethra may explain differential adherence and thus infection. Another anatomic difference between males and females that may have an impact on adherence of pathogens is that pooling of sperm in the vaginal vault may allow organisms more time to adhere to receptive epithelium. Finally, the concurrent presence of sperm and pathogens in the vaginal vault may predispose women to infection. Sperm have a neutralizing effect on immunologic parameters that repel foreign antigens. This may make the female genital tract more responsive to both sperm and bacteria. In both men and women, the finding that chlamydia adhere to spermatozoa in vitro may account for transport of pathogens throughout their genital tracts. Sperm may transport pathogens from the cervix into the endometrium and fallopian tubes in women and may transport pathogens from seminal vesicles to the epididymis in men.[84]

Anatomy and Symptomatology

Asymptomatic disease, particularly for chlamydia, is common among both women and men. But this may be a more common problem for women. The opening of the male urethra is amenable to direct examination, whereas the cervix opens to the vagina. Discharge from the urethra can be readily detected as indicative of infection, whereas discharge from the cervix admixes with the physiologic vaginal discharge from local glands and may be hard to detect as abnormal. Differential detection probably has a substantial impact on disease progression. Delaying treatment for symptoms of PID for more than 3 days increases the probability of experiencing infertility by threefold.[85]

Immunology and Ascension

Differential rigor in the immunologic response for women versus men may affect the greater propensity for pathogens to ascend up the genital tract. Specifically, it is possible that women's more rigorous immunologic responses inadvertently select for more pathogenic organisms, i.e., those organisms that ascend into the upper genital tract and cause the inflammation that results in later infertility. There is current evidence that bacterial diseases exhibit antigenic variation in concert with the immunologic pressure to mutate or be eradicated. Chlamydia has been shown to evade eradication and to remain within the genital tract for periods of months. Chlamydia has also been shown to exhibit, over time, increasingly complex antigenic variation within the genital tracts of women. Only specific variants of chlamydia will ascend into the upper genital tract.[86] It is therefore possible that the very efficiency of the female immune system selects for a broader range of antigenic variation in the pathogen and thereby increases the probability of selecting for variants that can ascend into the upper genital tract and cause infection and inflammation.

Environment and Ascension

Only women are exposed to certain environmental factors that may enhance bacterial ascension. These factors include intrauterine device (IUD) use, hormonal contraception, and douching. IUDs were strongly implicated in the rise in PID occurrence that took place during the 1970s.[87–89] A number of case–control studies showed that IUDs increased the risk of PID (see Chapter 17). Subsequent analyses have established that the highest risk period is in the few weeks[90] after the IUD insertion and that the risk for PID probably involved IUD placement through an infected cervix. These data imply that it is the process of moving a foreign object through an infected cervix and lodging it into the endometrium that promotes bacterial ascension. Similarly, several observational studies have shown that douching increases the risk for PID.[91–94] Because these studies have been retrospective, it is not clear whether douching itself causes PID as a result of movement of bacteria from the lower to the upper genital tract or whether women with lower genital tract infection douche and coincidentally are also at higher risk of upper genital tract infection. Forthcoming randomized clinical trials will be illuminating in dissecting this temporal relationship. Finally, hormonal contraception appears to have a complicated relationship to cervicitis and PID. Oral contraceptive (OC) use, compared with other contraception, has been associated with an increase in the prevalence of chlamydial cervicitis in most retrospective studies. In a meta-analysis it was estimated that twice as many women who used OCs, compared with other contraception, had chlamydial cervicitis.[95] Two cohort studies confirmed a twofold or higher increased risk of chlamydia cervicitis associated with OC use, even after adjustment for subjects' level of sexual activity.[96,97] Tissue culture and animal studies suggest that exogenous estrogen and progesterone enhance the growth and persistence of *C. trachomatis*,[98–100] although the effects of exogenous hormones on *N. gonorrhoeae* are less clear.[20] These findings are difficult to reconcile with the fact that OCs are negatively associated with symptomatic PID, even of chlamydial origin.[101–103] Further, among women with clinical signs and symptoms of PID, fewer women with salpingitis on laparoscopy used OCs compared with other forms of contraception. To complicate the matter even further, Ness et al. recently showed that women with unrecognized endometritis were 4.3 times (95% confidence interval 1.6 to 11.7) more likely than women with recognized endometritis to use OCs. The overall impact of OCs on PID and infertility is therefore unclear.[12]

SUMMARY

There is evidence that women are more likely than men to develop an upper genital tract infection once they have a lower genital tract infection. Women also appear to be more likely to develop infertility from PID than men are to develop infertility from epididymo-orchitis. However, epidemiologic studies in women have been larger and more methodologically sound, and they have benefited from having a more specific infertility end point. Therefore, caution is needed in interpreting these results.

Presuming a real difference between the rates of reproductive morbidity from sexually transmitted infections in men and women, there are several potential biologic explanations. If gender-specific differences are real and not the result of measurement, they shed light on mechanisms that may mediate the relationships among pathogens, upper-tract infection, and infertility. These mediating hypotheses may translate directly into health practice, as elements of mediation can be used to test for risk, modify behavior, and treat disease. First, for example, if only specific antigenic variants of chlamydia cause upper genital tract disease, then it would be most important to develop vaccines to these particular strains. Also, if immunologic factors select for particular variants, modulation of these immunologic factors may affect the occurrence of PID. Sociocultural environmental factors such as oral contraceptives and number of sexual partners may also interact with the potential for infection. These factors may also allow for targeted public health strategies. Future prospective studies comparing reproductive morbidity from sexually transmitted diseases in men and women are needed. Sound epidemiologic methods, employed in future studies, will need to consider measurement of bacterial exposures and infertility outcomes. Such studies will also need to consider selection and confounding factors, particularly those related to patterns of intercourse and use of contraception. Once more definitive epidemiologic data are available, biologic explanations for gender-specific differences in upper genital tract disease and infertility may help to define mechanisms by which pathogens cause reproductive morbidity.

REFERENCES

1. Cates W. Genital chlamydia infections: Epidemiology and reproductive sequelae. Am J Obstet Gynecol 1991;164:1771–1781.

2. Rees E, Tait A, Hobson D, Johnson FWA. Chlamydia in relation to cervical infection and pelvic inflammatory disease. In: D Hobson, KK Holmes, eds. Nongonococcal Urethritis and Related Infections. Washington, DC: American Society of Microbiology, 1977, pp. 67–76.

3. Brunham RC, Paavonen J, Stevens CE, Kiviat N, Kuo CC, Critchlow CW. Mucopurulent cervicitis: The ignored counterpart of urethritis in the male. N Engl J Med 1984;311:1–12.

4. Swinker ML, Young SA, Cleavenger RL, Neely JL, Palmer JE. Prevalence of *Chlamydia trachomatis* cervical infection in a college gynecology clinic: Relationship to other infections and clinical features. Sex Transm Dis 1988;15:133–136.

5. Paavonen J, Critchlow CW, DeRouen T, et al. Etiology of cervical inflammation. Am J Obstet Gynecol 1986;154:556–564.

6. Aral SO, Mosher WD, Cates W Jr. Self-reported pelvic inflammatory disease in the United States, 1988. JAMA 1991;266:2570–2573.

7. Rolfs RT, Galaid EI, Zaidi AA. Pelvic inflammatory disease: Trends in hospitalizations and office visists, 1979 through 1988. Am J Obstet Gynecol 1992;166:989–990.

8. Sweet RL. Pelvic inflammatory disease and infertility in women. Infect Dis Clin North Am 1987;1:199.

9. Jones HW, Toner JP. The infertile couple. N Engl J Med 1993; 329:1710–1715.

10. Wolner-Hanssen P, Kiviat NB, Holmes KK. Atypical pelvic inflammatory disease: Subacute, chronic, or subclinical upper genital tract infection in women. In: Holmes KK, Mardh PA, Sparling PF, eds. Sexually Transmitted Diseases, 2nd ed. New York: McGraw-Hill, 1989, pp. 615–620.

11. Paavonen J, Kiviat N, Brunham RC, et al. Prevalence and manifestations of endometritis among women with cervicitis. Am J Obstet Gynecol 1985;152:280–286.

12. Ness RB, Keder LM, Soper DE, et al. Oral contraception and the recognition of endometritis. Am J Obstet Gynecol 1997;176:580–585.

13. Cates W, Rolfs RT, Aral SO. Sexually transmitted diseases, pelvic inflammatory disease, and infertility: An epidemiologic update. Epidemiol Rev 1990;12:199–220.

14. Eschenbach DA, Hillier S, Critchlow C, Stevens C, DeRouen T, Holmes KK. Diagnosis and clinical manifestations of bacterial vaginosis. Am J Obstet Gynecol 1988; 158:819–828.

15. Soper DE, Brockwell NJ, Dalton HP. Microbial etiology of urban emergency department acute salpingitis: Treatment with ofloxacillin. Am J Obstet Gynecol 1992; 167:653–660.

16. Platt R, Rice PA, McCormack WM. Risk of acquiring gonorrhea and prevalence of abnormal adnexal findings among women recently exposed to gonorrhea. JAMA 1983;250:3205–3209.

17. Stamm WE, Guinan ME, Johnson C, Starcher T, Holmes KK, McCormack WM. Effect of treatment regimens for *N. gonnorrhoea* on simultaneous infection with *C. trachomatis*. N Engl J Med 1984;310:545–549.

18. Scholes D, Stergachis A,Heidrich FE, Andrilla H, Holmes KK, Stamm WE. Prevention of pelvic inflammatory disease by screening for cervical chlamydial infection. N Engl J Med 1996;334:1362–1366.

19. Westrom L. Decrease in incidence of women treated in hospital for acute salpingitis in Sweden. Genitourin Med 1988;64:59–63.

20. Rice PA, Schachter J. Pathogenesis of pelvic inflammatory disease. What are the questions? JAMA 1991;266:2587–2593.

21. Westrom LV. Sexually transmitted diseases and infertility. Sex Transm Dis 1994;21:532–537.

22. Westrom L, Joesoef R, Reynolds G, Hogdu A, Thompson SE. Pelvic inflammatory disease and fertility. A cohort study of 1,844 women with laparoscopically verified disease and 657 control women with normal laparoscopic results. Sex Transm Dis 1992;19:185–192.

23. Moore DE, Foy HM, Daling JR, et al. Increased frequency of serum antibodies to *Chlamydia trachomatis* in infertility due to distal tubal disease. Lancet 1982;2(8298): 574–577.

24. Conway D, Caul EO, Hull MGR, et al. Chlamydial serology in fertile and infertile women. Lancet 1984;1(8370):191–193.

25. Guderian AM, Trobough GE. Residues of pelvic inflammatory disease in intrauterine device users: A result of the intrauterine device or *Chlamydia trachomatis* infection? Am J Obstet Gynecol 1986;154:497–503.

26. Gump DW, Gibson M, Ashikaga T. Evidence of prior pelvic inflammatory disease and its relationship to *Chlamydia trachomatis* antibody and intrauterine contraceptive device use in infertile women. Am J Obstet Gynecol 1983;146:153–159.

27. Anestad G, Lunde O, Moen M, Dalaker K. Infertility and chlamydial infection. Fertil Steril 1987;48:787–790.

28. Kane JL, Woodland RM, Forsey T, Darougar S, Elder MG. Evidence of chlamydial infection in infertile women with and without fallopian tube obstruction. Fertil Steril 1984;42:843–848.

29. Jones RB, Ardery BR, Hui SL, Cleary RE. Correlation between serumantichlamydial antibodies and tubal factor as a cause of infertility. Fertil Steril 1982;38: 553–558.

30. Punnonen R, Terho P, Nikkanen V, Meurman O. Chlamydial serology in infertile women by immunofluorescence. Fertil Steril 1979;31:656–659.

31. Miettinen A, Heinonen PK, Teisala K, Hakkarainen K, Punnonen R. Serologic evidence for the role of *Chalmydia trachomatis, Neisseria gonorrhoeae,* and *Mycoplasma hominis* in the etiology of tubal factor infertility and ectopic pregnancy. Sex Transm Dis 1990;17:10–14.

32. Sellors JW, Mahony JB, Chernesky MA, Rath DJ. Tubal factor infertility: An association with prior chlamydial infection and asymptomatic salpingitis. Fertil Steril 1988;49:451–457.

33. World Health Organization Task Force on the Prevention and Management of Infertility. Tubal infertility: Serologic relationship to past chlamydial and gonococcal infection. Sex Transm Dis 1995;22:71–77.

34. Kiviat NB, Wolner-Hanssen P, Eschenbach DA, et al. Endometrial histopathology in patients with culture-proved upper genital tract infection and laparoscopically diagnosed acute salpingitis. Am J Surg Pathol 1990;14(2):167–175.

35. Walrath J, Fayerweather WE, Spreen KA. A survey of the prevalence of epididymitis in an industrial setting. J Occup Med 1992;34:170–172.

36. Krieger JN. Epididymitis, orchitis, and related conditions. Sex Transm Dis 1984;11:173–181.

37. U.S. Public Health Service. Sexually Transmitted Diseases 1980 Status Report, NIAID Study Group. National Institutes of Health publ. 81–2213. Washington, DC: Government Printing Office, 1981.

38. Drotman DP. Epidemiology and treatment of epididymitis. Rev Infect Dis 1982;4:S788–S791.

39. Berger RE, Alexander R, Monda GD, Ansell J, McCormick G, Holmes KK. *C. trachomatis* as a cause of acute "idiopathic" epididymitis. N Engl J Med 1978;298: 301–304.

40. Melekos MD, Asbach HW. Epididymitis: Aspects concerning etiology and treatment. J Urol 1987;138:83–86.

41. Colleen S, Mardh PA. Complicated infections of the male genital tract with emphasis on *C. trachomatis* as an etiological agent. Scand J Infect Dis Suppl 1982; 32:93–99.

42. Mulcahy FM, Bignell CJ, Rajakumar R, et al. Prevalence of chlamydial infection in acute epididymo-orchitis. Genitourin Med 1987;63:16–18.

43. Bowie WR. Nongonococcal urethritis. Urol Clin North Am 1984;11:45–53.

44. Pelouze PS. Epididymitis. In: Pelouze PS, ed. Gonorrhea in the Male and Female. Philadelphia: W.B. Saunders, 1941, pp. 240–253.

45. Stamm WE, Kontsky L, Jourden J, Bruhan R, Holmes KK. Prospective screening for urethral infection with *C. trachomatis* and *N. gonorrhoeae* in men attending a clinic for sexually transmitted disease. Clin Res 1981;29:51A.

46. Moller BR, Mardh PA. Experimental epididymitis and urethritis in grivet monkeys provoked by *C. trachomatis.* Fertil Steril 1980;34:275–279.

47. Campbell MF. Surgical pathology of epididymitis. Ann Surg 1928;88:98.

48. Osegbe DN. Testicular function after unilateral bacterial epididymo-orchitis. Eur Urol 1991;19:204–208.

49. Auroux MR, De Mouy DM, Acar JF. Male fertility and positive chlamydial serology: A study of 61 fertile and 82 subfertile men. J Androl 1987;8:197–200.

50. Hellstrom WJ, Schachter J, Sweet RL, McClure RD. Is there a role for *C. trachomatis* and genital mycoplasma in male infertility? Fertil Steril 1987;48:337–339.

51. Quinn PA, Petric M, Barkin M, et al. Prevalence of antibody to *Chlamydia trachomatis* in spontaneous abortion and infertility. Am J Obstet Gynecol 1987;156(2): 291–296.

52. Gregoriou O, Vitoratos N, Papadias C, Gregoriou G, Zourlas PA. The role of chlamydial serology in fertile and subfertile men. Eur Obstet Gynecol Redprod Biol 1989;30(1):53–58.

53. Greendale GA, Haas ST, Holbrook K, Walsh B, Schachter J, Phillips RS. The relationship of *C. trachomatis* infection and male infertility. Am J Public Health 1993; 83:996–1001.

54. Samra Z, Soffer Y, Pansky M. Prevalence of genital chlamydia and mycoplasma infection in couples attending a male infertility clinic. Eur J Epidemiol 1994; 10:69–73.

54a. Ness RB, Tharkovic N, Carlson CL, Coughlin MT. Do men become infertile after having sexually transmitted disease? Fertil Steril 1997;68(2).

55. Witkin SS, Toth A. Relationship between genital tract infections, sperm antibodies in seminal fluid, and infertility. Fertil Steril 1983;40:805–808.

56. Naessens A, Fonlon W, Delmaker P, Devroey P, Lauwers S. Recovery of microorganisms in semen and relationship to semen evaluation. Fertil Steril 1986;45(1): 101–105.

57. Close CE, Wang SP, Roberts PL, Berger RE. The relationship of infection with *C. trachomatis* to the parameters of male fertility and sperm autoimmunity. Fertil Steril 1987;48:880–883.

58. Gregoriou O, Botsis D, Papadias K, Kassanos D, Liapis A, Zourlas PA. Culture of seminal fluid in infertile men and relationship to semen evaluation. Int J Gynaecol Obstet 1989;28:149–153.

59. Bornman MS, Mahomed MF, Boomker D, Schulenburg GW, Reif S, Crewe-Brown HH. Microbial flora in semen of infertile African men at Garankuwa hospital. Andrologia 1990;22:118–121.

60. Nagy B, Corradi G, Vajda Z, Gimes R, Csomor S. The occurrence of *C. trachomatis* in the semen of men participating in an IVF programme. Hum Reprod 1989; 4:54–56.

61. Custo GM, Lauro V, Saitto C, Frongillo RF. Chlamydial infection and male infertility: An epidemiological study. Arch Androl 1989;23:243–248.

62. DeJong Z, Pontonnier F, Plante P, et al. Comparison of the incidence of *U. urealyticum* in infertile men and in donors of semen. Eur Urol 1990;18:127–131.

63. Eggert-Kruse W, Gerhard I, Naher H, Tilgen W, Runnebaum B. Chlamydial infection—a female and/or male infertility factor? Fertil Steril 1990;53:1037–1043.

64. Micic S, Petrovic S, Dotlic R. Seminal antisperm antibodies and genitourinary infection. Urology 1990;35:54–56.

65. Ruijs GJ, Kauer FM, Jager S, Schroder PF, Schirm J, Kremer J. Is serology of any use when searching for correlations between *C. trachomatis* infection and male infertility? Fertil Steril 1990;53:131–136.

66. Soffer Y, Ron-El R, Golan A, Herman A, Caspi E, Samra Z. Male genital mycoplasmas and *C. trachomatis* culture: Its relationship with accessory gland function, sperm quality, and autoimmunity. Fertil Steril 1990;53:331–336.

67. Wolff H, Neubert U, Zebhauser M, Bezold G, Korting HC, Meurer M. *C. trachomatis* induces an inflammatory response in the male genital tract and is associated with altered semen quality. Fertil Steril 1991;55:1017–1019.

68. Witkin SS, Jeremias J, Grifo JA, Ledger WJ. Detection of C. Trachomatis in semen by the polymerase chain reaction in male members of infertile couples. Am J Obstet Gynecol 1993;168:1457–1462.

69. Kahn JG, Walker CK, Washington AE, Landers DV, Sweet RL. Diagnosing pelvic inflammatory disease. A comprehensive analysis and considerations for developing a model. JAMA 1991;266:2594–2604.

70. Wasserheit JN, Bell TA, Kiviat NB, et al. Microbial causes of proven pelvic inflammatory disease and efficacy of clindamycin and tobramycin. Ann Intern Med 1986; 104:187–193.

71. Sellors J, Mahony J, Goldsmith C, et al. The accuracy of clinical findings and laparoscopy in pelvic inflammatory disease. Am J Obstet Gynecol 1991;164:113–120.

72. Harwood-Nuss A. Genitourinary disease. In: Rosen P, Baker FJ, Barkin RM, Braen GR, Dailey RH, Levy RC, eds. Emergency Medicine Concepts and Practice, 2nd ed. St. Louis: Mosby, 1988.

73. MacLeod J. Semen quality in 1,000 men of known fertility and in 800 cases of infertile marriages. Fertil Steril 1951;2:15.

74. David G, Jouannet P, Martin-Boyce A, Smira M, Schwartz D. Sperm counts in fertile and infertile men. Fertil Steril 1979;31:453–455.

75. Rehan NE, Sobrero A, Fertig JW. The semen of fertile men: Statistical analysis of 1300 men. Fertil Steril 1975;26:492–502.

76. Worm AM, Petersen CS. Transmission of chlamydia infections to sexual partners. Genitourin Med 1987;63:19–21.

77. Ramstedt K, Forssman L, Giesecke J, Johannisson G. Epidemiologic characteristics of two different populations of women with *Clamydia tracomatis* infection and their male partners. Sex Transm Dis 1991;18:205–210.

78. Lycke E, Lowhagen GB, Hallhagen G, Johannisson G, Ramstedt K. The risk of transmission of genital *Chlamydia trachomatis* infection is less than that of genital *Neisseria gonorrhoeae* infection. Sex Transm Dis 1980;7:6–9.

79. Katz BP, Caine VA, Jones RB. Estimation of transmission probabilities for chlamydial infection. In: Bowie WR, Caldwell HD, Jones RB, et al, eds. Chlamydia Infections. New York: Cambridge University Press, 1990, pp. 567–570.

80. Padian N, Shiboski S, Glass S, Hessol N, Vittinghoff E. Heterosexual transmission of HIV in California. Presented at the eleventh meeting of the International Society for STD Research. New Orleans, LA, August 27–30, 1995. Abstract #052.

81. Royce RR, Sena A, Cates W, Cohen MS. Sexual transmission of HIV. N Engl J Med 1997;336:1072–1078.

82. Quinn TC, Gaydos C, Shepherd M, et al. Epidemiologic and microbiologic correlates of *Chlamydia trachomatis* infection in sexual partnerships. JAMA 1996;276:1737–1742.

83. Washington AE, Aral SO, Wolner-Hanssen P, Grimes DA, Holmes KK. Assesing risk for pelvic inflammatory disease and its sequelae. JAMA 1991;266:2581–2586.

84. Wolner-Hanssen, Mardh PA. In vitro tests of the adherence of *C. trachomatis* to human spermatozoa. Fertil Steril 1984;42:102–107.

85. Hillier SD, Joesoef R, Marchbanks PA, Wasserheit JN, Cates W Jr, Westrom L. Delayed care of pelvic inflammatory disease as a risk factor for impaired fertility. Am J Obstet Gynecol 1993;168:1503–1509.

86. Dean D, Oudens E, Bolan G, Padian N, Schachter J. Polymorphism in the major outer membrane protein of *Chlamydia trachomatis* is associated with severe upper genital tract infections and histopathology in San Francisco [Abstract]. Presented at the eleventh meeting of the International Society for STD Research. New Orleans, LA August 27–30, 1995. Abstract #007.

87. Lee NC, Rubin GL, Ory HW, Burkman RT. Type of intrauterine device and the risk of pelvic inflammatory disease. Obstet Gynecol 1983;62:1–6.

88. Vessey MP, Yeates D, Flavel R, McPherson K, et al. Pelvic inflammatory disease and the intrauterine device: Findings in a large cohort study. BMJ 1981;282:855–857.

89. Kessel E. Pelvic inflammatory disease with intrauterine device use: A reassessment. Fertil Steril 1989;51:1–11.

90. Edelman DA. The use of intrauterine contraceptive devices, pelvic inflammatory disease, and *Chlamydia trachomatis* infection. Am J Obstet Gynecol 1988;158:956–959.

91. Wolner-Hanssen P, Eschenbach DA, Paavonen J, et al. Association between vaginal douching and acute pelvic inflammatory disease. JAMA 1990;263:1936–1941.

92. Forrest KA, Washington AE, Daling JR, Sweet RL. Vaginal douching as a possible risk factor for pelvic inflammatory disease. J Natl Med Assoc 1989;81:159–165.

93. Neumann HH, DeCherney A. Douching and pelvic inflammatory disease [Letter]. N Engl J Med 1976;295:789.

94. McGregor JA, Spencer NE, French JI, et al. Psychosocial and behavioral risk factors for acute salpingitis. Presented at the Sixth Annual Meeting of the International Society for STD Research, Brighton, England, August 1, 1985. Abstract #14.

95. Cottingham J, Hunter D. *Chlamydia trachomatis* and oral contraceptive use: A quantitative review. Genitourin Med 1992;68:209–216.

96. Louv WC, Austin H, Perlman J, Alexander WJ. Oral contraceptive use and the risk of chlamydial and gonoccal infection. Am J Obstet Gynecol 1989;160:396–402.

97. Avonts D, Sercu M, Heyerick P, Vandermeeren I, Meheus A, Piot P. Incidence of uncomplicated genital infections in women using oral contraception or an intrauterine device: A prospective study. Sex Transm Dis 1990;17:23–29.

98. Mardh PA, Paavonen J, Puolakkainen M. Chlamydia. New York: Plenum Press, 1989.

99. Rank RG, White HJ, Hough AJ Jr, Pasley JN, Barron AL. Effect of estradiol on chlamydial genital infection of female guinea pigs. Infect Immun 1982;38:699–705.

100. Tuffrey M, Taylor-Robinson D. Progesterone as a key factor in the development of a mouse model for genital tract infection with *Chlamydia trachomatis*. FEMS Microbiol Lett 1981;12:111–115.

101. Washington AE, Gove S, Schachter J, Sweet RL. Oral contraceptives, *Chlamydia trachomatis* infection, and pelvic inflammatory disease. A word of caution about protection. JAMA 1985;253:2246–2250.

102. Wolner-Hanssen P, Eschenbach DA, Paavonen J, et al. Decreased risk of symptomatic chlamydial pelvic inflammatory disease associated with oral contraceptive use. JAMA 1990;263:54–59.

103. Senanayake P, Kramer DG. Contraception and the etiology of pelvic inflammatory disease: New perspectives. Am J Obstet Gynecol 1980;138:852–860.

15

AUTOIMMUNE DISEASES

Susan Manzi and Rosalind Ramsey-Goldman

Under normal conditions, the immune system distinguishes the body's own tissues from external invaders. In autoimmune diseases the immune system inappropriately targets the body and this results in tissue injury. Autoimmune responses may be directed toward a specific organ or towards components of cells. Organ-specific autoimmune conditions include autoimmune thyroiditis and bullous dermatologic conditions, including pemphigoid. In contrast, systemic lupus erythematosus (SLE) is characterized by the production of autoantibodies directed against the nucleus, cytoplasm, or membrane of cells.[1,2] This generalized autoreactivity in SLE results in multi-organ involvement.

Sex hormones have been implicated in the pathogenesis of autoimmune diseases on the basis of both animal and human data.[3–11] Animal models show that estrogens stimulate and androgens suppress the immune system,[4,8,11] and many autoimmune diseases show marked gender predilections with women more commonly afflicted than men (Table 15–1).[3] Therefore, the gender inequity in autoimmune diseases may be the result of a relatively stimulated or "turned on" immune response.

This chapter will review the evidence that currently implicates hormones in the pathogenesis of autoimmunity. The discussion will focus on rheumatoid arthritis (RA) and systemic lupus erythematosus (SLE) since they have been the most thoroughly investigated autoimmune diseases with regard to sex hormone metabolism.

Table 15–1. Female Preponderance of Autoimmune Diseases

DISEASE	FEMALE/MALE RATIO
Thyroid diseases:	
Diffuse lymphocytic thyroiditis	
Goitrous, struma lymphomatosa (Hashimoto),	
Hypercellular variant, adult onset	25–50:1
Hypercellular variant, juvenile onset	4–7:1
Fibrous variant	4:1
Non goitrous	
Severe atrophic (myxedema)	6:1
Mild atrophic (asymptomatic)	8:1
Primary hyperthyroidism (Graves Basedow disease)	
With benign or no exophthalmos	4–8:1
With progressive ophthalmopathy	2:1
Systemic lupus erythematosus	9:1
Rhematoid arthritis	2–4:1
Sjögren's syndrome	9:1
Idiopathic adrenal insufficiency (autoimmune adrenal disease)	2–3:1
Scleroderma	3–4:1
Myasthenia gravis	2:1
Multiple sclerosis	1–5:1

[Reprinted with permission from International Journal of Fertility and Women's Medicine, Vol. 41, No. 2, Lahita, page 41, 1996[3]]

INFLUENCE OF GENDER AND SEX HORMONES ON AUTOIMMUNITY

Autoimmunity results from a breakdown or failure of the mechanisms that are normally responsible for maintaining self-tolerance, or the inability of the immune system to recognize self-antigens.[12–14] The most effective mechanism of self-tolerance is the deletion of T and B lymphocytes that recognize self-antigens and would therefore attack the host.[15,16] Concepts concerning the depletion of these self-recognizing lymphocytes are currently changing. Previously, it was believed that all self-reactive T cells were eliminated during fetal development. Now it is has been shown that reactivity to self by T cells during childhood and adulthood is physiologic and important to the formation of normal immune responses.[17,18] Similarly, B cells that have the potential to make autoantibodies are also not completely deleted prior to maturation.[19] Thus if everyone has T and B cells capable of reacting to self and ultimately inducing autoimmunity, it becomes important to determine the mechanism whereby this normal physiologic process becomes pathogenic. One theory is that in autoimmune diseases, T cells that are normally quiescent become activated and induce

B cells to produce pathogenic autoantibodies.[20–22] These antibodies, which are typically IgG and, unlike the low-affinity IgM antibodies produced during nonspecific activation, are high-affinity pathogenic antibodies directed at specific antigens. It is hypothesized that patients with some autoimmune diseases also lack the ability to regulate hyperactivated B and T cells. This overproduction of pathogenic autoantibodies, coupled with impairment of the normal downregulation of B and T cell hyperactivity, likely leads to immune complex (antigen/antibody) formation, inflammation, and tissue injury.

Multiple interacting factors contribute to the development of autoimmune disease. These include immunologic abnormalities, genetic predisposition to autoimmunity, hormonal influences, and possibly microbial infections or other environmental stimuli that may lead to aberrant lymphocyte stimulation. One or many of these factors may be operative in different autoimmune diseases; this results in a wide variety of clinical conditions.

Observations in animal models and humans with autoimmune conditions indicate that sex hormones influence autoimmune reactions.[3–11] Physiological levels of estrogens are thought to stimulate the immune response and male hormones to suppress it.[4,8,11] Estrogens have been demonstrated in vitro to stimulate B cell response and decrease suppressor T cell reactivity which can lead to an increase in autoantibody production.[23] Current evidence suggests that sex hormones influence the immune system through several mechanisms, such as the presence of intracellular sex steroid receptors in a variety of tissues and cells, including lymphocytes.[24,25] Estrogens likely account in part for the higher immune reactivity in females against a variety of antigens and the more rapid rejection of allografts.[26] The greater immune responses in females might also increase their susceptibility to autoimmune diseases.[4]

In addition to estrogens, dehyroepiandrosterone (DHEA) and DHEA sulfate (DHEAS) may play a role in immunity and autoimmunity. DHEA and DHEAS are weak androgens largely secreted by the adrenal glands. Their direct contribution to sex hormone physiology is believed to be small.[27,28] The major physiologic function of DHEA and DHEAS is still largely unknown,[27–29] however, studies in animal models and humans have shown that DHEA is capable of altering cytokine secretion and regulating cytokine production, both of which would have an impact on immune responsiveness. DHEA stimulates the production of the cytokine interleukin 2 (IL-2) (a TH 1 product) in human CD4+ T cells and suppresses the production of inteleukin 6 (IL-6) (a TH 2 product).[30,31] Both of these actions suggest a role for this androgen in the regulation of autoimmunity. TH 1 and TH 2, which are subsets of CD4+ T cells, produce cytokines that activate cellular immunity and humoral (antibody-mediated) immunity, respectively.

Sex steroids can modulate various autoimmune and rheumatic diseases in animals. In the nonobese diabetic mouse, the incidence of autoimmune diabetes is much higher in females than in males (80% vs. 20%). Ovariectomy decreases and orchiectomy increases the incidence of diabetes in female and male mice, respectively.[32] Similarly, in the rat model of autoimmune thyroiditis, testosterone can inhibit the development of thyroid disease.[33,34]

Rheumatoid arthritis (RA) and systemic lupus erythematosus (SLE) are two autoimmune disorders in which hormones influence pathogenesis. Although these two autoimmune conditions share a female gender predilection, they differ in their response to manipulation of hormone levels. For example, estrogens tend to ameliorate the incidence and severity of type II collagen-induced arthritis in mice and rats.[35] This T cell–dependent experimental model of arthritis is similar to human RA. In contrast, estrogens accelerate the disease process in some animal models of SLE. One of the most widely studied animal models of autoimmunity is a mouse model of SLE. These mice spontaneously develop a disease similar to human SLE, including developing antibodies to DNA and glomerulonephritis at 3 to 6 months, which progresses to death by 12 months.[36] Onset of lupus in mice is earlier and the disease is more severe in females than males. Males of this strain have a significantly longer survival than females and castration in males accelerates mortality to the rate found in female mice.[37,38] In addition, treatment of females with androgens postpones death.[37,39] These observations in both animal models and humans with RA and SLE have led to intensive inquiry and investigation into the relationship between hormonal milieu and disease state.

EPIDEMIOLOGY OF SEX HORMONES AND AUTOIMMUNE DISEASE

Observational studies in humans have helped to assess the relationships between steroid hormones and autoimmune diseases such as RA and SLE. For example, how each disease behaves during premenopause versus postmenopause, during the menstrual cycle or pregnancy, and under the influence of exogenous hormones provides clues about these relationships.

RHEUMATOID ARTHRITIS

Clinical Features

Rheumatoid arthritis (RA) is a systemic autoimmune disorder of unknown etiology.[40] Its major feature is a destructive, chronic arthritis and it is characterized by inflammation of the synovium, a thin vascular membrane that lines the joint capsule. Synovial inflammation contributes to the joint stiffness, swelling, and pain that patients with RA experience. Deformity may develop over time as the articular surface and supporting structures become damaged by the inflammatory process. Patients with RA may have clinical features beyond joint inflammation, including subcutaneous nodules, vasculitis, pericarditis, pulmonary nodules, interstitial pulmonary fibrosis, mononeuritis multiplex, and inflammatory eye disease such as episcleritis and scleritis. Table 15–2 shows the 1987 revised classification criteria for RA.[41] These criteria have been established primarily for epidemiologic research purposes to ensure uniform classification of patients across centers and not for the purpose of diagnosing RA in individual cases. However, they do provide useful guidelines for making a diagnosis of RA.

Immune Abnormalities and Pathophysiology

The histopathology of inflamed synovium suggests a local immune response.[40] The rheumatoid synovium is characterized by the presence of diffuse or nodular mononuclear inflammatory cell infiltrates. The cellular infiltrate is composed primarily of lymphocytes, macrophages, and plasma cells. Although the focus of much investigation into the pathogenesis of RA has been on T cells present in the synovium, there are also B cells that contribute to the local production of immune complexes. Numerous cytokines, including interleukin-1 (IL-1), tumor necrosis factor (TNF), and interferon-gamma (IFN-γ), have been detected in the joint fluid. Many of these cytokines play a role in the initiation of joint de-

Table 15–2.   1987 American College of Rheumatology Criteria
for the Classification of Rheumatoid Arthritis[a]

1. Morning stiffness in and around the joints, lasting at least 1 hour before maximal improvement.
2. At least 3 joint areas simultaneously have had soft tissue swelling or fluid (not bony overgrowth alone) observed by a physician. The 14 possible areas are right or left PIP, MCP, wrist, elbow, knee, ankle, and MTP joints.
3. At least 1 area swollen (as defined above) in a wrist, MCP, or PIP joint.
4. Simultaneous involvement of the same joint areas (as defined in no. 2) on both sides of the body (bilateral involvement of PIPs, MCPs, or MTPs is acceptable without absolute symmetry.
5. Subcutaneous nodules, over bony prominences, or extensor surfaces, or in juxta-articular regions, observed by a physician.
6. Demonstration of abnormal amounts of serum rheumatoid factor by any method for which the result has been positive in less than 5% of normal control subjects.
7. Radiographic changes typical of rheumatoid arthritis on posteroanterior hand and wrist radiographs, which must include erosions or unequivocal bony decalcification localized in or most marked adjacent to the involved joints (osteoarthritis changes alone do not qualify).

[a]For classifying a patient as having RA, four of the seven criteria are required. MCP, metacarpophalangeal; MTP, metatarsophalangeal; PIP, proximal interphalangeal.

[Reprinted with permission from Arthritis and Rheumatism, Vol. 31, No. 3, page 319, Arnett, et al., March 1988[41]]

struction and are produced as a result of local T cell and macrophage activation. The antigens initiating immune cell activation are unknown.

Epidemiology

The prevalence of RA increases with age for both males and females and has been reported to be most common in people over the age of 65. Males have a lower incidence of RA than women at any age, however, the gender differential decreases with increasing age.[42,43] Men under 45 years of age rarely develop RA. The female-to-male ratio is nearly 5:1 during the female reproductive years, but only 2:1 or less in young children and older adults.[5,45] Rheumatoid arthritis occurs in all races and in all parts of the world. There have been consistent estimates of the prevalence of RA in both North America and Europe ranging from 0.5 to 1.0%.[46,47] Considerably fewer studies examining the incidence of RA have reported rates ranging from 0.2 to 0.4 cases per 1,000 adults per year.[43,48,49]

Endogenous Hormones

Investigators have been unable to consistently show differences in levels of estradiol in men and women with RA compared with controls.[44,50] A reduction in male hormones is observed in males with RA when compared with age-matched controls who have osteoarthritis or ankylosing spondylitis or are healthy.[51-54] The source of the defect in men with RA may be a decrease in testosterone production from the testes.[42,55] One study reported lower testosterone levels in premenopausal women with RA compared with normal controls,[56] but other investigators have failed to show any differences in testosterone between women with RA compared with those having osteoarthritis or chronic low back pain.[50,57,58]

The MHC (major histocompatibility complex) or the HLA (human leukocyte antigen) region in humans is located on the short arm of chromosome 6 and contains the genes that regulate the immune response. HLA antigens detected on certain cells involved in the immune response are designated by the letter of the gene locus from which they are encoded, followed by a number. An association between RA and its severity and HLA-DR4/DW4 has been demonstrated in several studies.[59-61] Genes inside the HLA region, specifically HLA-B8 and HLA-B15, have been associated with significantly lower testosterone levels in women as well as in healthy and RA males.[62-64] These observations suggest that the association between RA and low testosterone concentrations may be mediated in part by the HLA-B locus.

A recent review examining sex hormones and rheumatoid arthritis[6] reported the results of several studies examining DHEAS levels in patients with

RA. There is evidence to suggest that women with RA have lower DHEA and DHEAS levels than normal women, women with osteoarthritis, and "HLA-identical" siblings without RA.[56,65–68] These lower levels of DHEAS were not consistently seen in men with RA.[54,55] The authors concluded that although these studies suggest hormonal differences in patients with RA, studies of early RA disease onset would help to address the dilemma of primary (present at disease onset) versus secondary (develops after disease onset) deficiencies, as well as other potential confounding factors. In a more recent study, serum levels of DHEAS in 21 new RA cases were analyzed a mean of 13 years before the onset of RA.[69] The sera were obtained in 1974 at entry into a community-wide, prospective study. Younger, premenopausal women who developed RA had lower DHEAS levels at study entry than women of similar age, race, and menopausal status without RA. These results suggest that low DHEAS levels may be a risk factor for the development of RA in young, premenopausal women. The authors concluded that if normal or elevated androgen levels are somehow protective in the development of RA or other autoimmune diseases, the incidence of RA should be studied in populations with hyperandrogenism, such as women with polycystic ovary disease or hirsutism.

Pregnancy

Fertility (ability to conceive) is not decreased, but fecundity (probability of conception) may be impaired in patients with RA. Several explanations have been proposed to explain this combination including ovulatory dysfunction or insufficient progesterone secretion by the corpus luteum, abnormalities of tubal transport or implantation, antibodies to spermatozoa, or an imbalance in the hypothalamic–pituitary–adrenal axis.[70] There is no evidence to suggest that having RA has an adverse effect on fetal outcome.

The majority of patients with RA show improved signs and symptoms of RA during pregnancy. This observation has been noted consistently in studies during the last 50 years.[71–75] Symptoms ameliorate during the first trimester and can continue to improve during the second and third trimesters and up to 65% of patients have a complete remission during pregnancy.[70] Pre-eclampsia may be decreased in patients with RA.[70] Exacerbation of disease in almost 100% of patients is noted by 4 months postpartum in many studies.[74–76]

The clinical course of pregnancy in a patient with RA is clearly in contrast to SLE patients who may experience flares in disease activity or develop clinically active disease for the first time during pregnancy. The reasons for disease remission in RA with pregnancy are not clearly understood. During normal pregnancy, the maternal immune system is altered in some way to tolerate the presence of the foreign paternal antigens that are inherited by the fetus. Specifically, there is a maternal immune response to paternally inherited fetal HLA antigens,[77] yet the fetus is not rejected by the mother. Recently, investigators have reported that disease remission in pregnant women with RA most often occurred when the fetal and maternal HLA class II antigens differed.[78] These findings suggest that the maternal immune response to fetal HLA class II antigens may play a role in the disease remission in pregnant women with RA. Several theories have been postulated to explain this phenomenon. Fetal HLA may affect maternal self-reactivity by inducing regulatory T cells in the maternal circulation.[79–81] Increased production of TH2 cytokines[82] and interactions between the neuroendocrine and immune systems during pregnancy may also be important.

Exogenous Hormones

The incidence of RA reportedly declined during the 1970s when there was an increased use of oral contraceptives.[83] This suggested that exogenous estrogen use might have a protective effect on the development of RA and led to further investigation. The decline in RA incidence previously reported is not uniformly accepted.[84] There are conflicting reports about the use of oral contraceptives (OCs) or hormone replacement therapy (HRT) and the subsequent risks of RA.[85] One study from The Netherlands reported a protective effect of HRT on the development of RA.[86] This conclusion was based on a case–control study using a postal questionnaire of 148 patients with RA and 186 women with either osteoarthritis or soft tissue rheumatologic disorders. A negative association was found between the onset of RA and previous use of HRT with an odds ratio of 0.22 (95% CI 0.08–0.60). There were several methodologic problems with this study, including a high percentage of incomplete questionnaires and the potential for recall bias in reporting the timing of estrogen use and first symptoms of RA. In a large case–control study of postmenopausal women selected from a registry of new patients attending a rheumatology clinic in Quebec City, Canada, cases were defined as those patients who met criteria for definite or classical RA and controls were patients with either osteoarthritis or soft tissue rheumatism.[87] Information on hormone exposure was obtained by telephone interview. There were 111 cases with RA and 305 controls available for analysis. In comparison to women who had never used postmenopausal hormones before onset of rheumatologic symptoms, the adjusted relative risk for past and current users was 0.95 (95% CI 0.56–1.60) and 0.89 (95% CI 0.49–1.63), respectively. This study provided little support for the hypothesis that postmenopausal hormones protect against the development of RA. Similarly, a study examining the incidence rates of RA from 1982 to 1986 among 4,326 women who attended a walk-in menopause clinic and a general practice registry in London failed to show a reduction in RA incidence in HRT users (relative risk for HRT use was 1.62, 95% CI 0.56–4.74).[88] In one large prospective study, the use of exogenous sex hormones in relation to risk of RA was examined in a cohort of married nurses 30–55 years of age who had been followed since 1976 in the Nurses' Health Study.[89] When compared with women who had never used oral contraceptives, the age-adjusted relative risk was 1.0 (95% CI 0.7–1.3) for past users. When compared with postmenopausal women who never used estrogens, the age-adjusted relative risk was 1.3 (95% CI 0.9–2.0) for current users, 0.7 (95% CI 0.5–1.2) for past users, and 1.0 (95% CI 0.7–1.4) for ever users. These three large studies from Canada, the United Kingdom, and the United States failed to confirm that estrogen therapy has a protective effect on the development of RA.

Summary

RA is a common disorder resulting in a destructive, inflammatory, chronic arthritis. The prevalence of RA increases with age in men and women, and in most populations studied it is most common in people over the age of 65. Males have a lower incidence of RA than women at any age. An association between RA, severity of RA disease, and genetic factors (HLA-DR4/DW4) has been well demonstrated. Although there are data to suggest that patients with RA may be relatively hypoandrogenic (have lower androgen levels) compared with those without RA, there are conflicting reports about the effects of exogenous hormones on disease expression. Some investigators found a protective effect of hormone replacement therapy in the development of RA, whereas others provided little support for this hypothesis. The reasons for pregnancy-induced disease remission in RA are not clearly understood. Disease remission in pregnant women with RA most often occurs when the fetal and maternal HLA class II antigens differ. These findings suggest that the maternal immune response to fetal HLA class II antigens, as opposed to the direct effects of changing sex hormone levels during pregnancy, plays a role in disease remission. Although RA is one of many autoimmune diseases predominantly affecting women, the role of sex hormones on pathogenesis and clinical course of the disease is still largely unknown.

SYSTEMIC LUPUS ERYTHEMATOSUS

Clinical Features

Systemic lupus is a chronic, inflammatory, autoimmune disease that targets various organs.[90–92] Criteria have been developed for the purpose of disease classification to ensure that large series of patients from different geographic locations are comparable to one another (Table 15–3).[93] Of the 11 criteria, the presence of four or more of them, either serially or simultaneously, is said to be sufficient for classification of a patient having SLE. Included are malar rash (nonscarring rash across the bridge of the nose and cheeks), discoid rash (scarring rash), photosensitivity, oral ulcers, arthritis, serositis (pleuritis or pericardi-

Table 15–3. 1982 Revised Criteria for Classification of
Systemic Lupus Erythematosus[a]

CRITERION	
1. Malar rash	Fixed erythema, flat or raised, over the malar eminences, tending to spare the nasolabial folds
2. Discoid rash	Erythematous raised patches with adherent keratotic scaling and follicular plugging; atrophic scarring may occur in older lesions
3. Photosensitivity	Skin rash as a result of unusual reaction to sunlight, by patient history or physician observation
4. Oral ulcers	Oral or nasopharyngeal ulceration, usually painless, observed by a physician
5. Arthritis	Non-erosive arthritis involving 2 or more peripheral joints, characterized by tenderness, swelling, or effusion
6. Serositis	a. Pleuritis: convincing history of pleuritic pain or rub heard by a physician or evidence of pleural effusion b. Pericarditis: documented by ECG or rub or evidence of pericardial effusion
7. Renal disorder	a. Persistent proteinuria >0.5 g/day or >3+ if quantitation not performed b. Cellular casts: may be red cell, hemoglobin, granular, tubular, or mixed
8. Neurologic disorder	a. Seizures: in the absence of offending drugs or known metabolic derangements, e.g., uremia, ketoacidosis, or electrolyte imbalance b. Psychosis: in the absence of offending drugs or known metabolic derangements; e.g., uremia, ketoacidosis, or electrolyte imbalance
9. Hematologic disorder	a. Hemolytic anemia: with reticulocytosis b. Leukopenia: <4,000/mm³ total on 2 or more occasions c. Lymphopenia: <1,500/mm³ on 2 or more occasions d. Thrombocytopenia: <100,000/mm³ in the absence of offending drugs
10. Immunologic disorder	a. Positive LE cell preparation b. Anti-DNA: antibody to native DNA in abnormal titer c. Anti-Sm: presence of antibody to Sm nuclear antigen d. False-positive serologic test for syphilis known to be positive for at least 6 months and confirmed by *Treponema pallidum* immobilization or fluorescent treponemal antibody absorption test
11. Antinuclear antibody	An abnormal titer of antinuclear antibody by immunofluorescence or an equivalent assay at any point in time and in the absence of drugs known to be associated with "drug-induced lupus" syndrome

[a]The proposed classification is based on 11 criteria. For the purpose of identifying patients in clinical studies, a person is said to have systemic lupus erythematosus if any 4 or more of the 11 criteria are present, serially or simultaneously, during any interval of observation.

[Reprinted with permission from Arthritis and Rheumatism, Vol. 25, No. 11, page 1274, Tan, et al., November 1982[93]] tis), renal involvement, central nervous system involvement (seizures or psychosis), hematologic abnormalities (hemolytic anemia, leukopenia, thrombocytopenia), immunologic markers (positive LE prep, antibodies to native DNA and Smith antigen, or a false-positive serologic test for syphilis), and a positive antinuclear antibody (ANA). Although these criteria were established primarily for research purposes, they serve as useful reminders of those features that distinguish lupus from other related connective tissue diseases.

Immune Abnormalities and Pathophysiology

The central immunologic disturbance in patients with SLE is autoantibody production.[1,2] These autoantibodies are directed against a host of self-antigens found in the nucleus, cytoplasm, and membranes of cells. SLE is generally classified as a disease of generalized autoimmunity because of the wide range of antigenic targets. Some of the most frequent antibodies are to nuclear antigens including anti-native DNA antibodies. Immune complexes formed by these autoantibodies and their specific antigens can deposit in the blood vessels of various organs, resulting in an inflammatory response and tissue damage. In addition, autoantibody-mediated cellular dysfunction may be the mechanism for autoimmune cytopenias. Although SLE is characterized by autoantibodies, help from T cells is required for antibody production. In mouse models of SLE, depletion of CD4+ T cells blocks onset of disease[94] and athymic mice do not develop SLE.[95] At present, it is unclear whether SLE is the result of excessive T cell help or defective T cell suppression.[95]

Epidemiology

The average incidence of SLE in the United States has been estimated to be between 1.8 and 7.6 cases per 100,000 persons per year.[96–100] Prevalence of SLE in the continental United States has been reported to range from 14.6 to 50.8 cases per 100,000.[96–98] The differences in reported incidence and prevalence rates are largely a reflection of differing methods of ascertainment. The frequency of disease is much higher in women than men. The peak incidence occurs between the ages of 15 and 45, the childbearing years, when the female-to-male ratio is about 12:1. In pediatric and older-onset patients, the female-to-male ratio is closer to 2:1. SLE occurrence is nearly three to four times higher among African-American women than Caucasian women. SLE is thought to be caused by genetically determined immune abnormalities that are potentially triggered by hormonal factors and other environmental stimuli. An association between HLA DR2 and DR3 and SLE has been reported in some populations.[101–103] Inherited complement deficiencies, particularly homozygous C4a deficiency, confers a very high risk for SLE.[104,105] Recently, two additional genes have been identified in patients with lupus. One gene codes for the FcγRIIA receptor; African-American lupus patients that inherit a specific version of this gene have an increased risk of lupus kidney disease.[106] Impaired Fc receptors on IgG may contribute to susceptibility to lupus because of impaired clearance of immune complexes. A candidate gene, 1q41–q42 region on chromosome 1, has been suggested as one genetic factor that may confer an increased risk for lupus in all ethnic groups.[107]

Endogenous Hormones

Both male and female patients with SLE have been found to have abnormalities in estrogen metabolism[3,108–111] (Figure 15–1).[112] Researchers have shown elevated levels of 16α-hydroxyestrone and estriol and low levels of the 2-hydroxylated estrogens in patients with SLE.[7,9] In contrast to the 16-hydroxylated metabolites, which retain significant peripheral estrogenic activity, the 2-hydroxylated compounds do not.[113,114] These observations were initially made by Lahita et al. when they examined urinary metabolites and later confirmed that the increased 16α-metabolites in urine were due to increased production rather than increased excretion.[108] The elevated conversion of estradiol to 16-hydroxylated metabolites in SLE patients did not appear to be associated with age, use of corticosteroids, or obesity.[108] Lahita et al. failed to show an association between these metabolites and SLE disease activity. However, their study included small numbers of patients (8 men, 15 women) and lacked a quantitative measure of lupus disease activity. Patients with other illnesses, including breast cancer, endometrial cancer, chronic liver disease, or rheumatoid arthritis, failed to show elevations in the 16-hydroxylated metabolites as great as those identified in patients with SLE. There are also data suggesting that first-degree relatives of patients with SLE have similar elevations of 16-hydroxylated metabolites.[110]

Lower plasma testosterone levels were demonstrated in women with SLE compared with age-similar healthy controls by Jungers et al.[115] All of the SLE women in this study had regular menses and none were on oral contraceptives or had clinical liver disease. Low testosterone levels could not be explained by corticosteroid adrenal suppression since many of the SLE women had never been on corticosteroids and the others had been off corticosteroids for 6 months to 7 years prior to obtaining the hormone levels. Testosterone is largely bound to sex hormone–binding globulin (SHBG). It is not clear whether the differences seen in testosterone levels are a reflection of lower SHBG in women with SLE. Other investigators have confirmed lower androgen levels in women with SLE. Although testosterone levels appeared lower in 22 women with active SLE disease compared with 6 women without disease, this did not reach statistical significance, perhaps because of inadequate study power.[112] One explanation for low testosterone levels in women with SLE is thought to be accelerated metabolism of testos-

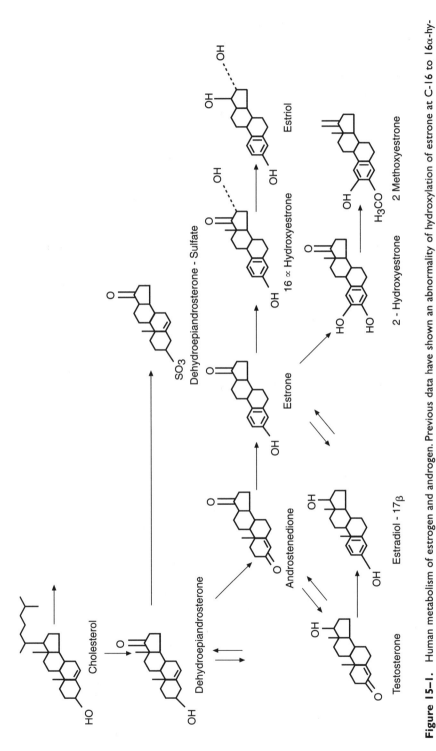

Figure 15–1. Human metabolism of estrogen and androgen. Previous data have shown an abnormality of hydroxylation of estrone at C-16 to 16α-hydroxyesterone and estriol, and abnormally rapid oxidation of testosterone to androstenedione at C-17. The latter finding is specific to female systemic lupus erythematosus patients. [Reprinted with permission from Arthritis and Rheumatism, Vol. 30, No. 3, page 246, Lahita, et al., March 1987[112]]

terone via oxidation to androstenedione at C-17.[112,116] Interestingly, men with SLE have not consistently been noted to have abnormalities in testosterone levels.[112]

In a later study, 26 nulliparous women with inactive SLE and not on corticosteroids had lower peak and 7-day postovulation serum progesterone concentrations than 21 healthy, nulliparous controls.[117] In all of the women studied, ovulation was confirmed by ultrasound. No differences were detected in serum concentrations of follicle-stimulating hormone (FSH), luteinizing hormone (LH), prolactin, estradiol-17β, testosterone, androstenedione, DHEAS, or cortisol. Very little attention has been given to progesterone in SLE and thus the significance of these findings in women with presumably inactive SLE is uncertain. Interestingly, progesterone is felt to have immunosuppressive properties and has been shown to depress cell-mediated immunity and enhance suppressor cell activity.[118,119]

During the normal menstrual cycle, progesterone levels rise during the luteal phase, which occurs after ovulation and prior to menses. Lower levels of progesterone found in women with lupus during the luteal phase may contribute to the increased symptoms reported by these women during the 2 weeks prior to menses. In addition, an inadequate production of progesterone in women may render them prone to autoimmune diseases such as SLE.

Although it is reported that SLE disease activity can be altered during pregnancy and postpartum, much less is known about the possible effects on SLE symptomatology during the normal menstrual cycle. Clinicians have recognized for some time that women with SLE often report increasing joint pain, fatigue, mouth ulcers, pleuritic chest pain, and other subjective symptoms at certain times during the menstrual cycle. Only a few investigators have actually examined this in detail.[120–122] In one report, 28 menstruating women were followed through 991 menstrual periods.[120] Increased signs or symptoms of SLE were reported in 172 (17%) of the cycles. Signs and symptoms consisted of pleurisy, pericarditis, arthritis or arthralgia, mucosal ulcers, increased rash, vasculitic lesions, and orthopnea. Most of these manifestations were confirmed by physical exam. Of the 172 periods with increased symptoms, 140 (81%) occurred in the 2 weeks prior to menstruation. These results suggest a possible relationship between SLE disease activity and the menstrual cycle, however, no sex hormone levels were measured. Thus, no conclusive statement about the association of sex hormones and SLE symptoms could be made. Other investigators have reported symptoms consistent with increased disease activity during the premenstrual period in 45%–60% of women with SLE.[121,122]

Pregnancy

Fertility does not appear to be decreased in lupus patients compared with the general obstetrical population,[123] except in the circumstances of very active systemic disease. There are no studies that evaluate fecundity in patients with lupus. Fetal outcome is adversely affected by maternal lupus. Approximately 50% of pregnancies in women with lupus result in a full-term, normal birth weight infant.[124–127] However, adverse fetal outcomes are common among mothers with lupus and include fetal death, preterm birth (before 37 weeks gestation), and intrauterine growth retardation. The manifestations of neonatal lupus include transient rash within the newborn period, permanent heart block, or both.[128] Fortunately, neonatal lupus is an extremely rare event. Less than 25% of infants have cutaneous neonatal lupus and less than 3% of infants have congenital heart block if their mothers with lupus also have the associated antibodies anti-SSA (Ro) or anti-SSB (La).[129] Maternal renal disease or hypertension, previous history of fetal death, or the presence of antiphospholipid antibodies adversely influence the risk of a poor fetal outcome in women with lupus.

During pregnancy, estrogen and progesterone levels rise, creating a natural state in which to explore the influence of sex hormones on the course of disease. Women with lupus frequently have symptoms of their disease during pregnancy. This is in contrast to the relatively benign pregnancy experience of women with RA. However, women with both RA and lupus can have active disease postpartum. These observations bring up several questions that have been debated in the literature for the last 50 years: Does pregnancy adversely affect lupus? When does flare occur? Are flares during pregnancy more severe than those occurring when women are not pregnant?

The lack of a consensus definition for lupus flare has been a major obstacle for investigators. The diagnosis of flare in the pregnant patient is even more difficult because common pregnancy-related symptoms can also be lupus symptoms. For example, arthralgia, facial and palmar erythema, thrombocytopenia, proteinuria, and anemia all occur in women with SLE who are not pregnant. Reliable indicators of active disease in pregnant lupus patients include rising levels of anti-DNA antibody, alternative-pathway hypocomplementemia, true arthritis, true rash, mucosal ulcers, and lymphadenopathy.[92] The results of six recent studies are split, with three supporting the increased occurrence of lupus flares during pregnancy[130–132] and three showing no increase in the occurrence of lupus flares during pregnancy.[133–135] However, most series agree that lupus symptoms are not more severe during pregnancy than the nonpregnant state and that disease activity can occur during any trimester and postpartum. Several methodologic issues also confound the results of these studies; these include selection of appropriate control populations for comparison, patients first diagnosed with lupus during pregnancy who may be sicker than patients with established lupus, clinical populations with a large percentage of African-American patients who have more severe lupus, a count of multiple pregnancies in the same woman, and in some studies, prophylactic use of prednisone. In conclusion, lupus symptoms are present during pregnancy and after delivery. Whether flare is increased and more severe during pregnancy than the nonpregnant state is still unclear.

Recently, a role for prolactin as an immunomodulator has been postulated. Estrogens stimulate prolactin production, prolactin receptors are similar to cytokine receptors, and prolactin receptors are expressed on T and B cells.[136] An increased risk of RA has been noted in association with breast-feeding and this suggests a role for prolactin.[137] This observation in humans is also supported by animal models in which the postpartum exacerbation of the collagen-induced arthritis model has been suppressed by treatment with bromocriptine, an inhibitor of prolactin.[138] In one study, prolactin levels were higher in pregnant patients with flare than in pregnant controls.[139] However, there has been no agreement on the relationship between prolactin levels and lupus disease activity in nonpregnant patients.[140, 141]

Exogenous Hormones

The effects of oral contraceptives (OCs) and hormone replacement therapy (HRT) in women with SLE are not well characterized because these exposures are usually avoided.[142] Several retrospective studies have shown that young women with SLE use OCs less often than healthy women of similar age.[143,144] This may reflect the concerns of the treating physicians with regard to potential worsening of SLE activity with hormone use. A retrospective, multicenter survey of 404 women with SLE reported that 55 (14%) used OCs after SLE diagnosis.[144] Only seven (13%) of the 55 women reported an increase in disease activity after OC use, which predominantly took the form of musculoskeletal symptoms. Isolated case reports have described disease flares in women with SLE who are on OCs containing estrogen.[145,146] Disease flares occurred within 8 weeks of instituting oral contraceptives. Other investigators have suggested that exogenous hormones may unmask subclinical SLE; they reported two cases of asymptomatic women with a biological false-positive test for syphilis (one of the serologic criteria for SLE) who developed signs and symptoms of clinical SLE 3–4 weeks after starting OCs.[147,148] One of the women had dramatic improvement in her symptoms within days of discontinuing the oral contraceptive.[148]

One study reported an association between OC use in healthy women seen in a birth control clinic and the presence of antinuclear antibodies (ANA).[149] The frequency of ANA positivity was 13.4% in 210 women on OCs versus 8.5% in women who never used OCs. None of these women reported symptoms consistent with a rheumatic disease. Other studies examining healthy women attending birth control clinics have shown no association between the presence of ANA and OC use.[150, 151]

Researchers have compared exacerbations of SLE disease activity in women on combination oral contraceptives (estrogen–progesterone) and those on progestin-only regimens. In one study, 9 (43%) of 20 women experienced initial manifestations or flare of SLE within 3 months of starting the combination pills.[152] Among the 11 women on pure progestins, including 5 women who had previously developed lupus exacerbation while receiving estrogen, none developed signs or symptoms of lupus exacerbation during a follow-up period of 5–30 months. The authors concluded that progestin-only oral contraceptives did not have as great a potential to induce disease flares as the combination pill. This study is flawed by its retrospective design the underlying disease severity of SLE (all of the women had renal disease), and concomitant use of corticosteroids in these women. Other investigators have also reported a decrease in SLE disease flares with progestin-only pills, but menstrual irregularities and other intolerable side effects have dampened the enthusiasm for these oral contraceptives.[145,153,154]

The administration of OCs among women with SLE have been associated with thromboembolic complications and chorea.[155–158] This risk may even be greater in patients with antiphospholipid antibodies.[156,157] Antibodies to phospholipids are found in 40%–50% of patients with lupus and are associated with recurrent fetal loss and thromboembolic events.[159–161] Oral contraceptives are generally not recommended for those SLE women with high levels of antiphospholipid antibodies, previous thrombotic events, and those who have currently active SLE and require high doses of corticosteroids or other immunosuppressive agents.

With the increased life expectancy of women with SLE due to improved therapy, there are emerging concerns about the safety of hormone replacement therapy in postmenopausal women. Examples of SLE flares in postmenopausal women taking estrogen replacement for osteoporosis prevention have been published.[162] Symptoms resolved when estrogen was discontinued and promptly recurred upon reinstitution of estrogen. An increased relative risk of developing SLE was reported in postmenopausal nurses exposed to HRT.[163] In this study, 69,435 postmenopausal women aged 30–55 without a diagnosis of SLE were followed from 1976 to 1990. Forty-eight percent of participants had either been current or past users of HRT. Compared with never-users, the age-adjusted relative risk for SLE was 2.1 (95% CI, 1.1–4.0) for ever-users, 2.5 (95% CI 1.2–5.0) for current users and 1.8 (95% CI 0.8–4.1) for past users. A proportional increase in risk for SLE was related to duration of HRT use. This study has several potential limitations. All hormone use was self-reported. It is possible that an increased opportunity to diagnose lupus was available to the women on estrogen replacement because of more active medical follow-up. The reasons why some women were given HRT and others were not is unclear. Subtle symptoms of SLE including fatigue, facial flushing, myalgia and arthralgia may have been misinterpreted as postmenopausal symptoms leading to the initiation of HRT. Although the results of this study are intriguing, they should be interpreted with caution. In two smaller retrospective studies of postmenopausal women with SLE, HRT appeared to be well tolerated with no increase in disease flares.[144,164] Thirty of the 60 SLE women in one study on HRT had the same rate of flare as the 30 women who never used HRT.[164] Moreover, the HRT group had an improved sense of well-being with less depression and migraine headaches.[164] In the other study, 48 (51%) of the 94 postmenopausal women surveyed had been on HRT after SLE diagnosis.[144] Only four of these women reported exacerbation of SLE disease activity.

While there are concerns regarding the use of exogenous hormones in women with SLE, there are also many potential benefits, including effective birth control with OCs, prevention of osteoporosis, reduction in coronary artery disease risk, and treatment of bothersome postmenopausal symptoms, such as hot flashes, depression, headaches, and decreased libido with HRT. There are now ongoing prospective, double-blinded, placebo-controlled trials examining the risks and benefits of exogenous hormone use in women with SLE.

Cardiovascular disease has been reported to be a major cause of both morbidity and mortality in women with SLE.[165-168] Rates of myocardial infarction have been reported to be nearly 50 times greater than those expected in women aged 35–44 years.[168] The pathogenesis of premature cardiovascular disease in women with lupus is likely multifactorial related to the underlying vascular inflammation and arterial wall injury, adverse effects of corticosteriods, the high prevalence of renal disease and hypertension, and increased risk of thrombosis in the setting of antiphospholipid antibodies. The role of estrogen in cardiovascular disease is of particular interest for women with SLE. Estrogen replacement therapy is thought to have beneficial effects on the prevention of cardiovascular disease in postmenopausal women. In young women with lupus, the relative hyperestrogenism may possibly have prothrombotic effects, particularly in combination with hypertension, renal disease, and antiphospholipid antibodies. The effects of estrogen on vascular disease in SLE are currently unknown.

Several studies have documented both cortical bone loss[169-171] and trabecular bone loss[171,172] in patients with lupus. Prevalence estimates of low bone mineral density (BMD) in a few studies that have measured BMD in lupus patients range from 4.5% to 25%.[171-173] There are several theoretical reasons why women with lupus may have low BMD. The candidate risk factors include *(1)* reproductive history (nulliparity);[174] *(2)* premature menopause due to the toxic effects of immunosuppressive medications on ovarian function;[175] *(3)* avoidance of oral contraceptives and/or hormone replacement therapy because of concerns about precipitating disease flare,[176,152] *(4)* decreased physical activity because of fatigue,[177] *(5)* cytokine imbalance resulting in elevated levels of interleukin-6 which have been implicated in the pathogenesis of accelerated bone remodeling;[178,179] *(6)* renal disease[180]; *(7)* decreased vitamin D levels due to sun exposure avoidance to prevent flare of lupus[181]; and *(8)* corticosteroid therapy.[182] Since estrogens clearly modulate bone mass,[179] the role of estrogens in osteoporosis is of particular interest in women with lupus.

Hormonal Therapy

There is interest in hormonal manipulation as a potentially effective treatment in SLE because of the strong evidence that hormones may induce or exacerbate disease activity. Danazol, a synthetic attenuated androgen, has been successfully used to treat immune-mediated thrombocytopenia[183] and several reports have also documented its efficacy in the treatment of autoimmune hemolytic anemia.[184] The mechanism of action of danazol is unclear. Six of eight patients tested in one series had elevated levels of IgG anti-platelet antibodies and in all six a marked decrease in these antibodies was noted following danazol treatment.[185] Clinical benefit has been noted in women, but not men, treated with danazol for lupus-like disease associated with hereditary C1-inhibitor deficiency.[185,186] Masculinizing side effects also limit the use of danazol.

Reduced levels of androgens (androstenedione, DHEA, DHEAS, and testosterone) have been observed in women with active lupus.[116,117] These observations were extended in animal experiments that explored the effect of DHEA treatment on the development of lupus. Indeed, these studies showed delayed formation of anti-DNA antibodies and improved survival.[39] A proposed mechanism of action for DHEA is suggested by experiments regulating IL-2 secretion by activated T cells.[31]

DHEA has been studied in patients with mild to moderate lupus and results of the open-label study have been published.[187] After 3 to 6 months of DHEA treatment, 10 women with lupus showed an improvement in disease activity index and reduced corticosteroid requirements. Of three patients with significant proteinuria, two showed marked and one showed modest reductions in protein excretion. DHEA was well tolerated and the only frequently noted side effect was acne. On the basis of this preliminary study, several double-blind, randomized, placebo-controlled studies are currently in progress to assess the efficacy of DHEA in reducing lupus disease activity and in decreasing corticosteroid doses. These promising studies represent the first clinical trials in lupus conducted in the last 30 years.

Summary

Systemic lupus is a multisystem, autoimmune disease resulting in chronic inflammation. It affects women during the childbearing ages at rates nearly 12 times greater than men. The pathogenesis of lupus is likely multifactorial, including genetic, hormonal, and environmental factors. Associations with HLA antigens, complement deficiencies, and other candidate genes, including those encoding for Fc receptors on IgG, have been reported. Much of the research on endogenous hormones in SLE has been done in animal models. Several human studies have reported increased levels of 16-hydroxylated estrogen metabolites as well as lower testosterone levels resulting in a relative "hyperestrogenic" state. Although women with lupus report increased symptoms of their disease at certain times during the menstrual cycle (usually within 2 weeks of the menses), no studies have looked at the corresponding hormone levels at the time of reported symptoms. The effect of pregnancy on lupus disease activity has been an area of some controversy. Most investigators will agree that lupus disease activity can occur during any trimester and postpartum, but whether disease activity is increased and more severe during pregnancy compared with nonpregnant controls is uncertain. While there are concerns regarding the use of exogenous hormones in women with lupus because of anecdotal reports of worsening disease activity in women taking oral contraceptives and hormone replacement therapy, there are clearly many potential benefits including prevention of premature cardiovascular disease and osteoporosis, which are common problems in these young women. There are ongoing, national clinical trials to examine the effects of exogenous hormone use in women with lupus.

CONCLUSIONS

Sex hormones have the capacity to regulate the immune system. We have provided evidence that implicates sex hormones in the pathogenesis and clinical course of two autoimmune diseases, rheumatoid arthritis and systemic lupus erythematosus. Whether a relative androgen deficiency or an estrogen excess contributes to the pathogenesis of these autoimmune diseases remains unknown. Nevertheless, it is believed that the proper balance of these sex hormones is somewhat protective in the development of these diseases.

RA and SLE share a female predilection as well as an exaggerated female predominance during the reproductive years. Similarly, in both diseases, patients have been reported to have lower androgen levels (testosterone and DHEAS) than age-matched controls. If a relative androgen deficiency or estrogen excess were the only factors involved in the pathogenesis of these diseases, one would expect there to be many more similarities between RA and SLE. There are, however, many differences that cannot be fully explained. Although the peak age-specific incidence in SLE is between the ages of 15 and 45 years, the incidence of disease in RA continues to rise well into the 7th and 8th decade. This late onset of disease in RA does not correlate with the time when female sex hormone levels are at their highest. Similarly, pregnancy commonly induces remission in RA, but not in SLE, and exogenous hormones may have a protective effect on the development of RA but a disease-inducing effect in SLE. We have provided data that highlight the controversy and uncertainty about the conflicting effects of hormones on both RA and SLE. Part of the answer to the questions about these diseases may lie in the complex interplay between TH2 cytokines, which are responsible for humoral immunity, and TH1 cytokines, which enhance cellular immunity. The fetoplacental unit up-regulates the secretion of TH2 cytokines, mainly IL-4, IL-6, IL-10, which have an inhibitory action on the production of TH1 cytokines. In this way, a new state is created of relative cellular immunosuppression and humoral immunostimulation. The main effect of the increased prolactin concentration that exists during pregnancy is to drive this system towards TH2 immunity. It is not difficult to understand the improvement of cell-mediated autoimmune diseases (RA) and the worsening of antibody-mediated autoimmune diseases (SLE) during pregnancy. However, these observations do not explain why both RA and SLE patients have increased disease activity postpartum when immunity shifts towards TH1. Recently, there has been growing support for the theory that the maternal immune response to fetal HLA class II antigens has a significant role in the pregnancy-induced disease remission in RA. This suggests that other nonhormonal factors, including genetic and environmental factors, may explain the apparent differences observed between RA and SLE.

Given the clinical heterogeneity of rheumatoid arthritis and systemic lupus erythematosus, it is conceivable that there are subsets of patients in which hormonal influences are greater. This may explain some of the conflicting data in large epidemiologic studies looking at the role of sex hormones on autoimmunity in which all patients who meet classification criteria for either systemic lupus or rheumatoid arthritis are analyzed as a group with no attempt to tease out the different clinical subsets based on various disease manifestations. A clearer understanding of the interactions among hormones, genetic predisposition, environmental factors, and the immune system may lead to new therapies for patients afflicted with these diseases.

REFERENCES

1. Klinman DM. B-cell abnormalities characteristic of systemic lupus erythematosus. In: Wallace DJ, Hahn BH, eds. Dubois' Lupus Erythematosus, 5th ed. Baltimore, MD: Williams & Wilkins, 1997, pp. 195–206.

2. Theofilopoulos AN, Dixon FJ. Etiopathogenesis of murine systemic lupus erythematosus. Immunol Rev 1981;55:179–216.

3. Lahita RG. The connective tissue diseases and the overall influence of gender. Int J Fertil 1996;41:156–165.

4. Cutolo M, Sulli A, Seriolo B, et al. Estrogens, the immune response and autoimmunity. Clin Exp Rheumatol 1995;13:217–226.

5. Masi AT, Feigenbaum SL, Chatterton RT. Hormonal and pregnancy relationships to rheumatoid arthritis: Convergent effects with immunologic and microvascular systems. Semin Arthritis Rheum 1995;25:1–27.

6. Masi AT. Sex hormones and rheumatoid arthritis: Cause or effect relationships in a complex pathophysiology. Clin Exp Rheumatol 1995;13:227–240.

7. Schuurs AHWM, Verheul HAM. Effects of gender and sex steroids on the immune response. J Steroid Biochem 1990;35:157–172.

8. Sthoeger ZN, Chiorazzi RG, Lahita RG. Regulation of the immune response by sex steroids. J Immunol 1988;141:91–98.

9. Ahmed SA, Penhale WJ, Talal N. Sex hormones and autoimmune diseases: Mechanisms of sex hormone action. Am J Pathol 1985;121:531–559.

10. Lahita RG. Sex steroids and the rheumatic diseases. Arthritis Rheum 1985;28: 121–126.

11. Grossman CJ. Interaction between the gonadal steroids and the immune system. Science 1985;227:257–261.

12. Theofilopoulos AN. The basis of autoimmunity: Part I. Mechanisms of aberrant self-recognition. Immunol Today 1995;16:90–98.

13. Theofilopoulos AN. The basis of autoimmunity: Part II. Genetic predisposition. Immunol Today 1995;16:150–159.

14. Hahn BH. An overview of the pathogenesis of systemic lupus erythematosus. In: Wallace DJ, Hahn BH, eds. Dubois' Lupus Erythematosus, 5th ed. Baltimore, MD: Williams & Wilkins, 1997, pp. 69–75.

15. Von Boehmer H, Kisielow P. Self-nonself discrimination by T cells. Science 1990;248:1368–1373.

16. Adelstein S, Pritchard-Briscoe H, Anderson TA, Crosbie J, Gammon G, Loblay RH, et al. Induction of self-tolerance in T cells but not B cells of transgenic mice expressing little self antigen. Science 1991;251:1223–1225.

17. Horowitz D, Stahl W, Gray JD. T lymphocytes, natural killer cells, cytokines and immune regulation. In: Wallace DJ, Hahn BH, eds. Dubuois' Lupus Erythematosus, 5th ed. Baltimore, MD: Williams & Wilkins, 1997, pp. 155–194.

18. Burkly LC, Lo D, Flavell RA. Tolerance in transgenic mice expressing major histocompatibility molecules extrathymically on pancreatic cells. Science 1990;248: 1364–1368.

19. Goodnow CC, Adelstein S, Basten A. The need for central and peripheral tolerance in the B cell repertoire. Science 1990;248:1373–1379.

20. Gharavi AE, Chu JL, Elkon KB. Autoantibodies to intracellular proteins in human SLE are not due to random polyclonal B cell activation. Arthritis Rheum 1988;31: 1337–1345.

21. Takeuchi T, Abe T, Koide J, Hosono O, Morimotos C, Homma M. Cellular mechanism of DNA-specific antibody synthesis by lymphocytes from systemic lupus erythematosus patients. Arthritis Rheum 1984;27:766–773.

22. Shivakumar S, Tsokos GC, Datta SK. T cell receptor alpha/beta expressing double negative (CD4$^-$/CD8$^-$) and CD4$^+$ T helper cells in humans augment the production of pathogenic anti-DNA autoantibodies associated with lupus nephritis. J Immunol 1989;143:103–112.

23. Carlsten H, Nilsson N, Jonsson R, Backman K, Holmdahl R, Tarkowski A. Estrogen accelerates immune complex glomerulonephritis but ameliorates T cell–mediated vasculitis and sialoadenitis in autoimmune MRL lpr/lpr mice. Cell Immunol 1992;144: 190–202.

24. Danel L, Souweine G, Monier JC, et al. Specific estrogen binding sites in human lymphoid cells and thymic cells. J Steroid Biochem 1983;18:559–563.

25. Cohen JHM, Danel L, Cordier G, et al. Sex steroid receptors in peripheral T

cells: Absence of androgen receptors and restriction of estrogen receptors to OKT8-positive cells. J Immunol 1983;131:2767–2771.

26. Graff RJ, Lappe MA, Snell GD. The influence of the gonads and adrenal glands on the immune response to skin grafts. Transplantation 1969;7:105–111.

27. Masi AT, Feigenbaum SL, Chatterton RT, Cutolo M. Integrated hormonal-immunological-vascular (H-I-V triad) systems interactions in the rheumatic diseases. Clin Exp Rheumatol 1995;13:203–216.

28. Grumbach MM, Styne DM. Puberty: Ontogeny, neuro-endocrinology, physiology and disorders. In: Wilson JD, Foster DW, eds. Williams Textbook of Endocrinology, 8th ed. Philadelphia: W.B. Saunders, 1992, pp. 1139–1221.

29. Kalimi M, Regelson W, eds. The Biological Role of Dehydroepiandrosterone (DHEA). Berlin: Walter de Gruyter, 1990.

30. Van Vollenhoven RF, McGuire JL. Estrogen, progesterone, and testosterone: Can they be used to treat autoimmune diseases? Cleve Clin J Med 1994;61:276–284.

31. Suzuki T, Suzuki N, Daynes RA, Engelman EG: Dehydroepiandrosterone enhances IL2 production and cytotoxic effector function of human T cells. Clin Immunol Immunopathol 1991;61:202–211.

32. Makino S, Kunimoto K, Muraoka Y, Katagiri K. Effect of castration on the appearance of diabetes in NOD mouse. Jikken Dobutsu. Exp Animals 1981;30:137–140.

33. Ahmed SA, Young PR, Penhale WJ. Beneficial effect of testosterone in the therapy of chronic autoimmune thyroiditis in rats. J Immunol 1986;136:143–148.

34. Ahmed SA, Penhale WJ. The influence of testosterone on the development of autoimmune thyroiditis in thymectomized and irradiated rats. Clin Exp Immunol 1982; 48:367–374.

35. Holmdahl R, Carlsten H, Jansson L, Larsson P. Oestrogen is a potent immunomodulator of murine experimental rheumatoid disease. Br J Rheumatol 1989;28 (suppl 1):54–58.

36. Theofilopoulos AN. Murine models of lupus. In: Lahita RG, ed. Systemic Lupus Erythematosus, 2nd ed. New York: Churchill Livingstone, 1992, pp. 121–194.

37. Roubinian JR, Papoian R, Talal N. Androgenic hormones modulate autoantibody responses and improve survival in murine lupus. J Clin Invest 1977;59:1066–1070.

38. Roubinian JR, Talal N, Greenspan JS, et al. Effect of castration and sex hormone treatment on survival, antinucleic acid antibodies and glomerulonephritis in NZB × NZW F1 mice. J Exp Med 1978;147:1568–1583.

39. Roubinian JR, Talal N, Greenspan JS, et al. Delayed androgen treatment prolongs survival in murine lupus. J Clin Invest 1979;63:902–911.

40. Harris ED Jr. Mechanisms of disease: Rheumatoid arthritis—pathophysiology and implications for therapy. N Engl J Med 1990;332:1277–1289.

41. Arnett FC, Edworthy SM, Bloch DA, et al. The American Rheumatism Association 1987 revised criteria for the classification of rheumatoid arthritis. Arthritis Rheum 1988;31:315–324.

42. Cutolo M, Accardo S. Sex hormones, HLA and rheumatoid arthritis. Clin Exp Rheumatol 1991;9:641–646.

43. Linos A, Worthington JW, O'Fallon MW, Kurland LT. The epidemiology of rheumatoid arthritis in Rochester, Minnesota: A study of incidence, prevalence and mortality. Am J Epidemiol 1980;1:87–98.

45. Masi AT. Incidence of rheumatoid arthritis: Do the observed age-sex interaction patterns support a role of androgenic-anabolic (AA) steroid deficiency in its pathogenesis? Br J Rheumatol 1994;33:697–699.

46. Felson DT. Epidemiology of the rheumatic diseases. In: Koopman WJ, ed. Arthritis and Allied Conditions: A Textbook of Rheumatology, 13th ed. Baltimore, MD: Williams & Wilkins, 1997, pp. 3–34.

47. Silman A, Hochberg MC. Epidemiology of the Rheumatic Diseases. New York: Oxford University Press, 1993.

48. O'Sullivan JB, Catchcart ES. The prevalence of rheumatoid arthritis. Follow-up evaluation of the effect of criteria on rates in Sudbury, Massachusetts. Ann Intern Med 1972;76:573–577.

49. Symmons DPM, Barrett EM, Bankhead CR, et al. The incidence of rheumatoid arthritis in the United Kingdom: Results from the Norfolk Arthritis Register. Br J Rheumatol 1994;33:735–739.

50. Cutolo M, Balleari E, Giusti M, et al. Sex hormone status in women suffering from rheumatoid arthritis. J Rheumatol 1986;13:1019–1023.

51. Spector TD, Ollier W, Perry LA, et al. Free and serum testosterone levels in 276 males: A comparative study of rheumatoid arthritis, ankylosing spondylitis and healthy controls. Clin Rheumatol 1989;8:37–41.

52. Cutolo M, Balleari E, Accardo S, et al. Preliminary results of serum androgen level testing in men with rheumatoid arthritis. Arthritis Rheum 1984;27:958–960.

53. Gordon D, Beastall GH, Thomson JA, Sturrock RD. Androgenic status and sexual function in males with rheumatoid arthritis and ankylosing spondylitis. Br J Rheumatol 1986;60:671–679.

54. Spector TD, Perry LA, Tubb G, Silman AJ, Huskisson EC. Low free testosterone levels in rheumatoid arthritis. Ann Rheum Dis 1988;47:65–68.

55. Cutolo M, Balleari E, Giusti M, Monachesi M, Accardo S. Sex hormone status of male patients with rheumatoid arthritis: Evidence of low serum concentrations of testosterone at baseline and after human chorionic gonadotropin stimulation. Arthritis Rheum 1988;31:1314–1317.

56. Fehér KG, Fehér T, Merétey K. Interrelationship between the immunological and steroid hormone parameters in rheumatoid arthritis. Exp Clin Endocrinol 1986; 87:38–42.

57. Arnalich F, Benito-Urbina S, Gonzalez Gancedo P, et al. Elévations des androgènes plasmatiques chez les femmes menopausées atteintes de polyarthrite rhumatoide. Rev Rhum Mal Osteoartic 1990;57:509–512.

58. Spector TD, Perry LA, Tubb G, et al. Androgen status of females with RA. Br J Rheumatol 1987;26:316–318.

59. Van Zeben D, Hazes JM, Zwinderman AH, et al. Association of HLA-DR4 with a more progressive disease course in patients with rheumatoid arthritis: Results of a follow up study. Arthritis Rheum 1991;34:822–830.

60. Winchester R, Dwyer E, Rose S. The genetic basis of rheumatoid arthritis: The shared epitome hypothesis. Rheum Dis Clin North Am 1992;18:761–783.

61. Weyand CM, Hicok KC, Conn DL, Goronzy JJ. The influence of HLA-DRB1 genes on disease severity in rheumatoid arthritis. Ann Intern Med 1992;117:801–806.

62. Ivanyi P, Hampl R, Starka L, Mickova M. Genetic association between H-2 gene and testosterone metabolism in mice. Nat New Biol 1972;238:281–282.

63. Ollier W, Spector T, Silman A, et al. Are certain HLA haplotype responsible for low testosterone levels in males? Dis Markers 1989;7:139–143.

64. Gerencer M, Tajic M, Kerhin-Brkljacic V, Kastelan A. An association between serum testosterone level and HLA phenotype. Immunol Lett 1982;4:152–155.

65. De La Torre B, Hedman M, Nilsson E, Olesen O, Thörner A. Relationship between blood and joint tissue DHEAS levels in rheumatoid arthritis and osteoarthritis. Clin Exp Rheumatol 1993;11:597–601.

66. Hedman M, Nilsson E, De La Torre B. Low blood and synovial fluid levels of sulpho-conjugated steroids in rheumatoid arthritis. Clin Exp Rheumatol 1992;10:25–30.

67. Sambrook PN, Eisman JA, Champion GD, Pocock NA. Sex hormone status and osteoporosis in postmenopausal women with rheumatoid arthritis. Arthritis Rheum 1988;31:973–978.

68. Deighton CM, Watson MJ, Walker DJ. Sex hormones in postmenopausal HLA-identical rheumatoid arthritis discordant sibling pairs. J Rheumatol 1992;19:1663–1667.

69. Masi AT, Chatterton RT, Comstock GW, Malamet RL, Hochberg MC. Decreased serum dehydroepiandrosterone sulfate (DHAS) levels before onset of RA in younger, premenopausal women: A controlled prospective study. Arthritis Rheum 1994;37:S315.

70. Nelson JL, Ostensen M. Pregnancy and rheumatoid arthritis. Rheum Dis Clin North Am 1997;23:195–212.

71. Hench PS. The ameliorating effect of pregnancy on chronic atrophic (infectious rheumatoid) arthritis, fibrositis, and intermittent hydrarthrosis. Mayo Clin Proc 1938;13:161–167.

72. Morris WIC. Pregnancy in rheumatoid arthritis and systemic lupus erythematosus. Aust N Z J Obstet Gynaecol 1969;9:136–144.

73. Oka M. Effect of pregnancy on the onset and course of rheumatoid arthritis. Ann Rheum Dis 1953;12:227–229.

74. Ostensen M, Aune B, Husby G. Effect of pregnancy and hormonal changes on the activity of rheumatoid arthritis. Scand J Rheumatol 1983;12:69–72.

75. Ostensen M, Husby G. A prospective clinical study of the effect of pregnancy on rheumatoid arthritis and ankylosing spondylitis. Arthritis Rheum 1983;26:1155–1159.

76. Persellin RH. The effect of pregnancy on rheumatoid arthritis. Bull Rheum Dis 1977;27:922–928.

77. Redman CWG, Arenas J, Mason DY, Sargent IL, Sutton L. Maternal alloimmune recognition of the fetus in human pregnancy. In: Gill TJ III, Wegmann TG, eds. Immunoregulation and Fetal Survival. New York: Oxford University Press, 1987, pp. 210–219.

78. Nelson JL, Hughes KA, Smith AG, Nisperos BB, Branchaud AM, Hansen JA. Maternal-fetal disparity in HLA class II alloantigens and the pregnancy-induced amelioration of rheumatoid arthritis. N Engl J Med 1993;329:466–471.

79. Nelson JL. Maternal-fetal immunology and autoimmune disease. Is some autoimmune disease auto-alloimmune or allo-autoimmune? Arthritis Rheum 1996;39: 191–194.

80. Salgame P, Convit J, Bloom B. Immunological suppression by human CD8+ T-cells is receptor dependent and HLA-DQ restricted. Proc Natl Acad Sci USA 1991;88:2598–2602.

81. Hirayama K, Matsushita S, Kikuchi I, Iuchi M, Ohta N, Sasazuki T. HLA-DQ is epistatic to HLA-DR in controlling the immune response to schistosomal antigen in humans. Nature 1987;327:426–430.

82. Wegman TG, Lin H, Builbert L, Mosmann TR. Bidirectional cytokine interactions in the maternal-fetal relationship: Is successful pregnancy a TH2 phenomenon? Immunol Today 1993;14:353–356.

83. Wingrave SJ, Kay CR. Reduction in incidence of rheumatoid arthritis associated with oral contraceptives. Lancet 1978;569–571.

84. Silman AJ. Is pregnancy a risk factor in the causation of rheumatoid arthritis? Ann Rheum Dis 1986;45:1031–1034.

85. Esdaile JM, Horwitz RI. Observational studies of cause–effect relationships: An example of methodologic problems as illustrated by the conflicting data for the role of oral contraceptives in the etiology of rheumatoid arthritis. J Chronic Dis 1986;39:841–852.

86. Vandenbroucke JP, Witteman JCM, Valkenburg HA, et al. Noncontraceptive hormones and rheumatoid arthritis in perimenopausal and postmenopausal women. JAMA 1986;255:1299–1303.

87. Carette S, Marcoux S, Gingras S. Postmenopausal hormones and the incidence of rheumatoid arthritis. J Rheumatol 1989;16:911–913.

88. Spector TD, Brennan P, Harris P, Studd JWW, Silman AJ. Does estrogen replacement therapy protect against rheumatoid arthritis? J Rheumatol 1991;18:1473–1476.

89. Hernandez-Avila M, Liang MH, Willett WC, et al. Exogenous sex hormones and the risk of rheumatoid arthritis. Arthritis Rheum 1990;33:947–953.

90. Mills JA. Systemic lupus erythematosus. N Engl J Med 1994;330:1871–1879.

91. Boumpas DT, Austin HA III, Fessler BJ, Balow JE, Klippel JH, Lockshin MD. Systemic lupus erythematosus: Emerging concepts. Part I: Renal, neuropsychiatric, cardiovascular, pulmonary and hematologic disease. Ann Intern Med 1995;122:940–950.

92. Boumpas DT, Fessler BJ, Austin HA, Balow JE, Klippel JH, Lockshin MD. Systemic lupus erythematosus: Emerging concepts. Part 2: Dermatologic and joint disease, the antiphospholipid antibody syndrome, pregnancy and hormonal therapy, morbidity and mortality and pathogenesis. Ann Intern Med 1995;123:42–53

93. Tan EM, Cohen AS, Fries JF, et al. The 1982 revised criteria for the classification of systemic lupus erythematosus (SLE). Arthritis Rheum 1982;25:1271–1277.

94. Wofsy D, Seaman WE. Reversal of advanced murine lupus in NZB/NZW F1 mice by treatment with monoclonal antibody to L3T4. J Immunol 1987;138:3247–3253.

95. Mihara M, Ohsugi Y, Saito K, et al. Immuologic abnormality in NZB/NZW F1 mice. Thymus-independent occurrence of B cell abnormality and requirement for T cells in the development of autoimmune disease, as evidenced by an analysis of the athymic nude individuals. J Immunol 1988;141:85–90.

96. Michet CJ Jr, McKenna CH, Elveback LR, Kaslow RA, Kurland LT. Epidemiology of systemic lupus erythematosus and other connective tissue disease in Rochester, Minnesota, 1950 through 1979. Mayo Clin Proc 1985;60:105–113.

97. Fessel WJ. Systemic lupus erythematosus in the community. Incidence, prevalence, outcome and first symptoms; The high prevalence in black women. Arch Intern Med 1974;134:1027–1035.

98. Siegel M, Lee SL. The epidemiology of systemic lupus erythematosus. Semin Arthritis Rheum 1973;3:1–54.

99. Hochberg MC. The incidence of systemic lupus erythematosus in Baltimore, Maryland, 1970–1977. Arthritis Rheum 1985;28:80–86.

100. McCarty DJ, Manzi S, Medsger TA Jr, Ramsey-Goldman R, LaPorte RE, Kwoh CK. Incidence of systemic lupus erythematosus: Race and gender differences. Arthritis Rheum 1995;38:1260–1270.

101. Reinertsen JL, Klippel JH, Johnston AH, Steinberg AD, Decker JL, Mann DL. B-lymphocyte alloantigens associated with systemic lupus erythematosus. N Engl J Med 1978;299:515–518.

102. Schur PH, Meyer I, Garovoy M, Carpenter CB. Associations between systemic lupus erythematosus and the major histocompatibility complex: Clinical and immunological considerations. Clin Immunol Immunopathol 1982;24:263–275.

103. Gibofsky AM, Winchester RJ, Patarroyo M, Fotino M, Kunkel HG. Disease association of the Ia-like human alloantigens: Contrasting patterns in rheumatoid arthritis and systemic lupus erythematosus. J Exp Med 1978;148:1728–1732.

104. Howard PF, Hochberg MC, Bias WB, Arnett FC, McLean RH. Relationship between C4 null genes, HLA-D region antigens, and genetic susceptibilities to systemic lupus erythematosus in Caucasians and black Americans. Am J Med 1986;81:187–1993.

105. Kemp ME, Atkinson JP, Skanes VM, Levine RP, Chaplin DD. Delection of C4A genes in patients with systemic lupus erythematosus. Arthritis Rheum 1987;30: 1015–1022.

106. Salmon JE, Milliard S, Schachter LA, et al. FcγRIIA alleles are heritable risk factors for lupus nephritis in African Americans. JCI 1996;97:1348–1354.

107. Tsao BP, Cantor RM, Kalunian KC, et al. Evidence for linkage of a candidate chromosome 1 region to human systemic lupus erythematosus. J Clin Invest 1997;99: 725–731.

108. Lahita RG, Bradlow HL, Kunkel HG, et al. Increased 16α-hydroxylation of estradiol in systemic lupus erythematosus. J Clin Endocrinol Metab 1981;53:174–178.

109. Lahita RG, Bradlow HL, Kunkel HG, et al. Alterations of estrogen metabolism in SLE. Arthritis Rheum 1979;22:1195–1198.

110. Lahita RG, Bradlow HL, Fishman J, et al. Estrogen metabolism in systemic lupus erythematosus: Patients and family members. Arthritis Rheum 1982;25:843–846

111. Inman RD, Jovanovic L, Markenson JA. Systemic lupus erythematosus in men: Genetic and endocrine features. Arch Intern Med 1982;142:1813–1815.

112. Lahita RG, Bradlow HL, Ginzler E, et al. Low plasma androgens in women with systemic lupus erythematosus. Arthritis Rheum 1987;30:241–248.

113. Martucci C, Fishman J. Direction of estradiol metabolism as a control of its hormonal action-uterotrophic activity of estradiol metabolites. Endocrinology 1977; 101:1709.

114. Fishman J, Martucci C. Biological properties of 16-alpha hydroxyestrone: Implications in estrogen physiology and pathophysiology. J Clin Endocrinol Metab 1980; 51:611–615.

115. Jungers P, Nahoul K, Pelissier C, et al. Low plasma androgens in women with active or quiescent systemic lupus erythematosus. Arthritis Rheum 1982;25:454–457.

116. Lahita RG, Kunkel HG, Bradlow HL. Increased oxidation of testosterone in systemic lupus erythematosus. Arthritis Rheum 1983;26:1517–1521.

117. Arnalich F, Benito-Urbina S, Gonzalez-Gancedo P, et al. Inadequate production of progesterone in women with systemic lupus erythematosus. Br J Rheumatol 1992;31:247–251.

118. Grossman C. Regulation of the immune system by sex steroids. Endocrinol Rev 1984;5:435–455.

119. Holdstock GI, Chastenay BF, Krawitt EL. Effects of testosterone, estradiol and progesterone on immune regulation. Clin Exp Immunol 1982;47:449–456.

120. Steinberg AD, Steinberg BJ. Lupus disease activity associated with menstrual cycle. J Rheumatol 1985;12:816–817.

121. Rose E, Pillsbury DM. Lupus erythematosus (erythematoides) and ovarian function: Observations in a possible relationship with a report of 6 cases. Ann Intern Med 1944;21:1022–1034.

122. Lim GS, Petri M, Goldman D. Menstruation and systemic lupus erythematosus (SLE). Arthritis Rheum 1993;36:R23.

123. Fraga A, Mintz G, Orozco J, Orozco JH. Sterility and fertility rates, fetal wastage and maternal morbidity in systemic lupus erythematosus. J Rheumatol 1974;1: 293–298.

124. Lockshin MD, Harpel PC, Druzin ML, et al. Lupus pregnancy. II. Unusual pattern of hypocomplementemia and thrombocytopenia in the pregnant lupus patients. Arthritis Rheum 1985;28:58–66.

125. Ramsey-Goldman R, Kutzer JE, Kuller LH, et al. Pregnancy outcome and anti-cardiolipin antibody in women with systemic lupus erythematosus. Am J Epidemiol 1993;138:1057–1569.

126. Julkunen T, Jouhikainen T, Kaaja R, et al. Fetal outcome in lupus pregnancy: A retrospective case-control study of 242 pregnancies in 112 patients. Lupus 1993;2: 125–131.

127. Petri M, Allbritton J. Fetal outcome of lupus pregnancy: A retrospective case–control study of the Hopkins Lupus Cohort. J Rheumatol 1993;20:650–656.

128. Lee LA. Neonatal lupus erythematosus. J Invest Dermatol 1993;100:9S–13S.

129. Buyon JP, Winchester RJ, Slade SG, et al. Identification of mothers at risk for congenital heart block and other neonatal lupus syndromes in their children. Comparison of enzyme-linked immunosorbent assay and immunoblot for measurement of anti-SSA/Ro and anti-SS-B/La antibodies. Arthritis Rheum 1993;36:1263–1273.

130. Petri M, Howard D, Repke J. Frequency of lupus flare in pregnancy. The Hopkins Lupus Pregnancy Center experience. Arthritis Rheum 1991;34:1538–1545.

131. Wong KL, Chan FY, Lee CP. Outcome of pregnancy in patients with systemic lupus erythematosus. A prospective study. Arch Intern Med 1991;151:269–273.

132. Ruiz-Irastorza G, Lima F, Alves J, et al. Increased rate of lupus flare during pregnancy and the puerperium. Br J Rheumatol 1996;35:133–135.

133. Mintz G, Niz J, Gutierrez G, et al. Prospective study of pregnancy in systemic lupus erythematosus. Results of a multidisciplinary approach. J Rheumatol 1986;13: 732–739.

134. Lockshin MD, Reinitz D, Druzin ML, et al. Lupus pregnancy. Case–control prospective study demonstrating absence of lupus exacerbation during or after pregnancy. Am J Med 1984;77:893–898.

135. Urowitz MB, Gladman DD, Farewell VT, et al. Lupus and pregnancy studies. Arthritis Rheum 1993;36:1392–1397.

136. Walker SE, Allen SH, Hoffman RW, et al. Prolactin: A stimulator of disease activity in systemic lupus erythematosus. Lupus 1995;4:3–9.

137. Brennan P, Silman A. Breast-feeding and the onset of rheumatoid arthritis. Arthritis Rheum 1994;37:808–813.

138. Whyte A, Williams RO. Bromocriptine suppresses postpartum exacerbation of collagen-induced arthritis. Arthritis Rheum 1988;31:927–928.

139. Jara-Quezada L, Graef A, Lavalle C. Prolactin and gonadal hormones during pregnancy in systemic lupus erythematosus. J Rheumatol 1991;18:349–353.

140. McMurray RW, Weidensaul D, Allen SH, et al. Efficacy of bromocriptine in an open label therapeutic trial for systemic lupus erythematosus. J Rheumatol 1995;22: 2084–2091.

141. Pauzner R, Urowitz MB, Gladman DD, et al. Prolactin in systemic lupus erythematosus. J Rheuamtol 1994;21:2064–2067.

142. Buyon JP, Wallace DJ. The endocrine system, use of exogenous estrogens, and the urogenital tract. In: Wallace DJ, Hahn BH, eds. Dubois' Lupus Erythematosus, 5th ed. Baltimore, MD: Williams & Wilkins, 1997, pp. 817–834.

143. Julkunen HA, Kaaja R, Friman C. Contraceptive practice in women with systemic lupus erythematosus. Br J Rheumatol 1993;32:227–230.

144. Buyon JP, Kalunian KC, Skovron ML, et al. Can women with systemic lupus erythematosus safely use exogenous estrogens? J Clin Rheumatol 1995;1:205–212.

145. Pimstone BL. Systemic lupus erythematosus exacerbated by oral contraceptives. S Afr J Obstet Gynaecol 1966;4:62.

146. Chapel TA, Burns RE. Oral contraceptives and exacerbation of lupus erythematosus. Am J Obstet Gynecol 1971;110:366–369.

147. Travers RL, Hughes GRV. Oral contraceptive therapy and systemic lupus erythematosus. J Rheumatol 1978;5:448–451.

148. Garovich M, Agudelo C, Pisko E. Oral contraceptives and systemic lupus erythematosus. Arthritis Rheum 1980;23:1396–1398.

149. Kay DR, Bole GG, Ledger WJ. Antinuclear antibodies, rheumatoid factor and C-reactive protein in serum of normal women using oral contraceptives. Arthritis Rheum 1971;14:239–248.

150. McKenna CH, Wieman KC, Shulman LE. Oral contraceptives, rheumatic disease and autoantibodies. Arthritis Rheum 1969;12:313–314.

151. Tarzy BJ, Garcia CR, Wallach EE, Zweiman B, Myers AR. Rheumatic disease, abnormal serology and oral contraceptives. Lancet 1972$_\infty$:501–503.

152. Jungers P, Dougados M, Pelissier C, et al. Influence of oral contraceptive therapy on the activity of systemic lupus erythematosus. Arthritis Rheum 1982;25:618–623.

153. Mintz G, Gutierrez G, Deleze M, et al. Contraception with progestogens in systemic lupus erythematosus. Contraception 1984;30:29–38.

154. Julkunen HA. Oral contraceptives in systemic lupus erythematosus: Side-effects and influence on the activity of SLE. Scand J Rheumatol 1991;20:427–433.

155. Pulsinelli WA, Hamil HW. Chorea complicating oral contraceptive therapy. Case report and review of the literature. Am J Med 1978;65:557–559.

156. Asherson RA, Harris EN, Gharavi AE, et al. Complications of oral contraceptives and antiphospholipid antibodies: Reply to a letter by Bruneau et al. Arthritis Rheum 1988;31:575–576.

157. Asherson RA, Harris EN, Gharavi AE, et al. Systemic lupus erythematosus, antiphospholipid antibodies, chorea and oral contraceptives. Arthritis Rheum 1986;29:1535–1536.

158. Nausieda PA, Koller WC, Weiner WJ. Chorea induced by oral contraceptives. Neurology 1979;29:1605–1609.

159. Alarcon-Segovia D, Perez-Vazquez ME, Villa AR, et al. Preliminary classification criteria for the antiphospholipid syndrome within systemic lupus erythematosus. Semin Arthritis Rheum 1992;21:275–286.

160. Alarcon-Segovia D. Clinical manifestations of the antiphospholipid syndrome. J Rheumatol 1992;19:1778–1781.

161. Lockshin MD. Antiphospholipid antibody syndrome. JAMA 1992;268:1451–1453.

162. Barrett C, Neylon N, Snaith ML. Oestrogen-induced systemic lupus erythematosus. Br J Rheumatol 1986;25:300–301.

163. Sanchez-Guerrero J, Liang MH, Karlson EW, Hunter DJ, Colditz GA. Postmenopausal estrogen therapy and the risk for developing systemic lupus erythematosus (SLE). Ann Intern Med 1995;122:430–433.

164. Arden NK, Lloyd M, Spector TD, Hughes GRV. Safety of hormone replacement therapy (HRT) in systemic lupus erythematosus (SLE). Lupus 1994;3:11–13.

165. Shome GP, Sakauchi M, Yamane K, et al. Ischemic heart disease in systemic lupus erythematosus. A retrospective study of 65 patients treated with prednisolone. Jpn J Med 1989;28:599–603.

166. Gladman DD, Uroitz MB. Morbidity in systemic lupus erythematosus. J Rheumatol 1987;14(suppl 13):223–226.

167. Petri M, Perez-Gutthann S, Spense D, et al. Risk factors for coronary artery disease in patients with systemic lupus erythematosus. Am J Med 1992;93:513–519.

168. Manzi S, Meilahn EN, Rairie JE, et al. Age-specific incidence rates of myocardial infarction and angina in women with systemic lupus erythematosus: Comparison with the Framingham Study. Am J Epidemiol 1997;145:408–415.

169. Kalla AA, Meyers OL, Parkyn ND, Kotze TJVW. Osteoporosis screening: Radiogrammetry revisited. Br J Rheumatol 1989;28:511–517.

170. Kalla AA, Kotze TJVW, Meyers OL. Metacarpal bone mass in systemic lupus erythematosus. Clin Rheumatol 1992;11:1–8.

171. Kalla AA, Fataar AB, Jessop SJ, Bewerunge L. Loss of trabecular bone mineral density in systemic lupus erythematosis. Arthritis Rheum 1993;36:1726–1734.

172. Formiga F, Moga I, Nolla JM, Pac M, Mitjavila F, Roig-Escofet D. Loss of bone mineral density in premenopausal women with systemic lupus erythematosus. Ann Rheum Dis 1995;54:274–276.

173. Dhillon VB, Davies MC, Hall ML, et al. Assessment of the effect of oral corticosteroids on bone mineral density in systemic lupus erythematosus: A preliminary study with dual energy X-ray absorptiometry. Ann Rheum Dis 1990;49:624–626.

174. Ramsey-Goldman R. Pregnancy in systemic lupus erythematosus. Rheum Dis Clin North Amer 1988;14:169–185.

175. Boumpas DT, Austin HA, Vaughn EM, Yarboro CH, Klippel JH, Balow JE. Risk of sustained amenorrhea in patients with systemic lupus erythematosus receiving intermittent pulse cyclophosphamide therapy. Ann Intern Med 1993;119:366–369.

176. Lahita R. The importance of estrogens in systemic lupus erythematosus. Clin Immunol Immunopathol 1992;6:17–18.

177. Krupp LB, LaRocca NG, Muir J, Steinberg AD. A study of fatigue in systemic lupus erythematosus. J Rheumatol 1990;17:1450–1450.

178. Linker-Israeli M, Deans RJ, Wallace DJ, Prehn J, Ozeri-Chen T, Klinenberg JR. Elevated levels of endogenous IL-6 in systemic lupus erythematosus. A putative role in pathogenesis. J Immunol 1991;147:117–123.

179. Manolagas SC, Jilka RL. Emerging insights into the pathophysiology of osteoporosis. N Engl J Med 1995;332:305–311.

180. Boumpas DT, Austin HA, Fessler BJ, Balow JE, Klippel JH, Lockshin MD. Systemic lupus erythematosus: Emerging concepts. Part 1: Renal, neuropsychiatric, cardiovascular, pulmonary and hematologic disease. Ann Intern Med 1995;122:940–950.

181. Sontheimer RD, Gilliam JN. Systemic Lupus Erythematosus and the Skin. In: Lahita RG, ed. Systemic Lupus Erythematosus, 2nd ed. New York: Churchill Livingstone, 1992, pp. 657–681.

182. Luckert BP, Raisz LG. Glucocorticoid induced osteoporosis. Pathogenesis and management. Ann Intern Med 1990;112:352–364.

183. Ahn YS, Harrington WJ, Simon SR, et al. Danazol for the treatment of idiopathic thrombocytopenia purpura. N Engl J Med 1983;308:1396–1399.

184. Ahn YS, Harrington WJ, Mylvaganam R, et al. Danazol therapy for autoimmune hemolytic anemia. Ann Intern Med 1985;102:298–301.

185. Masse R, Youinou P, Dowal JC, et al. Reversal of lupus-erythematosus-like disease with danazol. Lancet 1980;2:651.

186. Fretwell MD, Altman LC. Exacerbation of a lupus-erythematosus-like syndrome during treatment of non-C1-esterase-inhibitor-dependent angioedema. J Allergy Clin Immunol 1982;69:306–310.

187. Van Vollenhoven RF, Engleman EG, McGuire JL. An open study of dehydroepiandrosterone in systemic lupus erythematosus. Arthritis Rheum 1994;37: 1305–1310.

IV

EFFECTS OF REPRODUCTION AND CONTRACEPTION ON WOMEN'S HEALTH

16

ORAL CONTRACEPTIVES AND HORMONE REPLACEMENT THERAPY

Lewis H. Kuller and Roberta B. Ness

Women in the United States commonly take medications containing estrogens, progestogens, or both in order to benefit from the physiologic effects of elevated blood hormonal levels. The two most common types of hormonal medications, otherwise known as exogenous hormones, are oral contraceptives (OCs) and hormone replacement therapy (HRT). Oral contraceptives are generally used to prevent pregnancy by eliminating the gonadotropin alterations that induce ovulation (see Chapters 6, 17). In the past, hormone replacement therapy was generally prescribed to reduce the annoying symptoms associated with the menopause such as hot flashes and vaginal dryness. Currently, HRT is most often used to reduce the risk of coronary heart disease and osteoporosis (see Chapters 7,8). In this chapter, we will review the pharmacology of OC and HRT formulations and discuss the range of protective effects and risks arising from these exogenous hormonal preparations.

PHARMACOLOGY OF HORMONAL CONTRACEPTIVES

Oral contraceptives contain either a combination of estrogen and progestin (combination OCs) or progesterone alone (progestin-only agents). When estrogen and progesterone are given in combination, the doses can be fixed for 21 days out of a 28-day menstrual cycle (monophasic combination OCs) or the doses can be altered in a combined fashion over the course of the cycle (multiphasic OCs). Multiphasic OCs were formulated to more accurately mirror the hormonal changes that occur over the menstrual cycle and have a slightly lower progestin content than monophasic preparations. Sequential OCs, a formulation of OCs that is now unavailable in the U.S., consist of 2 weeks of estrogen without progestin, followed by combined estrogen/progestin dosing for 7 days. Sequential OCs were removed from the American market because they were associated with endometrial cancer (see below). The goal of all current OC formulations is to achieve the lowest possible doses of estrogen and progestin so as to reduce adverse metabolic effects while maintaining contraceptive efficacy and minimizing side effects, such as break-through bleeding (menstrual bleeding occurring outside of the timing of the normal menses).

Two synthetic estrogens comprise the estrogenic component of all combination OCs: ethinyl estradiol and mestranol.[1] Ethinyl estradiol is a derative of naturally occurring estradiol; the addition of an ethinyl group to estradiol allows for potent oral activity. Mestranol is the 3-methyl ether of ethinyl estradiol and is converted to the active ethinyl estradiol in women's bodies. Mestranol, perhaps because it needs to be converted to an active form, has been shown in animal models to be less potent than ethinyl estradiol. Original formulations of OCs frequently contained 50–500 μg of mestranol. For instance, Enovid® (Searle), the first OC marketed in the U.S. in 1960, contained 150 μg of mestranol. [2,3] By 1972, about one-third of OC prescriptions were for each of high-, medium- and low-dose (<50 μg/ml estrogen) pills, and thereafter, low dose pills have made up the preponderance of this type of contraception. Today, OCs generally contain no more than 50 μg of estrogen, with some containing as little as 20 μg.

The progestin component of combined OCs is more variable than the estrogen component. The first progestin constituents of OCs came from the norethindrone family, deratives of the orally potent androgen, ethisterone.[1] Conversion of ethisterone to norethindrone decreased, although did not entirely eliminate, androgenic activity, while producing progestational activity. Chemically related members of the norethindrone family include norethindrone, norethynodrel, norethindrone acetate, ethynodiol diacetate, lynestrenol, norgestrel (comprised of a racemic mixture of d-norgestrel and l-norgestrel or levonorgestrel), norgestimate, desogestrel, and gestodene. The last three members of this group constitute the newest, or third generation, of progestins and were specifically formulated to have the least androgenic effect. However, there is some evidence that third generation progestins may be more potent promoters of venous thromboembolism than earlier formulations (see below). A second group of progestins derive from substitutions to hydroxy progesterone and include a popular progestin, medroxyprogesterone acetate, the brand name for which is Provera. There is no standardly accepted ranking of the potency of various progestational agents. This is because progestins act in a variety of ways on a variety of target organs and the potency varies by the action and target. However, from a functional, reproductive perspective, all of the currently available OCs contain similar potencies of progestins. (See Appendix 16–1 for a comprehensive listing of OCs available in the U.S. and their pharmacologic components.)

Progestin-only mini-pills consist of low doses of a variety of progestins as single contraceptive agents. The low dose does not consistently interfere with gonadotropins; these agents rely more on their maintenance of thick cervical mucus and thin endometrium then on their suppression of ovulation. They must be taken at the same time of the day each day in order to be as effective in preventing pregnancy as combined OCs.

Another form of hormonal contraception consists of long-acting progestins that are injected or implanted under the skin. Two long-acting progestins are currently available in the U.S. Norplant uses levonorgestrel sealed inside silastic tubing which is permeable to steroid molecules. Because the drug delivery rate is determined by the surface area and thickness of the tubing, a small and sustained medication release is achieved. Blood levels of progestin are one-fourth to one-tenth the level of those attained by OCs, yet progestins are equally effective in preventing pregnancy. Norplant can provide stable levels of progestin for up to 5 years. Depoprovera consists of an injection of medroxyprogesterone acetate. Like Norplant, it delivers low-dose, continuous levels of progestin. Its effectiveness lasts for 3 to 6 months.

HORMONAL CONTRACEPTIVES, CONTRACEPTION, AND ACCEPTANCE

Hormonal contraception is one of the most effective means of pregnancy prevention. The lowest expected rate of pregnancy with the use of a combination pill is 0.1% and with a progestin-only agent it is 0.5% (see Chapter 17). In actual use, pregnancy rates approximate 3% in a compliant population, but may be much higher in groups of women at risk for stopping medications and continuing to have unprotected intercourse.[4] In high-risk populations, the use of long-acting progestins has been more effective at preventing pregnancy. For long-acting progestins, the theoretical and actual pregnancy rates are equivalent.

Both the estrogenic and progestational components of OCs interfere with reproduction. The estrogen component suppresses follicle-stimulating hormone (FSH) secretion and thus prevents the emergence of a dominant follicle (see Chapters 6, 11). It also stabilizes the endometrium so that shedding is not haphazard and it potentiates the action of the progestin so that a lower dose can be used. The progestin component of the OC suppresses luteinizing hormone (LH) secretion and thus ovulation. It also produces thick cervical mucous, atrophied endometrium, and perhaps effects on the fallopian tubes, all of which create an environment hostile to sperm transport and to ovum implantation.

Hormonal contraceptives appear to have some continued suppressive effect on reproduction after they are discontinued. Prospective studies from the

Appendix 16–1. Combination Monophasic Oral Contraceptives
Available in the United States[a]

ORAL CONTRACEPTIVE	PROGESTIN	PROGESTIN DOSE (MG)	ESTROGEN	ESTROGEN DOSE (μG)
Brevicon 21 day	Norethindrone	0.50	Ethinyl estradiol	35.0
Brevicon 28 day	Norethindrone	0.50	Ethinyl estradiol	35.0
Brevicon 1–35 28 day	Norethindrone	1.00	Ethinyl estradiol	35.0
C-Quens Variation (Seq) 20 day	Chlormadinone	2.00	Mestranol	80
Demulen 1/35 21 day	Ethynodiol diac	1.00	Ethinyl estradiol	35.0
Demulen 1/35 28 day	Ethynodiol diac	1.00	Ethinyl estradiol	35.0
Demulen 1/50 21 day	Ethynodiol diac	1.00	Ethinyl estradiol	50.0
Demulen 1/50 28 day	Ethynodiol diac	1.00	Ethinyl estradiol	50.0
Desogen 28 day	Desogestrel	0.15	Ethinyl estradiol	30
Enovid 5	Norethynodrel	5.00	Mestranol	75.0
Enovid 10	Norethynodrel	9.85	Mestranol	150.0
Enovid E 20 day	Norethynodrel	2.50	Mestranol	100
Enovid E 21 day	Norethynodrel	2.50	Mestranol	100
Gencept 1/35 28 day	Norethisterone	1.00	Ethinyl estradiol	35
Gencept .5/35	Norethisterone	0.50	Ethinyl estradiol	35
Genora 0.5/35E 21 day	Norethindrone	0.50	Ethinyl estradiol	35
Genora 1/35	Norethindrone	1.00	Ethinyl estradiol	35.0
Genora 1/50	Norethindrone	1.00	Mestranol	50.0
Jenest-28	Norethindrone	0.54	Ethinyl estradiol	35
Levlen 21 day	Levonorgestrel	0.15	Ethinyl estradiol	30.0
Levlen 28 day	Levonorgestrel	0.15	Ethinyl estradiol	30.0
Lo/Ovral 21 day	Norgestrel	0.30	Ethinyl estradiol	30.0
Lo/Ovral 28 day	Norgestrel	0.30	Ethinyl estradiol	30.0
Loestrin 1.5/30 21 day	Norethindrone A	1.50	Ethinyl estradiol	30.0
Loestrin 1.5/30 FE 28 day	Norethindrone A	1.50	Ethinyl estradiol	30.0
Loestrin 1.5/30 FE 28 day V1	Norethindrone A	1.50	Ethinyl estradiol	30.0
Loestrin 1.5/30 FE 28 day V2	Norethindrone A	1.50	Ethinyl estradiol	30.0
Loestrin 1/20 21 day	Norethindrone A	1.00	Ethinyl estradiol	20.0
Loestrin 1/20 FE 28 day V1	Norethindrone A	1.00	Ethinyl estradiol	20.0
Loestrin 1/20 FE 28 day V2	Norethindrone A	1.00	Ethinyl estradiol	20.0
Modicon 21 day V1	Norethindrone	0.50	Ethinyl estradiol	35.0
Modicon 21 day V2	Norethindrone	0.50	Ethinyl estradiol	35.0
Modicon 21 day V3	Norethindrone	0.50	Ethinyl estradiol	35.0
Modicon 28 day	Norethindrone	0.50	Ethinyl estradiol	35.0
N.E.E. 1/35 21 day	Norethindrone	1.00	Ethinyl estradiol	35.0
N.E.E. 1/35 28 day	Norethindrone	1.00	Ethinyl estradiol	35.0
N.E.E. 1/50	Norethindrone	1.00	Mestranol	50

(Continued)

Appendix 16–1. Combination Monophasic Oral Contraceptives
Available in the United States[a] *(Continued)*

ORAL CONTRACEPTIVE	PROGESTIN	PROGESTIN DOSE (MG)	ESTROGEN	ESTROGEN DOSE (μG)
Nelova 1/50M-28	Norethindrone	1.00	Mestranol	50
Nelova 0.5/35E	Norethindrone	0.50	Ethinyl estradiol	35.0
Nelova 1/35E	Norethindrone	1.00	Ethinyl estradiol	35.0
Neocon 21 day	Norethisterone	1.00	Ethinyl estradiol	35
Norcept-E 1–35 28 pack	Norethindrone	1.00	Ethinyl estradiol	35
Nor Q.D. Seq	Norethindrone	0.35	Not applicable	0.0
Nordette 21 day	Levonorgestrel	1.50	Ethinyl estradiol	30.0
Nordette 28 day	Levonorgestrel	1.50	Ethinyl estradiol	30.0
Norethin 1/35E 21 day	Norethindrone	1.00	Ethinyl estradiol	35
Norethin 1/35E 28 day	Norethindrone	1.00	Ethinyl estradiol	35
Norethin 1/50 21 day	Norethindrone	1.00	Ethinyl estradiol	50
Norethin 1/50 28 day	Norethindrone	1.00	Mestranol	50
Noriday 28 day	Norethindrone	1.00	Mestranol	50
Norinyl 2MG 20 day	Norethindrone	2.00	Mestranol	100
Norinyl 1+35 21 day	Norethindrone	1.00	Ethinyl estradiol	35.0
Norinyl 1+35 28 day	Norethindrone	1.00	Ethinyl estradiol	35.0
Norinyl 1+50 21 day V1	Norethindrone	1.00	Mestranol	50.0
Norinyl 1+50 21 day V2	Norethindrone	1.00	Mestranol	50.0
Norinyl 1+50 28 day V1	Norethindrone	1.00	Mestranol	50.0
Norinyl 1+50 28 day V2	Norethindrone	1.00	Mestranol	50.0
Norinyl 1+80 21 day	Norethindrone	1.00	Mestranol	80.0
Norinyl 1+80 28 day	Norethindrone	1.00	Mestranol	80.0
Norinyl 1+80 FE 28 day	Norethindrone	1.00	Mestranol	80
Norinyl-1 20 day	Norethisterone	1.00	Mestranol	50.0
Norinyl-1 21 day	Norethindrone	1.00	Mestranol	50.0
Norinyl-1 28 day	Norethindrone	1.00	Mestranol	50.0
Norlestrin 1MG 20 day	Norethindrone A	1.00	Ethinyl estradiol	50.0
Norlestrin 1MG 21 day V1	Norethindrone A	1.00	Ethinyl estradiol	50.0
Norlestrin FE 1/50	Norethindrone A	1.00	Ethinyl estradiol	50
Norlestrin 1/50 21 day V2	Norethindrone A	1.00	Ethinyl estradiol	50.0
Norlestrin 1/50 28 day V1	Norethindrone A	1.00	Ethinyl estradiol	50.0
Norlestrin 1/50 28 day V2	Norethindrone A	1.00	Ethinyl estradiol	50.0

(Continued)

Appendix 16–1. Combination Monophasic Oral Contraceptives
Available in the United States[a] *(Continued)*

ORAL CONTRACEPTIVE	PROGESTIN	PROGESTIN DOSE (MG)	ESTROGEN	ESTROGEN DOSE (μG)
Norlestrin 1/50 FE 28 day	Norethindrone A	1.00	Ethinyl estradiol	50.0
Norlestrin 2.5/50 20 day	Norethindrone A	2.50	Ethinyl estradiol	50.0
Norlestrin 2.5/50 21 day V1	Norethindrone A	2.50	Ethinyl estradiol	50.0
Norlestrin 2.5/50 21 day V2	Norethindrone A	2.50	Ethinyl estradiol	50.0
Norlestrin 2.5/50 FE 28 day	Norethindrone A	2.50	Ethinyl estradiol	50.0
Norlestrin 2.5/50 FE 28 day V1	Norethindrone A	2.50	Ethinyl estradiol	50.0
Norlestrin 2.5/50 FE 28 day V2	Norethindrone A	2.50	Ethinyl estradiol	50.0
Norlutate 2.5MG 21 day	Norethindrone A	2.50	Not applicable	0.0
Nor-Q-D SEQ	Norethindrone	0.35	Not applicable	0.0
Norinyl 10MG 20 day	Norethindrone	10.0	Mestranol	60.0
Norquen Seq 20 day	Norethindrone	2.00	Mestranol	80.0
Oracon Seq 21 day V1 & V2	Dimethisterone	25.0	Ethinyl estradiol	100.0
Oracon Seq 28 day	Dimethisterone	25.0	Ethinyl estradiol	100.0
Ortho-Cept 21 day	Desogestrel	0.15	Ethinyl estradiol	30
Ortho-Cept 28 day	Desogestrel	0.15	Ethinyl estradiol	30
Ortho-Cyclen 21 day	Norgestimate	0.25	Ethinyl estradiol	35
Ortho-Cyclen 28 day	Norgestimate	0.25	Ethinyl estradiol	35
Ortho-Novum 1/35 21 day	Norethindrone	1.00	Ethinyl estradiol	35.0
Ortho-Novum 1/35 28 day	Norethindrone	1.00	Ethinyl estradiol	35.0
Ortho-Novum 1/50 21 day V1	Norethindrone	1.00	Mestranol	50.0
Ortho-Novum 1/50 21 day V2	Norethindrone	1.00	Mestranol	50.0
Ortho-Novum 1/50 28 day V1	Norethindrone	1.00	Mestranol	50.0
Ortho-Novum 1/50 28 day V2	Norethindrone	1.00	Mestranol	50.0
Ortho-Novum 1/80 21 day V1	Norethindrone	1.00	Mestranol	80.0
Ortho-Novum 1/80 21 day V2	Norethindrone	1.00	Mestranol	80.0

(Continued)

Appendix 16–1. Combination Monophasic Oral Contraceptives
Available in the United States[a] *(Continued)*

ORAL CONTRACEPTIVE	PROGESTIN	PROGESTIN DOSE (MG)	ESTROGEN	ESTROGEN DOSE (μG)
Ortho-Novum 1/80 28 day V1	Norethindrone	1.00	Mestranol	80.0
Ortho-Novum 1/80 28 day V2	Norethindrone	1.00	Mestranol	80.0
Ortho-Novum 1/80 28 day V3	Norethindrone	1.00	Mestranol	80.0
Ortho-Novum 10MG 20 day	Norethindrone	10.0	Mestranol	60
Ortho-Novum 2MG 21 day	Norethindrone	2.00	Mestranol	100
Ortho-Novum Seq 20 day	Norethindrone	2.00	Mestranol	80.0
Ovcon-35 21 day	Norethindrone	0.40	Ethinyl estradiol	35.0
Ovcon-35 28 day V1	Norethindrone	0.40	Ethinyl estradiol	35.0
Ovcon-35 28 day V2	Norethindrone	0.40	Ethinyl estradiol	35.0
Ovcon-50 21 day	Norethindrone	1.00	Ethinyl estradiol	50.0
Ovcon-50 28 day V1	Norethindrone	1.00	Ethinyl estradiol	50.0
Ovcon-50 28 day V2	Norethindrone	1.00	Ethinyl estradiol	50.0
Ovral 21 day	Norgestrel	0.50	Ethinyl estradiol	50.0
Ovral 28 day V1	Norgestrel	0.50	Ethinyl estradiol	50.0
Ovral 28 day V2	Norgestrel	0.50	Ethinyl estradiol	50.0
Ovral FE 28 day	Norgestrel	0.50	Ethinyl estradiol	50.0
Ovrette 28 day	Norgestrel	0.07	Not applicable	0.0
Ovulen 20 day	Ethynodiol diac	1.00	Mestranol	100
Ovulen 21 day	Ethynodiol diac	1.00	Mestranol	100
Ovulen 28 day	Ethynodiol diac	1.00	Mestranol	100.0
Ovulen 50	Ethynodiol diac	1.00	Ethinyl estradiol	50.0
Provest 20 day	Medroxiprogeste	10.0	Ethinyl estradiol	50
Zorane 1.5/30.0 28 day	Norethindrone A	1.50	Ethinyl estradiol	30.0
Zorane 1/20 28 day 28 day	Norethindrone A	1.00	Ethinyl estradiol	20.0
Zorane 1/50 28 day	Norethindrone A	1.00	Ethinyl estradiol	50

[a]Includes all drugs for which progestin and estrogen type and dose were available.

United States and from England show that women who recently stopped using OCs took longer to conceive than women who stopped using other methods of birth control. Linn et al.[5] reported that almost a quarter of women took at least 13 months to conceive after the cessation of OCs compared with about 10% after the cessation of other methods of birth control. Bracken et al.[6] confirmed these findings and showed that higher-dose preparations resulted in longer delays. Despite these consistent findings, there is no evidence that OCs produce irreversible infertility nor is there evidence that OCs are associated with spontaneous abortion or adverse birth outcomes.[7-10]

Although progestins alone provide perfectly acceptable contraception, progestin-only agents are likely to cause a variety of often unacceptable side effects. These effects are thought to be the result of *(1)* the destabilized endometrium in the absence of estrogen and *(2)* the androgenic qualities of synthetic progestins. Unwanted side effects include break-through bleeding or variable patterns of menstrual bleeding, weight gain and bloating, breast tenderness, headache, and mood alterations such as anxiety and depression. These side effects are common among long-dose progestin and mini-pill users and are the most common reasons for discontinuation of use. Although these same side effects occur in OC users, their frequency is much less common and is more likely to be self-limited.

OTHER METABOLIC IMPACTS OF HORMONAL CONTRACEPTION

Exogenous hormones in the form of hormonal contraception affect a broad range of organs. This is understandable, given that almost every organ in the body has estrogen receptors. Of particular clinical importance, and the focus of these next sections, are the effects on the cardiovascular system and on a variety of cancers. Because the relationship between OCs and breast cancer is reviewed in Chapter 9, we will confine the following discussion to OCs and endometrial cancer and OCs and ovarian cancer.

Cardiovascular Effects of Oral Contraceptives

Previous prospective studies and case–control studies indicated that current OC use increased the risk of venous thromboembolism, myocardial infarction, and stroke. Soon after the introduction of oral contraceptives there were clinical reports of an association with the risks of venous thrombosis, stroke, and myocardial infarction.[11,12] Case–control studies from the early 1960s documented a substantial excess risk of thromboembolism associated with oral contraceptive use.[13,14] These early reports suggested that the dose of estrogen in oral contraceptives was associated with the excess risk of thromboembolism.[15] Prospective studies subsequently verified the results shown in these case-control studies.[16] The association between oral contraceptives and myocardial infarction and stroke was thought to be linked to the androgenicity of the progestin in the oral contraceptives and possibly, to cofactors, such as cigarette smoking and older age of users. These early studies led to efforts to reduce the estrogen dose to <50 µg of estradiol and to try to identify less androgenic progestin compounds.

In 1995 a World Health Organization (WHO) study suggested that the third generation progestins used in oral contraceptives (because they were believed to be less androgenic) might actually be associated with an increased risk of venous thromboembolism, although there might be a decrease in myocardial infarction.[17] Several other studies support these initial observations. A large study based on 540,000 premenopausal women in the United Kingdom reported that the crude rate per 10,000/year was 4.1 in OC users, 3.1 in second generation users, and 5.0 in third generation progestin users. The risks, surprisingly, appear to be greater in the women who are also on low-dose estradiol.[18]

Until recently, only about 5% of venous thromboembolism could be directly related to genetic abnormalities of clotting (i.e., host susceptibility), proteins C and S, and antithrombin III. This changed with the identification of a genetic abnormality of resistance to protein C (so-called Leiden factor V). Protein C is a natural inhibitor of clotting. Activated protein C (APC) with protein S inhibits clotting by blocking the activity of factor V. Resistance to protein C is the result of a mutation in the factor V gene (factor V Leiden).[19,20] It has been estimated that APC resistance is associated with about an eightfold increased risk of venous thrombosis in heterozygotes and an extremely high risk in the rare homozygotes. The third generation progestins in the oral contraceptives were also found to induce APC resistance at about the same magnitude as the effect of Leiden V,[20] whereas the second generation progestins in the oral contraceptives showed a lesser effect. The combination of third generation oral contraceptives in Leiden V results in a substantial excess risk for venous thrombosis, close to that of the homozygotes (about a 15- to 100-fold increase).

The relative risk confounded by Leiden V mutation alone, as noted, is about eightfold (five- to tenfold). The increased risk of third generation OCs may be in the range of six- to ninefold compared with a three- to fourfold increased risk for second generation OCs and the risk of venous thrombosis.[21] The combination of Leiden V mutation and OCs is believed to increase the risk of venous thrombosis to about 30-fold and probably to about 50-fold with the combination of third generation OCs and Leiden V. This is one of the best examples of host–environment associations that indicates the need to understand host–drug interactions when trying to evaluate the effects of a drug on a disease outcome. Similar drug or environmental gene interactions are important in understanding susceptibility to various diseases in relation to agent and environmental effects. The results strongly suggest that APC resistance may also be the mechanism for the increased risk of thromboembolism associated with oral contraceptives.[21]

The risk of venous thrombosis is about 1/10,000 among premenopausal women. A 30-fold increased risk would still result in a relatively low risk per year of use (about 30/10,000). However, 20 years of OC use among women with Leiden V abnormality might increase their risk to as high as 6% (i.e., 30/10,000 × 20 years of exposure). At the present time, there is no evidence that such a high risk exists, but it is important to further evaluate this association, given the large number of women on oral contraceptives. About 20% of the cases of venous thromboembolism are believed to be related to Leiden V abnormalities. The estimated prevalence of Leiden V heterozygosity is about 5% in the population. At least one report has suggested, however, that there is substantial ethnic variability (5.3% in Caucasian-Americans, 2.2% in Hispanic-Americans, 1.2% in African-Americans, 0.5% in Asian-Americans, and about 1% in Native-Americans).[22] These were not population samples, and further evaluation of the prevalence of Leiden V, APC resistance, and its relationship to venous thrombosis in different populations is underway.

There are several approaches used to evaluate the risk of APC resistance and oral contraceptives in a given woman. First, a history of previous venous thromboembolism[23] disease or a family history of venous thromboembolism should increase the likelihood of a woman having Leiden V abnormality and being at risk. Second, there are specific tests for APC resistance and DNA testing to identify this specific genetic abnormality. An important issue that is still unresolved is how to identify these higher-risk women and specifically, whether genetic testing of all women on OCs would be too costly. Therefore, at a minimum, a careful family history of venous thromboembolism, as well as a history of any possible venous thromboembolism in the index women, is of considerable importance.

Ovarian and Endometrial Cancers

Oral contraceptives have different effects on endometrial and ovarian cancers. Whereas sequential OCs are strongly related to endometrial cancer, combined OCs protect against endometrial cancer. In contrast, both sequential and combined OCs strongly protect against ovarian cancer. These epidemiologic observations suggest that the pathophysiology of these diseases differs and that their interaction with exogenous hormones also differs. Better understanding of the differential hormonal pathogenesis for these gynecologic cancers may lead to the development of innovative strategies for prevention.

Endometrial Cancer

A recent estimate of the relationship between combined OCs and endometrial cancer plotted the results of 11 studies involving 1,660 women with invasive endometrial cancer, 232 of whom used combined OCs.[24] The relative risk of endometrial cancer for women with 4 years of OC use was reduced by 56% and continued to decline with continued use, such that risk was reduced by 72% with 12 years of use. This protection persisted for 20 years or more and protected against all major types of endometrial cancer: adenocarcinoma, adenoacanthoma, and adenosquamous cancers. Key and Pike[25] predicted that 5 years of OC use beginning at age 28 would produce a 60% reduction in lifetime risk as a result of suppressing endometrial cell proliferation sufficiently to delay a risk in the age-specific incidence rate of cancer.

At the same time, sequential OCs have been strongly implicated in the genesis of endometrial cancer, probably because of the high-dose, unopposed estrogen that these drugs deliver for fully half the menstrual cycle. Also, data from a World Health Organization study[26] showed that endometrial cancer risk was neither reduced nor increased among users of high-dose estrogen, low-dose progestin OCs; however, risk was markedly reduced among high-dose progestin users, regardless of estrogen content. Although this study had a relatively small number of users of each type of hormonal contraceptive, and it was confirmed by some,[27, 28] but not all,[29] other case–control studies, these results are biologically consistent with the notion that unopposed estrogen is involved in the genesis of endometrial cancer.

Other epidemiologic observations support the biologic hypothesis that estrogen stimulation without adequate progesterone effect mediates the occurrence of endometrial cancer. In particular, estrogen replacement therapy (ERT) has been strongly related to endometrial hyperplasia and endometrial cancer; added progestin markedly reduces this risk.[30–43] Endometrial hyperplasia represents a spectrum of histologic changes in the endometrial glands and stroma that range from simple excess growth to complex rearrangement or distortion of the glands. These changes have variable probabilities of progressing to cancer, with simple changes being least likely (1%) and complex glandular changes with atypical cellular components being most likely (29%).[44] Endometrial hyperplasia is markedly more common in women using unopposed estrogen replacement therapy than in those using a regimen containing a progestin. For example, in the Postmenopausal Estrogen/Progestogen Interventions (PEPI) trial,[45] 62% of women randomized to unopposed ERT developed endometrial hyperplasia compared with 4% of women randomized to a regimen containing a progestogen and 2% randomized to placebo. Multiple case–control studies and prospective studies have shown a strong association between ERT and endometrial cancer after adjustment for major confounding factors. This association increased with increasing duration of use and with increasing estrogen dose.[24] It persisted for at least 10 years after stopping ERT. Schlesselman and Collins[24] estimated that the relative risk for endometrial cancer after just 1 year of ERT use was 1.7, after 4 years was 3.6, after 8 years was 5.8, and after 12 years was 7.7.

Nulliparity, obesity, early menarche, and late menopause are all factors that have been shown in epidemiologic studies to increase the risk of endometrial cancer.[29,46,47] Nulliparity and obesity produce a frequently anovulatory menstrual cycle dominated by unopposed estrogen. Early menarche and late menopause increase the number of menstrual cycles over a lifetime. Thus, both the epidemiologic data relating to exogenous hormones and that related to endogenous hormonal patterns suggest that estrogen stimulation of the endometrium, without sufficient progestin effect, mediates the occurrence of endometrial cancer.

Estrogen has been shown to be a potent stimulator of endometrial cell proliferation, an effect important in the natural progression of the menstrual cycle. However, as such, estrogen in the absence of adequate cyclic progesterone may promote the cancer potential of cells that have already suffered damage to DNA (been induced) by virtue of chemical, radiation, or viral exposures, or perhaps through spontaneous mutation.[48,49] Replication or promotion of induced cells is considered a common mechanism through which early tumors develop.

Ovarian Cancer

Malignant epithelial tumors, deriving from the surface epithelium of the ovary, account for about 90% of ovarian cancers.[50] Because the remaining ovarian tumors (sex cord–stromal tumors and germ-cell tumors) are so uncommon, almost all of the epidemiologic studies to date have focused on epithelial tumors.

Use of OCs has been consistently shown to decrease the risk of ovarian cancer, despite the comparison of cases to different control groups (hospital based or community based) and the study of populations in different countries. Of 21 studies referenced here,[51–71] 19 have shown a reduction in risk, with odds ratios (ORs) ranging from 0.3 to 0.8 (Table 16–1). A summary OR of 0.7 (confidence interval [CI] 0.6–0.7) was calculated by meta-analysis.[72] Although the great majority of these studies used a case–control design, more recent cohort studies[71,73] supported the finding of a protective effect for OCs. Only one study conducted in China by Shu et al.[64] found an increased risk (OR 1.8) among OC users, but it only included 21 OC users among 172 cases and 12 users among 172 controls. Additionally, the protective effect of OCs has been shown to be greater with longer duration of use[51–54,62–65,67–69] and to persist for 10 or more years after discontinuation of use.[52–54,65–69]

Nulliparity and single marital status have been consistently related to a high risk of cancer with ORs ranging from 1.1 to as high as 5. However, whether nulliparity/low parity or difficulty in conceiving facilitates the development of ovarian cancer remains controversial. In support of the former, most studies suggest that increased numbers of pregnancies reduce the risk of ovarian cancer. Of at least 20 studies[52,55–59,61,62,69,73–83] that have examined this, 17[55,57–58,61,62,69,73–81] (13 statistically significant) have demonstrated a further decline in risk associated with full-term pregnancies after the first pregnancy, with ORs ranging from 0.1 to 0.6 for 5 or more pregnancies. On the other hand, infertility itself may be a risk factor for ovarian cancer.[52,77,84–86] The fact that nulliparity and lack of OC use are both common in infertile women and are both risk factors for ovarian

Table 16-1. Studies of Oral Contraceptive Use and Ovarian Cancer

STUDIES NOT STATISTICALLY SIGNIFICANT			STUDIES REACHING STATISTICAL SIGNIFICANCE		
REFERENCE	TUMOR TYPE[a]	OR (95% CI)	REFERENCE	TUMOR TYPE	OR (95% CI)
Tzonou et al., 1984[57]	EP[a]	0.4 (0.1–1.1)	Vessey et al., 1987[71]	EP	0.3 (0.1–0.7)
Hildreth et al., 1981[58]	EP	0.5 (0.2–1.7)	Cramer et al., 1982[65]	EP, LMP	0.4 (0.2–1.0)
Newhouse et al., 1977[59]	All	0.6 (0.3–1.1)	Harlow et al., 1988[66]	LMP	0.4 (0.2–0.9)
Beral et al., 1988[60]	All	0.6 (0.1–2.3)	Booth et al., 1989[52]	EP	0.5 (0.3–0.9)
Wu et al., 1988[61]	EP	0.7 (0.5–1.1)	Gwinn et al., 1990[56]	EP, LMP	0.5 (0.4–0.7)
McGowan et al., 1979[55]	EP, LMP	0.7 LMP–0.6	Weiss et al., 1981[67]	EP, LMP	0.6 (0.4–1.0)
Casagrande et al., 1979[62]	EP	0.7 (0.4–1.1)	CASH, 1987[53]	All	0.6 (0.5–0.9)
Willett et al., 1981[63]	EP	0.8 (0.4–1.5)	La Vecchia et al., 1984[68]	EP	0.6 (0.3–1.0)
Hartge et al., 1989[51]	EP, LMP	1.0 (0.7–1.7)	Rosenberg et al., 1982[69]	EP	0.6 (0.4–0.9)
Shu et al., 1989[64]	All	1.8 (0.8–4.1)	Parazzini et al., 1991[70]	EP	0.7 (0.5–1.0)
			WHO Study, 1989[54]	EP, LMP	0.8 (0.6–1.0)

[a]EP, epithelial tumors; LMP, epithelial tumors of low malignant potential (borderline).

cancer suggests further exploration of the association between infertility and ovarian cancer.

Breast-feeding has consistently been shown to protect against ovarian cancer in a dose-related fashion.[85] Body size has not been a consistent risk factor. Findings have been completely mixed regarding the relationship between hormone replacement therapy (the vast majority of which was estrogen alone) and ovarian cancer. Several studies[58,61,66,87,88] showed a protective effect in women who have ever used estrogens in menopause, two of which were significant (ORs = 0.5 and 0.6 for Annegers[87] and Hartge,[88] respectively). Several other studies[52,57,75,89,90] showed no overall effect and/or a moderate increase in risk in certain subgroups, as in Booth et al.'s study[52] of hysterectomized women (OR 10.9), and studies by La Vecchia et al.,[91] and Weiss et al.[89] for the histologic subtype of endometroid tumors (OR 2.3 and 3.1, respectively). None of these studies found a trend with duration of use.

Two major competing hypotheses have been proposed to explain the array of factors that either offer protection against or increase the risk for ovarian cancer. The ovulation hypothesis suggests that ovulation exposes the ovarian epithelium to recurrent minor trauma which allows promotion of cells containing genetic damage (see above) and possibly inactivates genes that suppress developing tumors (tumor-suppressor genes).[92] Hence, factors that suppress ovulation are proposed to reduce the risk of ovarian tumors.[93,94] In support of this hypothesis, OC use and parity[52,55,56–58,61,62,69,73–81] have been shown to decrease the risk of ovarian cancer, whereas late menopause[52,57,58,61,64,78,95] and lifelong regular menstrual periods increase the risk of disease.[95]

The pituitary gonadotropin hormone hypothesis proposes that high levels of pituitary gonadotropin hormones increase the risk of ovarian cancer through their ability to stimulate follicular development.[96,97] In support of this hypothesis is the observation that pregnancy and OC use may protect against ovarian cancer by reducing total exposure to pituitary gonadotropin. The validity of each of these hypotheses is weakened by certain epidemiologic data. For example, the finding that there is greater ovarian cancer risk reduction per month of pregnancy than per month of OC use is inconsistent with the ovulation hypothesis. Counter to the pituitary gonadotropin hormone hypothesis, direct gonadotropin measurements are not higher in women destined to develop ovarian cancer.[98] There are also no consistent data showing protection from estrogen replacement therapy, which would reduce gonadotropin stimulation later in life.

An important methodologic consideration about studies relating OCs to ovarian and endometrial cancers is that those which have demonstrated the protective effect of OCs have all involved older, higher dose formulations. There has been some concern that lower-dose combination pills may not afford the same degree of protection as their high dose predecessors. Only a handful of studies involving a small number of women have assessed the risk of endometrial or ovarian cancers in relation to strength of combination OC formulations.[53,67] Weiss et al.[67] found no difference in the protection afforded by OCs of various potencies for ovarian cancer. Similarly, in the Cancer and Steroid Hormone (CASH) Study,[53] protection for ovarian and endometrial cancers were reported for ever use of the most frequently reported combined OC formulations, irrespective of type and dose of estrogen and progestin in the formulations. And in the World Health Organization study,[54] both women who used high-estrogen/high-progestin pills and those who used low-estrogen/low-progestin pills had reductions in endometrial cancer risk. However, as described above, pills with a high estrogen-to-progesterone ratio produced the opposite effect.

ESTROGEN THERAPY

Premarin, the most widely used estrogen (as noted), is approved for *(1)* moderate to severe vasomotor symptoms associated with the menopause (such as hot flashes), *(2)* atropic vaginitis, *(3)* prevention of osteoporosis, and *(4)* hypo estrogenism due to oophorectomy or primary ovarian failure. Prevention of cardiovascular disease is not a current indication for estrogen therapy.[99]

Several different approaches have been evaluated to determine the number of women in the United States using hormone replacement therapy and the characteristics of such women. The National Prescription Audit estimates the number of prescriptions dispensed by chain and independent pharmacies.[100] The National Disease and Therapeutic Index obtains information from a sample of physicians in private office-based medical practices. The Epidemiological Follow-up Study to the First National Health and Nutrition Examination Study has followed a representative cohort in the United States from the 1970s until 1992.[101] Other studies have estimated hormone use in specific population samples in different parts of the United States.[102]

Retail pharmacies dispensed 13.6 million prescriptions for oral menopausal estrogens in 1982, and by 1992 this figure had risen to 31.7 million (a 2.3-fold increase).[100] In 1992 Premarin was the most frequently dispensed brand-name pharmaceutical in the United States. Estraderm, a transdermal estrogen, also increased in use to 4.7 million prescriptions in 1992. Injectable estrogens remained fairly constant at about 0.1 million prescriptions from 1982 to 1992.[100] Prescriptions for oral medroxy-progesterone, Provera, increased from 2.3 million in 1982 to 11.3 million in 1992—this is mostly used in combination with Premarin. The majority of prescriptions were written by obstetricians and gynecologists.[100]

By 1992 an estimated 45% of U.S. women born between 1897 and 1950 and menopausal had used HRT for at least 1 month. Among women who experienced bilateral oophorectomy, use increased from 37% for the women who were menopausal prior to 1945 to 71% in women who were postmenopausal

1990–92. Among women with natural menopause, ever-users increased from 11% to 46% in 1990–92. Use of hormone therapy decreased in the 1970s because of the observation of an increased risk of endometrial cancer associated with unopposed estrogen therapy. Use began to rise again in the 1980s, especially in combination with an oral progesterone.[101]

The median length of use of HRT in the national sample was 36 months with a mean of 6.6 years, and 43% of women had been on hormone replacement therapy for at least 5 years. Twenty percent of all women in the national cohort who were postmenopausal had been on HRT for 5 or more years. The characteristics of long-term users (>5 years) included bilateral oophorectomy, higher levels of education, white race, not overweight, and consumers of alcoholic beverages. Other studies have also noted substantial selection for use of HRT, especially body weight, education, and oophorectomy/hysterectomy. In 1992 approximately one-third of women used progestins with estrogens. Women who had a "natural" menopause and an intact uterus were much more likely to use the combination of estrogen and progesterone.[101]

Administration of Estrogen

Any of the estrogens taken orally are converted primarily to estrone because of the "first pass" through the liver. There is a significant loss of bioavailability of estrogens following this first pass through the liver. The major metabolite is estrone-3 glucuronide. The glucuronidation of estrone can be modified by certain drugs and probably by genetic (host) and lifestyle factors. The peak levels of estrone occur about 4 hours after oral administration and these levels increase more than estradiol levels. The increase in both is directly related to the dose of oral estrogens.[103]

The blood levels of estradiol among women on oral HRT are higher than for women not on HRT, but they remain much lower than peak estradiol levels during the menstrual cycles. Thus, with a 0.625 mg standard dose of Premarin, estradiol levels may rise from about 10 pg/ml to perhaps 40 pg/ml but are still much lower than the 200 pg/ml of estradiol during the menstrual cycle. Oral estrogens have been taken primarily to relieve menopausal symptoms (such as hot flashes) and prevent osteoporosis—not to provide physiological replacement of estrogen levels found during the premenopause.[103] Levels of estradiol can be higher after use of a transdermal patch or by injection. Whether these higher levels result in reduced or increased risk of disease is unknown.[103]

The use of conjugated estrogen, such as Premarin, also results in a complex mixture of estrogens in the blood and it is difficult to measure the specific levels of estrogens among women on Premarin therapy.

Estrogen is absorbed from the skin, subcutaneous fat, and vagina. These methods are not associated with first-pass changes through the liver, thus levels of estradiol in the blood are higher than those for estrone. The transdermal method has been used more frequently in recent years and, as noted, increases estradiol levels to 40–80 pg/ml. The patch must be replaced every 3 days. At the present time, there is no evidence of whether the patch versus oral estrogens are associated with differences in risk benefits of disease.

The oral estrogens, such as Premarin, result in an increase in high-density lipoprotein cholesterol (HDLc) levels that is not observed by the transdermal or injectable estradiol approach. If the rise in HDLc has a cardioprotective effect (this is unknown at the present time), then the effects of oral estrogen (especially Premarin) may be preferable to transdermal approaches.[104,105] This increase in HDLc, which, as noted, may be cardioprotective, is not consistent with the small change in total HDLc seen at the time of natural menopause[106] and the substantial decreases in estradiol levels. The higher HDLc levels in women than in men are primarily due to a decrease in HDLc levels in men during adolescence and not to an increase in HDLc in women during the premenopausal years, nor can they be attributed to a substantial change in HDL at the time of menopause. The increase in HDLc is related both to the method of administration of the estrogen (greater increase with oral) and the type of estrogen (greater effect with Premarin).[103]

The effects of estrogen and estrogen–progestin regimes on heart disease risk factors were evaluated in the PEPI trial. Estrogen alone resulted in a substantial increase in HDLc (5.6 mg), a decrease in low-density lipoprotein cholesterol (LDLc) (14.5 mg), and an increase in triglycerides (13.7 mg). There was no substantial change in blood pressure, glucose-insulin metabolism, or body weight, but there was a small, significant decrease in fibrinogen levels. There were few changes in the placebo group.[104]

Premarin and continuous medroxy progesterone blunted the increase in HDLc (1.2 mg). The use of Premarin with micronized (natural) progesterone did not blunt the rise in HDLc (4.1 mg) compared with the use of medroxy progesterone. Further evaluation of micronized progesterone is continuing. The use of estrogen alone among postmenopausal women with an intact uterus has resulted in substantial risk of uterine hyperplasia and probably a premalignant lesion. Thus oral estrogen alone should not be prescribed for women with an intact uterus.[104]

The combination of estrogen with progesterone (usually medroxy progesterone) taken either continuously or sequentially, is the most widely used postmenopausal hormone therapy today. A major reason for women to discontinue hormone therapy is bleeding. In a 1-year double-blind, randomized study with 1,724 postmenopausal women, the effects of 2.5 or 5 mg of medroxy progesterone taken continuously or 5–10 mg cyclically (i.e., about 14 days) was evaluated along with 0.625 mg of conjugated estrogen (Premarin). The continuous regime resulted in 61.4% and 72.8% amenorrhea for the two doses for all months over the year. The incidence of amenorrhea increases with duration of therapy. However, complete amenorrhea was found for only 40% of women on the continuous low dose (2.5 mg) and 50% on the higher dose (5 mg) of progesterone during the last seven cycles of the study. Women who took the sequential regimes had good cycle control of their bleeding but had monthly bleeding. The problem of bleeding among women on HRT estrogens and progesterones remains a major problem and is associated with a greater likelihood of stopping hormone therapy.[107]

The dose of estrogens used for postmenopausal hormone replacement therapy is substantially lower than in oral contraceptives. There has been controversy as to whether postmenopausal hormone therapy is associated with an increased risk of venous thromboembolism (VTE). A case–control study in the Oxford Regional Health Authority of 81 women with VTE and 146 hospital controls found a 3.5-fold odds ratio of VTE associated with the use of hormone replacement therapy.[108] A similar case–control study from the Group Health Cooperative of Puget Sound also noted a 3.6-fold risk that was directly related to the dose of estrogen.[109] In a prospective study (the Nurses Study), the risk of pulmonary embolism alone was 16/100,000 in non-users, 13/100,000 in past users, and 20/100,000 in current users of HRT. The relative risk for heavy users, after adjustment for other risk factors, was 1.8-fold.[110]

The absolute risk of VTE among women on hormone replacement therapy is low. However, it is likely that much of the excess risk is in women who have activated protein C deficiency, which is probably related to a Leiden V genetic abnormality, and is similar to the situation of women on oral contraceptives. The risk of venous thrombosis could be substantial among women with Leiden V abnormalities and on HRT, especially if they also have other risk factors for venous thromboembolism (such as obesity, immobility, trauma, surgical treatment, and older age). The potential interaction of host susceptibility, postmenopausal hormone therapy, and risk of venous thromboembolism is an important and very high priority for further study.

Recently, a new class of drugs that have estrogen effects and may be useful for hormone replacement therapy have become available. These drugs are classified as specialized estrogen receptor modifiers (SERMs); they bind to the estrogen receptor but have different effects on post-translational activity in the estrogen response elements. The first drug in this class was tamoxifen, which was initially used for the treatment of both pre- and postmenopausal breast cancer, especially estrogen receptor–positive cancer. The drug was very effective in reducing mortality among women with breast cancer and in reducing the risk of breast cancer in the opposite breast.

Women on tamoxifen therapy were noted to have higher bone mineral density and decreased loss of bone. Tamoxifen also reduced LDLc but had little effect on HDLc, and also reduced fibrinogen levels.[111] Like estrogen, however, tamoxifen increased the risk of uterine hyperplasia and endometrial cancer. Women with an intact uterus on tamoxifen require repeated endometrial biopsies to determine the risk of endometrial hyperplasia and cancer. Because of its anti-estrogen effect, tamoxifen also increases the extent of hot flashes among postmenopausal women and has also been associated with an increased risk of a specific type of cataracts. Tamoxifen may be associated with decreased risk of cardiovascular disease.[112]

Several newer specialized estrogen receptor modifiers are currently being evaluated.[113,114] Apparently these newer drugs do not increase the risk of uterine hyperplasia (i.e., they're anti-estrogens to the uterus) or of endometrial cancer. They also prevent bone loss but are not as effective as estrogens. They have little effect on HDLc but do lower LDLc and fibrinogen levels, effects similar to those of postmenopausal estrogen therapy.

Tamoxifen is currently being tested in the primary prevention of breast cancer among high-risk pre- and postmenopausal women. The results of this trial would have major importance to the future selection of postmenopausal hormone therapy. The ideal drug would obviously reduce vasomotor symptoms (i.e., hot flashes, cardiovascular disease, prevent osteoporosis and breast cancer) without causing uterine hyperplasia, endometrial cancer, or other side effects. At present, several of the other SERMs are in phase II and III trials to measure bone density and possibly, fracture and cardiovascular risk and primary endpoints. There is some suggestion that these drugs may be beneficial in reducing the risk of breast cancer, although further studies are needed to evaluate the relationship of SERMs to this risk.

Currently, larger clinical trials of hormone replacement therapy, estrogen, and progesterone are evaluating the potential benefit of hormone replacement therapy (such as in the Women's Health Initiative) in terms of the primary prevention of cardiovascular disease, osteoporotic fractures, colon cancer, and total mortality. A secondary prevention trial of estrogens and progestins is being conducted in women who already have cardiovascular disease (HERS study). Several other studies continue to evaluate the effects of HRT and SERMS on endothelial function, subclinical vascular disease (especially measures of atherosclerosis), and bone metabolism.

Finally, an important new area of interest is whether estrogen therapy can reduce the risk of dementia, especially that due to Alzheimer's disease.[115,116] Since there are estrogen receptors on neurons in the brain, and estrogen stimulates nerve growth factors, it may reduce the loss of synopsis in the brain, which is a cardinal finding in Alzheimer's disease. Several observational case–control studies have suggested a lower odds ratio for Alzheimer's disease among women on HRT compared with controls. A large clinical trial (WHIMS) that is embedded in the Women's Health Initiative will evaluate whether estrogen–progesterone or estrogens alone, compared with placebo, can reduce the risk of dementia.

The results of these trials, as well as the development of newer drugs (SERMs), will provide the basis for a rational preventive treatment of disease for postmenopausal women. It is likely, however, that individualized approaches will still be required that are based on host susceptibility and genetic and lifestyle factors related to risk factors and specific diseases. It is unlikely that all postmenopausal women will require some type of hormonal preventive therapy to successfully survive the postmenopause. Menopause is not a disease and the medical treatment for all postmenopausal women for the prevention of disease may result in as many side effects as benefits. Some women, and perhaps a fairly large percentage, will need specific types of therapies to reduce their risks. Others can probably succeed using nonpharmacological approaches such as diet and increased exercise to prevent weight gain and thus reduce their risks of disease. Hormone therapy is not physiological replacement, and it will not make women live forever or even substantially increase life expectancy. Thus, a major goal of future research should be to carefully define the use of hormone therapy as efficacious drugs among selected samples of postmenopausal women.

REFERENCES

1. Sporoff C, Dorney P. Oral contraception. In: A Clinical Guide for Contraception. Baltimore, MD: Williams & Wilkins, 1992, pp. 21–108.

2. Dawson DA. Trends in use of oral contraceptives data from the 1987 National Health Interview Survey. Fam Plann Perspect 1990;22:169–172.

3. Piper JM, Kennedy DL. Oral contraceptives in the United States: Trends in content and potency. Int J Epidemiol 1987;16:215–221.

4. Polaneczky M, Slap G, Forhe C, Rappaport A, Sondheimer S. The use of levonorgestrel implants (Norplant) for contraception in adolescent mothers. N Engl J Med 1994;331:1201–1206.

5. Linn S, Schoenbaum SC, Monson RR, Rosner B, Ryan KJ. Delay in conception for former "pill users". JAMA 1982;247:629–632.

6. Bracken MB, Hellenbrand KG, Holford TR. Contraception delay after oral contraception use: The effect of estrogen dose. Fertil Steril 1990;53:21–27.

7. Rothman KJ. Fetal loss, twinning, and birth weight after oral contraceptive use. N Engl J Med 1977;297:468–471.

8. Vessey M, Doll R, Peto R, Johnson B, Wiggins P. A long term follow-up study of women using different methods of contraception—an interim report. J Biosoc Sci 1976;8:373–427.

9. Royal College of General Practitioners. The outcome of pregnancy in former oral contraceptive users. Br J Obstet Gynaecol 1976;83:608–616.

10. Magidor S, Poalti H, Harlap S, Baras M. Long-term follow-up of children whose mothers used oral contraceptives prior to contraception. Contraception 1984;29:203–214.

11. Ask-Upmark E. Thromboembolism and oral contraceptives: Post or propter? Acta Med Scand 1966;179:463–473.

12. Collaborative Group for the Study of Stroke in Young Women. Oral contraceptives and stroke in young women. Associated risk factors. JAMA 1975;231:718–722.

13. Sartwell PE, Masi AT, Arthes FG, Greene GR, Smith HE. Thromboembolism and oral contraceptives: An epidemiologic case–control study. Am J Epidemiol 1969;90: 365–380.

14. Inman WHW, Vessey MP, Westerholm B, Engelund A. Thromboembolic disease and the steroidal content of oral contraceptives: A report to the Committee on Safety of Drugs. BMJ 1970;25:203–209.

15. Stolley PD, Tonascia JA, Tockman MS, Sartwell PE, Rutledge AH, Jacobs MP. Thrombosis with low-estrogen oral contraceptives. Am J Epidemiol 1975;102:197–208.

16. Vessey M, Mant D, Smith A, Yeates D. Oral contraceptives and venous thromboembolism: Findings in a large prospective study. BMJ Clinical Research Edition 1986; 292(6519):526.

17. World Health Organization. WHO collaborative study of cardiovascular disease and steroid hormone contraception. Effect of different progestogens in low oestrogen oral contraceptives on venous thromboembolic disease. Lancet 1995;346: 1582–1588.

18. Farmer RDT, Lawrenson RA, Thompson CR, Kennedy JG, Hambleton IR. Population-based study of risk of venous thromboembolism associated with various oral contraceptives. Lancet 1997;3349:83–88.

19. Bloemenkamp KWM, Rosendaal FR, Helmerhorst FM, Büller HR, Vandenbroucke JP. Enhancement by factor V Leiden mutation of risk of deep-vein thrombosis associated with oral contraceptives containing a third-generation progestogen. Lancet 1995;346:1593–1596.

20. Rosing J, Tans G, Nicolaes GAF, et al. Oral contraceptives and venous thrombosis: Different sensitivities to activated protein C in women using second- and third-generation oral contraceptives. Br J Haematol 1997;97:233–238.

21. Vandenbroucke JP, Rosendaal FR. End of the line for "third-generation-pill" controversy? Lancet 1997;349:1113–1114.

22. Ridker PM, Miletich JP, Hennekens CH, Buring JE. Ethnic distribution of factor V Leiden in 4047 men and women. Implications for venous thromboembolism screening. JAMA 1997;227:1305–1307.

23. Simioni P, Prandoni P, Lensing AWA, et al. The risk of recurrent venous thromboembolism in patients with an Arg 506 Gln mutation in the gene for factor V (factor V Leiden). N Engl J Med 1997;336:399–403.

24. Schlesselman JJ, Collins JA. In: Fraser IS, Lobo RA, Jansen R, Whitehead M, eds. London: Churchill Livingstone. The influence of steroids on the incidence and severity of gynecologic cancers. Estrogens and Progestogens in Clinical Practice.

25. Key TJ, Pike MC. The dose–effect relationship between "unopposed" oestrogens and endometrial mitotic rate: Its central role in explaining and predicting endometrial cancer risk. Br J Cancer 1988;57:205–212.

26. Rosenblatt KA, Thomas DB, WHO Collaborative Study. Hormonal content of combined oral contraceptives in relation to the reduced risk of endometrial carcinoma. Int J Cancer 1991;49:870–874.

27. Weiss NS, Sayvetz TA. Incidence of endometrial cancer in relation to the use of oral contraceptives. N Engl J Med 1980;302:551–554.

28. Hulka BS, Chambless LE, Kaufman DG, Fowler WC, Greenberg BG. Protection against endometrial carcinoma by combined product oral contraceptives. JAMA 1982;247:475–477.

29. Henderson BE, Casagrande JT, Pike MC, Mack T, Rosario L, Duke A. The epidemiology of endometrial cancer in young women. Br J Cancer 1983;47:749–756.

30. Ziel HK, Fingle WD. Increased risk of endometrial carcinoma among users of conjugated estrogens. N Engl J Med 1975;293:1164–1170.

31. McDonald TW, Annegers JF, O'Gallon WM, Dockkerty MB, Malkasian GD, Kurland LT. Exogenous estrogen and endometrial carcinoma: Case-control and incidence study. Am J Obstet Gynecol 1977;127:572–579.

32. Weiss NS, Szekely DR, English DR, Schweid AI. Endometrial cancer in relation to patterns of menopausal estrogen use. JAMA 1979;242:261–264.

33. Folsone AR, Mink PJ, Sellers TA, Hong C, Zheng W, Potter JD. Hormonal replacement therapy and morbidity and mortality in a prospective study of postmenopausal women. Am J Public Health 1995;85:1128–1132.

34. Paganini-Hill A, Ross RK, Henderson BE. Endometrial cancer and patterns of use of oestrogen replacement therapy: A cohort study. Br J Cancer 1989;59:445–447.

35. Persson I, Adami H, Bergkvist L, et al. Risk of endometrial cancer after treatment with oestrogen alone or in conjunction with progesterone: Results of a prospective study. BMJ 1989;298:147–151.

36. Petitti D, Perlman J, Sidney S. Noncontraceptive estrogens and mortality: Long-term follow-up of women in the Walnut Creek study. Obstet Gynecol 1987;70: 289–293.

37. Antunes C, Stolley P, Rosenshein N, et al. Endometrial cancer and estrogen use: Report of a large case-control study. N Engl J Med 1979;300:9–13.

38. Brinton LA, Hoover RN, Endometrial Cancer Collaborative Group. Estrogen replacement therapy and endometrial cancer risk: Unresolved issues. Obstet Gynecol 1993;81:2:265–271.

39. Buring JE, Bain CJ, Ehrmann RL. Conjugated estrogen use and risk of endometrial cancer. Am J Epidemiol 1986;124:434–441.

40. Franks AL, Kendrick J, Tyler C, The Cancer and Steroid Hormone Study Group. Postmenopausal smoking, estrogen replacement therapy, and the risk of endometrial cancer. Am J Obstet Gynecol 1987;156:20–23.

41. Levi F, LaVecchia C, Gulie C, Granceschi S, Negri E. Oestrogen replacement treatment and the risk of endometrial cancer: Assessment of the role of co-variates. Eur J Cancer 1993;29A:1445–1449.

42. Spangler R, Clarke E, Woolever C, Newman A, Osborn R. Exogenous estrogens and endometrial cancer: A case–control study and assessment of potential biases. Am J Epidemiol 1981;114:497–506.

43. Voigt LF, Weiss NS, Chu J, Daling JR, McKnight B, Van Belle G. Progestogen supplementation of exogenous oestrogens and risk of endometrial cancer. Lancet 1991; 338(8762):274–277.

44. Kurman R, Kaminski P, Norris H. The behavior of endometrial hyperplasia: A long-term study of "untreated" hyperplasia in 170 patients. Cancer 1985;56:403–412.

45. PEPI Trial Writing Group. Effects of hormone replacement therapy on endometrial histology in postmenopausal women. JAMA 1996;275:370–375.

46. Kelsey JL, Whittemore AS. Epidemiology and primary prevention of cancers of the breast, endometrium, and ovary. A brief overview. Ann Epidemiol 1994;4:89–95.

47. Stanford JL, Brinton LA, Berman ML, et al. Oral contraceptives and endometrial cancer: Do other risk factors modify the association? Int J Cancer 1993;54:243–248.

48. Ziel HK. Estrogen's role in endometrial cancer. Obstet Gynecol 1982;60: 509–515.

49. King RJB. Biology of female sex hormone action in relation to contraceptive agents and neoplasia. Contraception 1991;43:527–542.

50. Scully R. Classification of human ovarian tumors. Environ Health Perspect 1987;73:15–24.

51. Hartge P, Schiffman MH, Hoover R, McGowan L, Lesher L, Norris HJ. A case–control study of epithelial ovarian cancer. Am J Obstet Gynecol 1989;161:10–16.

52. Booth M, Beral V, Smith P. Risk factors for ovarian cancer: A case–control study. Br J Cancer 1989;60:592–598.

53. The Cancer and Steroid Hormone (CASH) Study of the Centers for Disease Control and the National Institute of Child Health and Human Development. The reduction in risk of ovarian cancer associated with oral-contraceptive use. N Engl J Med 1987; 316:650–655.

54. The WHO Collaborative Study of Neoplasia and Steroid Contraceptives. Epithelial ovarian cancer and combined oral contraceptives. Int J Epidemiol 1989;18: 538–545.

55. McGowan L, Parent L, Lednar W, Norris HJ. The women at risk for developing ovarian cancer. Gynecol Oncol 1979;7:325–344.

56. Gwinn ML, Lee NC, Rhoses PH, Layde PM, Rubin GL. Pregnancy, breast feeding, and oral contraceptives and the risk of epithelial ovarian cancer. J Clin Epidemiol 1990;6:559–568.

57. Tzonou A, Day NE, Trichopoulos D, et al. The epidemiology of ovarian cancer in Greece: A case-control study. Eur J Cancer Clin Oncol 1984;20:1045–1052.

58. Hildreth NG, Kelsey JL, LiVolsi VA, et al. An epidemiology study of epithelial carcinoma of the ovary. Am J Epidemiol 1981;114:398–405.

59. Newhouse ML, Pearson RM, Fullerton JM, Boeson EA, Shannon HS. A case–control study of the ovary. Br J Prev Soc Med 1977;31:148–153.

60. Beral V, Hannaford P, Kay C. Oral contraceptive use and malignancies of the genital tract. Lancet 1988ii:1331–1334.

61. Wu ML, Whittemore AS, Paffengarger RS, et al. Personal and environmental characteristics related to epithelial ovarian cancer. I. Reproductive and menstrual events and oral contraceptive use. Am J Epidemiol 1988;128:1216–1227.

62. Casagrande JT, Louie EW, Pike MC, Roy S, Ross RK, Henderson BE. Incessant ovulation and ovarian cancer. Lancet 1979;II (8135):170–2.

63. Willett WC, Bain C, Hennekens CH, Rosner B, Speizer FE. Oral contraceptives and the risk of ovarian cancer. Cancer 1981;48:1684–1687.

64. Shu WO, Brinton LA, Gao YT, Yuan JM. Population-based case–control study in Shanghai. Cancer Res 1989;49:3670–3674.

65. Cramer DW, Hutchison GB, Welch WR, Scully RE, Knapp RC. Factors affecting the association of oral contraceptives and ovarian cancer. N Engl J Med 1982;307:1047–1051.

66. Harlow BL, Weiss NS, Roth GJ, Chu J, Daling JR. Case–control study of borderline ovarian tumors: Reproductive history and exposure to exogenous female hormones. Cancer Res 1988;48:5849–5852.

67. Weiss NS, Lyon JL, Liff JM, Vollmer WM, Daling JR. Incidence of ovarian cancer in relation to the use of oral contraceptives. Int J Cancer 1981;54:669–671.

68. La Vecchia C, Decarli A, Fasoli M. Oral contraceptives and cancers of the breast and of the female genital tract. Interim results from a case–control study. Br J Cancer 1986;54:311–317.

69. Rosenberg L, Shapiro S, Slone D, et al. Epithelial ovarian cancer and combination oral contraceptives. JAMA 1982;247:3210–3212.

70. Parazzini F, La Vecchia C, Negri E, Bocciolone L, Fedele L. Oral contraceptive use and the risk of ovarian cancer: Another Italian case–control study. Eur J Cancer 1991;27:594–598.

71. Vessey V, Metcalfe A, Wells C, McPherson K, Westhoff C, Yates D. Ovarian neoplasms, functional ovarian cysts, and oral contraceptives. Br Med J 1987;294: 1518–1520.

72. Stanford J. Oral contraceptives and neoplasia of the ovary. Contraception 1991;43:543–556.

73. Kvale G, Heuch I, Nilssen S, Beral V. Reproductive factors and risk of ovarian cancer: A prospective study. Int J Cancer 1988;42:246–251.

74. Mori M, Harabuchi I, Miyake H, Casagrande JT, Henderson BE, Ross RK. Reproductive, genetic, and dietary risk factors for ovarian cancer. Am J Epidemiol 1988; 128:771–777.

75. Cramer DW, Hutchison GS, Welch WR, Scully RE, Ryan KJ. Determinants of ovarian cancer risk. J Natl Cancer Inst 1983;71:711–716.

76. Joly DJ, Lilienfeld AM, Diamond El, Bross IDJ. An epidemiologic study of the relationship of reproductive experience to cancer of the ovary. Am J Epidemiol 1974;99:190–209.

77. Nasca PC, Greenwald P, Chorost S, Richarr R, Caputo T. An epidemiologic case–control study of ovarian cancer and reproductive factors. Am J Epidemiol 1974; 99:190–209.

78. Franceschi S, LaVecchia C, Helmrich SP, Mangioni C, Tognoni G. Risk factors for epithelial ovarian cancer in Italy. Am J Epidemiol 1982;119:705–713.

79. LaVecchia C, Cecarli A, Franceshi S, Regallo M, Tognoni G. Age at first birth and the risk of epithelial ovarian cancer. J Natl Cancer Inst 1984;73(3):663–666.

80. Risch HA, Weiss NS, Lyon JL, Daling JR, Liff JM. Events of reproductive life and the incidence of epithelial ovarian cancer. Am J Epidemiol 1983;117:128–139.

81. Voight LF, Harlow BL, Weiss NS. The influence of age at first birth and parity on ovarian cancer risk. Am J Epidemiol 1986;124:490–491.

82. Mori M, Kiyosawa H, Miyake H. Case–control study of ovarian cancer in Japan. Cancer 1984;53:2746–2752.

83. Wynder EL, Dodo H, Barber HRK. Epidemiology of cancer of the ovary. Cancer 1969;23(2):352–370.

84. Rossing MA, Daling JR, Weiss NS, Moore DE, Self SG. Ovarian tumors in a cohort of infertile women. N Engl J Med 1994;331:771–776.

85. Whittemore AS, Harris R, Intyre J, Collaborative Ovarian Cancer Group. Characteristics relating to ovarian cancer risk: Collaborative analysis of 12 U.S. case–control studies. Am J Epidemiol 1992;136:1184–1203.

86. Kaufman SC, Spirtas R, Alexander NJ. Do fertility drugs cause ovarian tumors? J Women's Health 1995;4:247–259.

87. Annegers JF, Strom H, Decker DG, Dockerty MD, O'Fallon WM. Ovarian cancer: Incidence and case–control study. Cancer 1979;43:729–732.

88. Hartge P, Hoover R, McGowan L, Lesher L, Norris HJ. Menopause and ovarian cancer. Am J Epidemiol 1988;127:990–998.

89. Weiss NS, Lyon JL, Krishnamurthy S, Dietert SE, Liff JM, Daling JR. Noncontraceptive estrogen use and the occurrence of ovarian cancer. J Natl Cancer Inst 1982;68:95–98.

90. Kaufman DW, Kelly JP, Welch WR, et al. Noncontraceptive estrogen use and the occurrence of ovarian cancer. Am J Epidemiol 1989;130:1142–1151.

91. La Vecchia C, Liberati A, Franceschi S. Noncontraceptive estrogen use and the occurrence of ovarian cancer. J Natl Cancer Inst 1982;69:1207.

92. Fathalla MF. Incessant ovulation—a factor in ovarian neoplasia? Lancet 1971ii:163.

93. Russell SEH, Hickey GI, Lowry WS, et al. Allele loss from chromosome 17 in ovarian cancer. Oncogene 1990;5:1581–1586.

94. Eccles DM, Cranston G, Steele CM, et al. Allele loss on chromosome 17 in human epithelial ovarian carcinoma. Oncogene 1990;5:1599–1601.

95. Parazzini F, La Vecchia C, Gentile A. Menstrual factors and the risk of epithelial ovarian cancer. J Clin Epidemiol 1989;42:443–448.

96. Weiss NS. Ovary. In: Schottenfeld D, Fraumeni JF Jr, eds. Cancer Epidemiology and Prevention. Philadelphia; W.B. Saunders, 1982, pp. 871–880.

97. Cramer DW, Welch WR. Determinants of ovarian cancer risk. Inferences regarding pathogenesis. J Natl Cancer Inst 1983;71:717–721.

98. Helzlsover KJ, Alberg AJ, Gordon GB, et al. Serum gonadotrophins and steroid hormones and the development of ovarian cancer. JAMA 1995;274:1926–1930.

99. Physicians Desk Reference, 1995, pp. 2722–2735.

100. Wysowski DK, Golden L, Burke L. Use of menopausal estrogens and medroxyprogesterone in the United States, 1982–1992. Obstet Gynecol 1995;85:6–10.

101. Brett KM, Madans JH. Use of postmenopausal hormone replacement therapy: Estimates from a nationally representative cohort study. Am J Epidemiol 1997;145: 536–545.

102. U.S. Congress, Office of Technology Assessment. Hormone products and prescription. In: The Menopause, Hormone Therapy, and Women's Health. OTA-BP-BA-88. Washington, DC: U.S. Government Printing Office, May 1992, pp. 63–72.

103. Lobo RA. Absorption and metabolic effects of different types of estrogens and progestogens. Obstet Gynecol Clin North Am 1987;14:143–167.

104. The Writing Group for the PEPI Trial. Effects of estrogen or estrogen/progestin regimens on heart disease risk factors in postmenopausal women. The Postmenopausal Estrogen/Progestin Interventions (PEPI) Trial. JAMA 1995;273:199–208.

105. Samaan SA, Crawford MH. Estrogen and cardiovascular function after menopause. J Am Coll Cardiol 1995;26:1403–1410.

106. Kuller LH, Meilahn EN, Lassila H, Matthews K, Wing R. Cardiovascular risk factors during first five years postmenopause in nonhormone replacement therapy users. In: Forte TM, ed. Hormonal, Metabolic, and Cellular Influences on Cardiovascular Disease in Women. Armonk, NY: Futura, 1997, pp. 273–287.

107. Archer DF, Pickar JH, Bottiglioni F, for the Menopause Study Group. Bleeding patterns in postmenopausal women taking continuous combined or sequential regimens of conjugated estrogens with medroxyprogesterone acetate. Obstet Gynecol 1994; 83:686–692.

108. Daly E, Vessey MP, Hawkins MM, Carson JL, Gough P, Marsh S. Risk of venous thromboembolism in users of hormone replacement therapy. Lancet 1996;348: 977–980.

109. Jick H, Derby LE, Myers MW, Vasilakis C, Newton KM. Risk of hospital admission for idiopathic venous thromboembolism among users of postmenopausal oestrogens. Lancet 1996;348:981–983.

110. Grodstein F, Stampfer MJ, Goldhaber SZ, et al. Prospective study of exogenous hormones and risk of pulmonary embolism in women. Lancet 1996;348: 983–987.

111. Love RR, Newcomb PA, Wiebe DA, et al. Effects of tamoxifen therapy on lipid and lipoprotein levels in postmenopausal patients with node-negative breast cancer. J Natl Cancer Inst 1990;82:1327–1332.

112. Costantino JP, Kuller LH, Ives DG, Fisher B, Dignam J. Coronary heart disease mortality and adjuvant tamoxifen therapy. J Natl Cancer Inst 1997;89:776–782.

113. Pennisi E. Drug's link to genes reveals estrogen's many sides. Science 1996; 273:1171.

114. Grainger DJ, Metcalfe JC. Tamoxifen: Teaching an old drug new tricks? [Commentary]. Nat Med 1996;2:381–385.

115. Kuller, LH. Hormone replacement therapy and its potential relationship to dementia [Commentary]. J Am Geriatr Soc 1996;44:878–880.

116. Birge SJ. Is there a role for estrogen replacement therapy in the prevention and treatment of dementia? J Am Geriatr Soc 1996;44:865–870.

17

CONTRACEPTIVE CHOICES AND SEXUALLY TRANSMITTED INFECTIONS AMONG WOMEN

Willard Cates, Jr.

Using contraception has two main benefits:[1-11] prevention of unplanned pregnancy and protection against sexually transmitted infections. Abstinence from sexual intercourse provides nearly absolute protection against both outcomes. For those choosing to be sexually active, contraception reduces but does not eliminate the risk of unintended pregnancy. Unfortunately, the contraceptives with the best record for pregnancy prevention provide minimal protection against sexually transmitted disease (STD). Some contraceptives may even raise the risk of certain infections.

The choice of contraception is further complicated by its longer-range reproductive implications. Contraceptive use has an influence on not only the acute risks of STD and unplanned pregnancy but also the eventual reproductive capacity of those making contraceptive decisions. Therefore, personal choices, community programs, and/or policy decisions made in the short run to prevent STD and unplanned pregnancy can simultaneously improve (or harm) chances of planned procreation in the long run.[12,13] This delicate balance of benefit and risk for pregnancy prevention versus STD prevention (including HIV) forms the basis for this chapter.

THE EFFECT OF CONTRACEPTIVE USE ON PREGNANCY

Our modern contraceptives have been portrayed as having both an ideal and an actual use effectiveness.[14] The ideal effectiveness describes the rate of pregnancy that occurs when a contraceptive is used correctly and consistently according to standard directions. The actual effectiveness describes the pregnancy

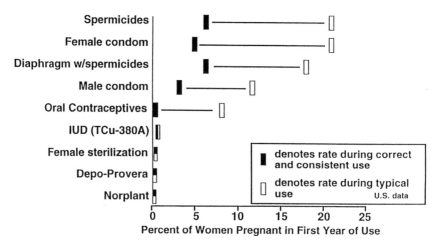

Figure 17–1. Contraceptive pregnancy rates [Source: Adapted by Family Health International from 1995 NSFG, Piccinino and Mosher, *Family Planning Perspectives*, 1998.[15]]

rates that occur when contraceptives are used under "typical" conditions. In general, barrier methods of contraception have lower ideal effectiveness and much lower actual effectiveness than nonbarrier methods. Oral contraceptives provide intermediate pregnancy prevention. Methods that are fixed and require no user action, such as IUDs, implantable or injectable hormones such as depoprovera and norplant, and tubal sterilization, have the highest level of effectiveness. Moreover, the actual use effectiveness depends upon a variety of factors that provide a large range of effectiveness in preventing unintended pregnancies (Fig. 17–1). For example, according to data from the National Survey of Family Growth, young, unmarried persons generally have higher contraceptive pregnancy rates using barrier methods than older, married individuals.[15] Many of the factors that produce the varying pregnancy rates for the compliance-dependent, coitally related barrier methods of contraception are the same ones that affect the degree of STD and HIV protection these methods provide under typical use (see below).

THE EFFECT OF CONTRACEPTIVE USE ON STD/HIV

Unraveling etiologic relationships among contraception, sexually transmitted diseases (STDs), pelvic inflammatory disease (PID), and sequelae is a complex exercise in causal reasoning (Fig. 17–2). We must examine correlations among variables with inconsistent use, varying definitions, imprecise diagnoses, and different microbial organisms.[1,11] The causal pathway includes four distinct links in the chain: contraceptive choice as the antecedent condition, lower geni-

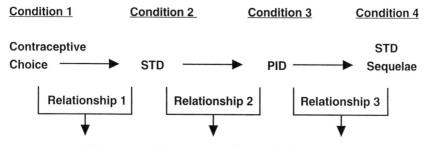

Figure 17–2. Etiologic relationships among contraceptive choice, STD, PID, and STD sequelae

tal tract STDs and upper genital tract PID as intermediate conditions, and eventual sequelae as the outcome. The conditions each have a temporal lag in clinical expression (contraceptive use affects STDs, STDs lead to PID, PID leads to sequelae). These relationships in turn are influenced by the overlapping effects of three environments: *(1)* the genital microbial environment, *(2)* the individual behavioral environment, (e.g., sexual behavior, contraceptive practice, and health care utilization patterns, and *(3)* the sociogeographic environment.[16]

The recent scientific literature has been replete with reviews of the effects of different contraceptives on the risk of STD and HIV.[1-11] In general, they all come to the same conclusion (Table 17–1). Male condoms used correctly and consistently provide good protection against most STDs, both bacterial and viral. Spermicides alone and combinations of mechanical and chemical methods can provide modest protection against bacterial STD but little protection against HIV. Hormonal contraception may enhance some cervical infections, but its impact on *upper* genital tract infection and HIV is still unresolved. The IUD is associated with acute PID, albeit primarily during the interval after its insertion.

Male Condoms

If men are willing and educated to use male condoms properly, they can protect themselves and their sex partners against transmission of STD by preventing direct contact with semen, genital discharge, some genital lesions, or infectious secretions.[17-19] To be effective, condoms must be applied prior to genital contact, must remain intact, and most importantly, must be used *consistently* and *correctly.*[17]

Laboratory studies confirm that latex and polyurethane condoms provide an impervious barrier to most STD pathogens. In experimental transmission

Table 17–1. Effects of Contraceptives on Bacterial and Viral
Sexually Transmitted Infections (STI)

CONTRACEPTIVE METHODS	BACTERIAL STI	VIRAL STI
Condoms	Protective	Protective
Spermicides	Modestly protective against cervical gonorrhea and anaerobic overgrowth	Undetermined in vivo chlamydia
Diaphragms	Protective against cervical infection; associated with vaginal anaerobic overgrowth	Protective against cervical infection
Hormonal	Associated with increased cervical chlamydia; protective against symptomatic PID	
IUD	Associated with PID in first month after insertion	Not protective
Natural family planning	Not protective	Not protective

[Reprinted with permission from Contraception, Unintended Pregnancies and STDs, American Journal of Epidemiology, Vol. 143., No. 4, Cates, page 315, February 1996[13]]

models, condoms have been shown to be effective barriers against herpes simplex virus (HSV),[20] *Chlamydia trachomatis,*[20] and human immunodeficiency virus (HIV).[21] "Natural membrane" condoms, made of sheep intestinal membrane, may not be as effective as synthetic condoms in preventing STD, since HIV, hepatitis B virus (HBV), and HSV can pass through natural membrane condoms. This permeability may be on account of the size of pores in the intestinal membranes.

Epidemiologic studies show that women are protected by male condoms against some STDs, but not all. This may be due in part to the wider variety of organisms studied and the varying consistency of the partner's condom use. For example, a study in Colorado of women attending STD clinics showed that those women whose partners had used condoms during the previous month were less likely to have gonorrhea or trichomoniasis, but just as likely to have chlamydia or bacterial vaginosis.[22] In Kenya,[23] sex workers who reported using condoms all the time had less than one-fifth the risk of acquiring genital ulcers than those who never used condoms. Because HIV infection confounded the association, the protective impact of condoms on genital ulcer disease was not readily apparent until the data were adjusted for HIV status.

Much recent work has evaluated the male condom's influence in protecting against HIV (Fig. 17–3). Although low prevalence of infection has reduced the power of many studies to demonstrate statistically "significant" associations,

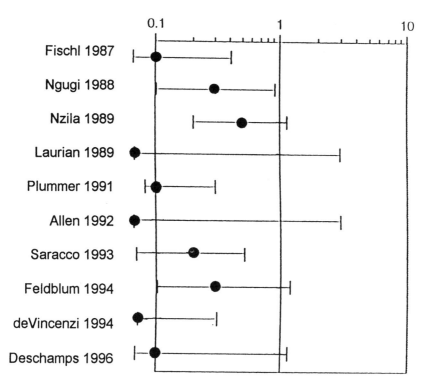

Figure 17–3. Condom use and HIV infection in heterosexuals, relative risk (log scale) and 95% confidence interval

the data are remarkably supportive. Regular use of male condoms reduces the risk of acquiring or transmitting HIV.[9] For example, in Kenya, consistent use of condoms by the clients of commercial sex workers led to lower HIV seroconversion rates in women.[24] In France, none of the female partners of HIV seropositive men with hemophilia who always used condoms became infected with the virus.[25] In Rwanda, the rate of HIV seroconversion declined in a population of urban women who increasingly used condoms.[26] Finally, in the most definitive examples, the European and Haitian studies of HIV discordant couples showed that those who reported consistent condom use had minimal or no HIV transmission after multiple years of observation.[27,28]

Taken together, these clinical studies strongly support the protective effect of consistent condom use against many STDs. However, the variation in the data implies that other factors also affect their impact. For example, the quality of partner communication is apparently the strongest predictor of consistent and correct use.[29] Couples who discussed the use of condoms prior to having initiated intercourse and who practiced using different types until they found a preferred brand, tended to use condoms more consistently.[30] Future investigations will help clarify the behavioral determinants of more effective condom use at the population level.[13]

Female Condoms

Several female condoms ("intravaginal pouches," "vaginal condoms") have been licensed in the U.S. and elsewhere.[31] Basically, these products are pouches made of polyurethane that line the vagina. As with male condoms, protection against STD is likely only if these products are used consistently and stay properly positioned during intercourse. In vitro testing of the Reality®female condom showed it to be an effective barrier to HIV and cytomegalovirus (CMV).[32] Moreover, it also provided significant in vivo protection against recurrent trichomonal infection.[33] However, the higher cost and lower acceptability of female condoms than male condoms are likely to limit usefulness, especially in developing countries.[34] Future products involving female physical barriers need to be less expensive and more widely available to help reduce birth rates and control STD on a population level.

Spermicides

In vitro studies have shown that contraceptive spermicides kill or inactivate most STD pathogens. The main spermicidal agent that has been evaluated in vivo is nonoxynol-9, a nonionic surfactant that damages the cell walls of sperm—and STD pathogens. Laboratory tests have documented activity against *Neisseria gonorrhoeae, Trichomonas vaginalis,* herpes simplex virus, HIV, and *Treponema pallidum.*[9] Reports on the effect of spermicides on *C. trachomatis* are conflicting: some[35] found that nonoxynol-9 inactivated chlamydial organisms, whereas others[36] found no such effect.

In vitro microbicide activity, however, does not mean that spermicides can provide reliable in vivo protection. Data from epidemiologic studies of humans have been inconsistent regarding both the efficacy and safety of N-9. These studies have used different formulations and concentrations of spermicide and have been conducted in disparate populations. Thus, drawing clinically meaningful conclusions has been difficult. The best studies are randomized controlled trials (RCTs). Through 1997, the three better-quality RCTs have compared three different products—a gel,[37,38] the sponge,[39] and the film.[40] Taken together, these studies have shown N-9 spermicide used alone reduces the risks of both gonorrhea and chlamydia infection, albeit at modest levels of protection (Fig. 17–4). In Alabama, regular use of N-9 gel by women attending an STD clinic reduced cervical gonorrhea by 24%, cervical chlamydial infection by 22%, trichomoniasis by 17%, and bacterial vaginosis by 14%.[37,38] In Kenya, a

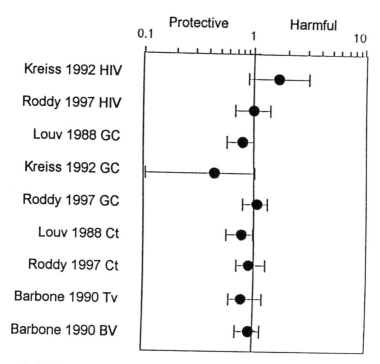

Figure 17–4. Spermicides and STDs among women, relative risk (log scale) and 95% confidence interval

sponge containing high doses of N-9 apparently protected against gonorrhea but raised the risks of HIV.[39] However, the authors' use of nonstandard denominator measures (number of examinations) limits comparison with other studies. In Cameroon, no protection was found for any of the STDs, including HIV.[40]

No data suggest that spermicides alone, without any mechanical barriers, protect against HIV.[39,40] Published observational studies have produced conflicting results.[9,41] Since current ethical standards require that randomized controlled trials encourage study populations to use condoms as their primary method of HIV prevention, the resulting design primarily assesses the marginal impact of adding spermicides to condoms as a means of protecting against HIV acquisition. Moreover, methodologic issues such as the type of delivery system (e.g., film versus gel) and the population studied (e.g., sex workers versus family planning clients) also play a crucial role in allowing correct interpretation of studies involving spermicides and barriers.

A potential risk of spermicide users is chemical irritation of the vaginal epithelium, caused by nonoxynol-9's membrane-disrupting properties.[9] In Thailand, nearly half of sexually inactive women randomized to receive 150 mg nonoxynol-9 suppositories four times a day suffered epithelial disruption of their vaginal or cervical mucosa;[42] none of those receiving placebo did. A second randomized clinical trial in Thailand showed that use of nonoxynol-9 vaginal film was associated with a small increase in genital irritation although this did not vary with number of inserts used, nor was it related to clinical signs.[43]

Combined Barrier Contraceptives

Combined mechanical and chemical barrier methods may have harmful effects on normal genital flora. Vaginal infection with *Candida albicans* was more likely in sponge users,[44] possibly because of disruption to the normal lactobacilli. In addition, a cohort study of foam-condom users and diaphragm-spermicide users showed that both methods were associated with vaginal colonization and bacteriuria with *Escherichia coli*.[45] Some studies have found that women using diaphragm-spermicides or spermicide-coated male condoms have higher risks of acute urinary tract infections.[46-48] Potential mechanisms for the *E. coli* colonization include alteration of the vaginal ecosystem by the spermicide and/or a mechanical effect of the diaphragm. Because domination of vaginal flora by facultative anaerobic microbes (e.g., bacterial vaginosis) has been associated with both urinary and upper genital tract infection,[47] the implications of this finding are of concern.

Hormonal Contraceptives

Combined oral contraceptives (OCs) have an array of noncontraceptive health benefits; however, their influence on STD, HIV, PID, and eventual reproductive sequelae remains unsettled. Most studies, though not all, have found an increased risk of cervical infections with *C. trachomatis* among users of OCs compared with nonusers.[49-51] In Birmingham, OC users had higher rates of both *C. trachomatis* and *N. gonorrhoeae* detected in the cervix.[52] The association between OC use and cervical infection may be mediated through the cervical ectopy commonly induced by OCs.[53,54] *C. trachomatis* has been isolated more frequently among women with ectopy than among women without ectopy, regardless of the method of birth control used.[50, 54]

The influence of OCs on the upper genital tract may be different from that on the lower genital tract. Studies from Europe and the United States[55,56] have revealed that women using OCs are half as likely to be hospitalized for PID, compared with sexually active women who do not use contraception. In a multicenter case–control study from the United States,[57] the protection from PID was observed only among women who had been using oral contraceptives for more than 12 months. Past use of OCs conferred no protection. In Lund, Sweden,[58] OC use was associated with a significant reduction in the risk of gonococcal PID; the protective effect was not as strong for chlamydial PID. However, in

Seattle, women using OCs apparently were differentially protected against chlamydial compared with gonococcal PID.[59]

Whether these findings are real, or represent an artifact of clinical detection of PID, is unclear. OC users tend to have milder upper genital tract infection with *C. trachomatis,* as manifested by antibody response and laparoscopy.[60] However, OC users have increased risks of unrecognized endometritis.[61] In addition, data on the impact of previous OC use on primary tubal infertility are conflicting. In the U.S.,[62] among former users of most current low-estrogen OCs, tubal infertility was not reduced as might be expected if their use led to an decreased risk of chlamydial PID. In fact, users of those OCs with estrogen levels higher than 50 μg had an increased risk of tubal infertility. In the Lund, Sweden cohort, women who had been using OCs at the time their salpingitis was diagnosed had a 70% lower risk of tubal infertility than women using other methods.[63] The reason for this discrepancy is unclear.

Possible mechanisms for the consistent protective effect of OCs on symptomatic PID remain speculative. The progestin component of combination OCs thickens the cervical mucus. Changes in either mucus composition or its immunologic properties might account for this protection. Likewise, the thinner endometrium and/or the decreased menstrual flow associated with pill use may play a role. Alternatively, if OC use tends to mask the symptoms of PID, they will appear protective even though unrecognized inflammation may be occurring.

Consistent with this latter explanation is the observation that use of hormonal contraception also seems to modify the acute clinical course of PID favorably. As judged by laparoscopic examination, women with PID who were using OCs had milder inflammation than women not using OCs.[64] Among women with chlamydial salpingitis, use of OCs protected against Fitz-Hugh-Curtis syndrome. In addition, pill users had a significantly lower titer of antibodies against *C. trachomatis* than did nonusers.[59] Moreover, an IUD with progesterone protected against histological salpingitis compared with non-hormonal IUDs.[65] In monkey models, however, OCs containing both estrogen and progesterone did not alter the course of experimentally induced chlamydial salpingitis.[66] Sex steroids can modify immunologic function,[67] so their impact on infectious inflammation is plausible, though still disputed.

The effect of hormonal contraception on HIV transmission, acquisition, or disease progression remains unsettled.[68,69] Both animal and epidemiologic studies since 1987 have produced equivocal results. The initial observational investigations examined use of combined oral contraceptives and HIV, while attempting to control for such intervening variables as cervical ectopy and infectious cervicitis and behavioral confounders such as condom use. At least four prospective studies of sex workers in Kenya have provided support for the hypothesis that use of hormonal contraception could facilitate HIV acquisition.[70–73] However, a variety of other studies in Africa and on other continents have found little or no association between OC use and HIV seropositivity.[7,68,69]

Animal models, using simian immunodeficiency virus (SIV) as the HIV surrogate, have raised concerns about progestin-only contraceptives.[74] In rhesus macaques, an increase in SIV acquisition occurred in monkeys with progesterone implants compared with monkeys in the follicular phase of a normal menstrual cycle. However, the risk of SIV acquisition was lower if the full menstrual cycle was used as the comparison group.[75] Whether these data translate to humans remains to be seen.

Potential biologic mechanisms by which hormonal contraception might facilitate HIV transmission include the following: *(1)* increased cervical ectopy (and associated friability) caused by OC use; *(2)* increased cervical chlamydial infection (and associated purulence), possibly associated with the ectopy; *(3)* systemic immunologic changes associated with some exogenous steroids; and *(4)* if long-acting hormonal contraception is used, irregular uterine bleeding and/or thinning of the vaginal epithelium. In addition, the particular type of estrogens and progestins contained in the OCs or other longer-term hormonal contraceptives may be important factors relating to any impact on HIV acquisition or transmission.[69]

A variety of biases could account for these inconsistent results. Many problems exist in these observational studies with the comparability either between cases (women infected with HIV) and controls (uninfected women) or between the exposed (users of hormonal contraception) and the unexposed (users or nonusers of other methods). Moreover, in most studies, a relatively small number of women used hormonal contraception. Thus, because of statistical power considerations, the risk estimates are imprecise. Finally, the myriad of existing observational studies covered different populations, used differing designs, applied crude definitions of hormonal contraceptive use, had different hormonal mixes, and were unable to control for crucial confounders. Creative experimental designs using randomized interventions will probably be needed to definitively answer the question of the hormonal contraceptive role in HIV transmission. Because of the crucial role that OC and other hormonal forms of contraception play in international family planning programs, and because the HIV pandemic is one of the world's most important health problems, scientists must assign the highest research priority to resolving this issue.

Intrauterine Devices

The precise risk of IUD use on STD is also unclear. Few publications have objectively examined the effect of the IUD on *lower* genital tract infections. One review article concluded that the IUD was unrelated to cervical chlamydial infection.[76] However, an analysis of cross-sectional data from a population-based sample of Seattle women found that those who had ever used an IUD had a significantly higher percentage of chlamydial antibodies than those who never used an IUD, even after stratifying for number of sex partners.[77] In contrast, a prospective study in Antwerp found that IUD users had ninefold lower rates of chlamydia than OC users;[78] however, the same study showed that women using IUDs had nearly eight times higher rates of bacterial vaginosis.

The possible association between IUD use and the development of *upper* genital tract infection remains a controversial topic. More recent epidemiologic evidence showed the initial association between IUD use and PID found in the 1970s to be overestimated.[79] Three particular methodologic problems in the early studies contributed to their overly pessimistic assessment. First, women using barrier or oral contraceptives served as the comparison group in most studies.[80] Since these methods *reduce* the risk of symptomatic PID, such comparisons artifactually elevated the apparent risk associated with IUD use. Second, the PID diagnosis often rests on highly subjective symptoms and signs that are difficult to assess.[81] Since the putative association between IUD use and PID has been recognized since the 1960s, PID "diagnostic bias" might occur among IUD users. Third, the early analyses did not adjust for type of IUD and the timing of its insertion. If either of these factors creates a disproportionate degree of PID risk, the overall crude risk for IUDs as a group is also spuriously elevated.

More sophisticated studies have revised our understanding of the IUD–PID association. Current evidence suggests that the small, but still measurable, increased risk of PID associated with IUD use occurs around the time of insertion.[82] Thus, contamination of the endometrial cavity at insertion may be more responsible for IUD-related PID than the device itself. Because of the association of PID to the timing of IUD insertion, short-term antibiotics might help reduce the risks. In Kenya,[83] Nigeria,[84] and the U.S.,[85] randomized clinical trials of prophylactic doxycycline at the time of IUD insertion found much lower than expected rates of IUD-associated PID, even among the placebo group. Because of the infrequency of IUD-related PID, even in the developing world, and because of the limited size of the studies, they had insufficient power to distinguish any statistically significant differences among treatment and placebo groups.

Many perceive the IUD's safety today as vastly different from that of a decade ago. With proper screening of clients, the IUD poses little, if any, added STD risk. For example, among women who used copper IUDs and who had only one sex partner, no increase occurred in the risk of either PID or tubal infertility.[86] Thus, the challenge for future researchers will be to establish criteria based on a combination of demographic, behavioral, and clinical factors that would expand the proportion of women for whom the IUD would be a good contraceptive choice. Moreover, because newer IUDs containing levonorgestrel apparently are associated with even lower rates of PID,[87] they may be more appropriate contraception in populations where the risk of STD is unknown.

Tubal Sterilization

Tubal sterilization protects against PID, but this protection is not absolute. Most typical cases of PID are thought to arise from ascent of cervical pathogens via the endometrial cavity; hence, disrupting the continuity of this passage should prevent inoculation of the distal fallopian tubes. Even though endometritis and proximal salpingitis are potentially possible, PID is rarely observed[88] among women after tubal sterilization. A more likely mechanism for post-sterilization PID is iatrogenic contamination of the tubes during the operative procedure.

Abortion

Women who have cervical infection with either *N. gonorrhoeae* or *C. trachomatis* have an increased risk of endometritis following induced abortion performed under proper hygienic conditions. The risk of endometritis appears to be at least tripled in the presence of either organism.[89] A number of studies suggest that use of prophylactic antibiotics at the time of the abortion procedure reduces the risk of infection by one-half to two-thirds.[90] While preoperative screening for infection with these organisms is desirable, a brief perioperative course of an antibiotic such as azithromycin seems both safe and cost effective. Women later found to be infected by *N. gonorrhoeae* and/or *C. trachomatis* can be followed up with a full course of recommended antibiotics.

The greatest risk of upper genital tract infection associated with induced abortion occurs in circumstances where sterile conditions are not maintained. In countries where abortion services are restricted by law or practice, and especially in resource-poor regions where, even if legal, access to sanitary procedures is limited, postabortion infection poses risks not only to future fertility but also to the woman's life.[91] More than half the estimated 100,000 abortion-related deaths worldwide occur in Southeast Asia, followed by sub-Saharan Africa, and then Latin America and the Caribbean.[92]

In both the developed and less developed world, carrying a pregnancy to term leads to greater risks of infection and death than terminating it through induced abortion.[93,94] Under sterile conditions, abortion is five to ten times safer than childbearing. Under less hygienic conditions, the risks of *both* pregnancy outcomes increase, and the gap between the infection risks from abortion and childbirth probably narrows. In these circumstances, use of any method of contraception to reduce pregnancy has simultaneous effects on reducing pregnancy-associated infection (see below).

CLINICAL AND POLICY IMPLICATIONS

Contraceptive/STD Prevention Trade-Offs

In ideal circumstances, consistent and correct use of male or female condoms can prevent *both* pregnancy and STD. However, in typical situations of inconsistent use, they provide lower rates of protection against these conditions. Moreover, if couples choose to use contraceptive methods other than condoms, those with the best record for pregnancy prevention provide little STD protection. Thus, trade-off choices are necessary.

For those whose families are not completed, yet who do not wish to currently become pregnant, hormonal contraceptives and the IUD remain the most effective reversible methods available to prevent unintended pregnancy. However, they provide no protection against vaginal or cervical infection and inserting the IUD carries temporary risks to the upper genital tract. Hence, for persons who are not mutually monogamous, addition of a barrier method such as a condom will help reduce the risk of STD, as well as unplanned pregnancy. Under typical conditions, however, barrier methods are substantially less effective in preventing conception than hormonal methods, yet they offer important protection against STD. To maximize protection against both unintended pregnancy and STD, a barrier method should be used in conjunction with a hormonal method or IUD.

Because both mechanical and chemical barrier prophylaxis are coitally dependent, their efficacy in preventing either infection or unplanned pregnancy depends entirely on compliance by the couple. Some populations have demonstrated high levels of barrier method use. For example, in Thailand, a "100% condom policy" in commercial sex facilities has led to widespread use among the workers and has been associated with marked reductions in HIV and other STDs.[95] In the United States, women working in Nevada brothels have had similar success.[96] Unfortunately, to date, most heterosexual populations worldwide have not reported the same magnitude of condom use and have not experienced decreases in the traditional STDs.[97]

Another important aspect of assessing trade-off concerns is whether conditions exist for safe, sterile childbirth and/or abortion. If pregnancy itself, regardless of whether it is terminated or continued, carries markedly high "iatrogenic" risks of genital infection, then the pregnancy prevention efficacy of the contraceptive choice takes on greater weight. By preventing undesired pregnancy, the contraceptive method(s) simultaneously protect against pregnancy-associated infections of the reproductive tract. In the developing world, postabortal and puerperal infections are important causes of tubal infertility. In Africa, where the infectious etiology of infertility was most evident,[98] genital infections occurring both before and after the first pregnancy were associated with tubal occlusion. In Asia, abortion appeared to play a larger role than childbirth in contributing to infectious infertility, whereas in Latin America the reverse was found.[99]

CONCLUSION

Because contraception affects not only the risk of unplanned pregnancy but also that of sexually transmitted infections, the choice of particular methods is important to future fertility. However, important trade-offs exist. Contraceptives with the best record of preventing pregnancy provide little protection against sexually transmitted diseases. Moreover, epidemiologic studies are equivocal about the value of either recommending dual methods of contraception or relying on the condom alone to prevent both unplanned pregnancy and STDs. Use of emergency contraception as a back-up to barrier methods is another approach that warrants evaluation.

Moreover, individual choices may conflict with public health needs. For example, a woman who perceives an unintended pregnancy to be a greater risk may choose her contraceptive method without regard to STD prophylaxis. However, the community in which she lives may be marketing condoms as the preferred contraceptive for their dual prophylactic effects against both pregnancy and infection. The ultimate impact of this dynamic benefit-to-risk relationship among contraceptives for pregnancy protection versus STD prophylaxis is to create trade-off choices for both individual women and public health policymakers. Continued biologic and behavioral research will be necessary to disentangle these complex relationships.

REFERENCES

1. Cates W Jr, Stone KM. Family planning, sexually transmitted diseases and contraceptive choice: A literature update—Part I and Part II. Fam Plann Perspect 1992;24 (2):75–84.

2. Harlap S, Kost K, Forrest JD. Preventing Pregnancy, Protecting Health: A New Look at Birth Control Choices in the United States. New York: The Alan Guttmacher Institute, 1991.

3. DaVanzo J, Parnell AM, Foege WH. Health consequences of contraceptive use and reproductive patterns. JAMA 1991;265:2692–2696.

4. Elias CJ, Leonard A. Family planning and sexually transmitted diseases: The need to enhance contraceptive choice. Curr Issues Public Health 1995;1:191–199.

5. Fox LJ, Williamson NE, Cates W Jr, Dallabetta G. Improving reproductive health: Integrating STD and contraceptive services. J Am Med Wom Assoc 1995;50: 129–136.

6. Carlin EM, Boag FC. Women, contraceptives and STDs including HIV. Int J STD AIDS 1995;6:373–386.

7. Daly CC, Helling-Giese GE, Mati JK, Hunter DJ. Contraceptive methods and the transmission of HIV: Implications for family planning. Genitourin Med 1994;70: 110–117.

8. Anderson DJ, Voeller B. AIDS and contraception. In: Soupe D, Haseltine FP, eds. Contraception. New York: Springer-Verlag, 1993, pp. 192–209.

9. Feldblum PJ, Morrison CS, Roddy RE, Cates W. The effectiveness of barrier methods of contraception in preventing the spread of HIV. AIDS 1995;9(suppl A): 585–593.

10. Howe JE, Minkoff HL, Duerr AC. Contraceptives and HIV. AIDS 1994;8: 861–871.

11. Cates W Jr. Contraceptive choice, sexually transmitted diseases, HIV infection, and future fecundity. J Br Fertil Soc 1996;1(1):18–22.

12. Forrest JD. Timing of reproductive life stages. Obstet Gynecol 1993;82: 105–111.

13. Cates W Jr. Contraception, unintended pregnancies, and sexually transmitted diseases: Why isn't a simple solution possible? Am J Epidemiol 1996;143(4):311–318.

14. Trussell J, Hatcher RA, Cates W Jr, et al. Contraceptive failure in the United States: An update. Stud Fam Plann 1990;21:51–54.

15. Piccinino LJ, Mosher WD. Trends in contraceptive use in the United States: 1982-1995. Fam Plann Perspect 1998;30:4–10,46.

16. Wasserheit JN. Effect of changes in human ecology and behavior on patterns of sexually transmitted diseases, including human immunodeficiency virus infection. Proc Natl Acad Sci USA 1994;91:2430–2435.

17. Centers for Disease Control and Prevention. Update: Barrier protection against HIV infection and other sexually transmitted diseases. MMWR 1993;42:589–591.

18. Roper WL, Peterson HB, Curran JW. Commentary: Condoms and HIV/STD prevention—clarifying the message. Am J Public Health 1993;83:501–503.

19. Consumer Reports. How reliable are condoms? Consumer Reports 1995;May: 320–325.

20. Judson FN, Ehret JM, Bodin GF, Levin MJ, Rietjmeijer CAM. In vitro evaluation of condoms with and without nonoxynol 9 as physical and chemical barriers against Chlamydia trachomatis, herpes simplex virus type 2 and human immunodeficiency virus. Sex Transm Dis 1989;16:51–56.

21. Conant M, Hardy D, Sernatinger J, Spicer D, Levy JA. Condoms prevent transmission of AIDS-associated retrovirus. JAMA 1986;255:1706.

22. Rosenberg MJ, Davidson AJ, Chen J-H, Judson FN, Douglas JM. Barrier contraceptives and sexually transmitted diseases in women: A comparison of female-dependent methods and condoms. Am J Public Health 1992;82:669–674.

23. Cameron DW, Ngugi EN, Ronald AR, et al. Condom use prevents genital ulcers in women working as prostitutes: Influence of human immunodeficiency virus infection. Sex Transm Dis 1991;18:188–191.

24. Ngugi EN, Plummer FA, Simonsen JN, et al. Prevention of transmission of human immunodeficiency virus in Africa: Effectiveness of condom promotion and health education among prostitutes. Lancet 1988;2:887–890.

25. Laurian Y, Peynet J, Verroust F. HIV infection in sexual partners of HIV seropositive patients with hemophilia. N Engl J Med 1989;320:183.

26. Allen S, Tice J, Van de Perre P, et al. Effect of serotesting with counseling on condom use and seroconversion among HIV discordant couples in Africa. Br Med J 1992;304:1605–1609.

27. de Vincenzi I. A longitudinal study of human immunodeficiency virus transmission by heterosexual partners. N Engl J Med 1994;334:341–346.

28. Deschamps M-M, Pape JW, Hafner A, Johnson WD Jr. Heterosexual transmission of HIV in Haiti. Ann Intern Med 1996;125:324–330.

29. Oakley D, Bogue EL. Quality of condom use as reported by female clients of a family planning clinic. Am J Public Health 1995;85:1526–1530.

30. Warner DL, Hatcher RA. Male condoms. In: Hatcher RA, Trussell J, Stewart FH, Cates W Jr, Stewart GK, Guest F, Kowal D, eds. Contraceptive Technology, 17th ed. New York: Irvington Publishers, 1998, pp. 437–454.

31. Gollub E, Stein Z. The new female condom—item 1 on a woman's AIDS prevention agenda. Am J Public Health 1993;83:498–500.

32. Drew WL, Blair M, Miner RC, Conant M. Evaluation of the virus permeability of a new condom for women. Sex Transm Dis 1990;17:110–112.

33. Soper DE, Shoupe D, Shangold GA, Shangold MM, Gutmann J, Mercer L. Prevention of vaginal trichomoniasis by compliant use of the female condom. Sex Transm Dis 1993;20:137–139.

34. Farr G, Gabelnick H, Sturgen K, Dorflinger L. Contraceptive efficacy and acceptability of the female condom. Am J Public Health 1994;84:1960–1964.

35. Benes S, McCormack WM. Inhibition of growth of *Chlamydia trachomatis* by nonoxynol-9 in vitro. Antimicrob Agents Chemother 1985;27:724–726.

36. Kappus EW, Quinn TC. The spermicide nonoxynol-9 does not inhibit Chlamydia trachomatis in vitro. Sex Transm Dis 1986;13:134–137.

37. Louv WC, Austin H, Alexander WJ, Stagno S, Cheeks J. A clinical trial of nonoxynol-9 as a prophylaxis for cervical *Neisseria gonorrhoeae* and *Chlamydia trachomatis* infections. J Infect Dis 1988;158:518–523.

38. Barbone F, Austin H, Louv WC, Alexander WJ. A follow-up study of methods of contraception, sexual activity, and rates of trichomoniasis, candidiasis, and bacterial vaginosis. Am J Obstet Gynecol 1990;163:510–514.

39. Kreiss J, Ngugi E, Holmes KK, et al. Efficacy of nonoxynol-9 contraceptive sponge use in preventing heterosexual acquisition of HIV in Nairobi prostitutes. JAMA 1992;268:477–482.

40. Roddy RE, Zekeng L, Ryan KA, et al. A randomized controlled trial of the effect of nonoxynyl-9 film use on male-to-female transmission of HIV-1 [Abstract]. Program from the National Conference on Women and HIV, Los Angeles, CA. 1997; page 135.

41. Roddy RE, Schulz KF, Cates W Jr. Microbicides, meta-analysis, and the N-9 question: Where's the research? Sex Transm Dis 1998;25:151–153.

42. Niruthisard S, Roddy RE, Chutivongse S. The effects of frequent nonoxynol-9 use on the vaginal and cervical mucosa. Sex Transm Dis 1991;18:176–179.

43. Roddy RE, Cordero M, Cordero C, Fortney JA. A dosing study of nonoxynol-9 and genital irritation. Int J STD AIDS 1993;4:165–170.

44. Rosenberg MJ, Rojanapithayakorn W, Feldblum PJ, Higgins JE. Effect of the contraceptive sponge on chlamydial infection, gonorrhea, and candidiasis. A comparative clinical trial. JAMA 1987;257:2308–2312.

45. Hooton RM, Hillier S, Johnson C, Roberts PL, Stamm WE. *Escherichia coli* bacteriuria and contraceptive method. JAMA 1991;265:64–69.

46. Foxman B, Geiger AM, Palin K, Gillespie B, Koopman JS. First-time urinary tract infection and sexual behavior. Epidemiology 1995;6:162–168.

47. Hooten TM, Scholes D, Hughes JP, et al. A prospective study of risk factors for symptomatic urinary tract infection in young women. N Engl J Med 1996;335:468–474.

48. Fihn SD, Boyko EJ, Normand EH, et al. Association between use of spermicide-coated condoms and Escherichia coli urinary tract infection in young women. Am J Epidemiol 1996;144:512–520.

49. Washington AE, Gove S, Schachter J, Sweet RL. Oral contraceptives, *Chlamydia trachomatis* infection, and pelvic inflammatory disease. JAMA 1985;253: 2246–2250.

50. Cottingham J, Hunter D. *Chlamydia trachomatis* and oral contraceptive use: A quantitative review. Genitourin Med 1992;68:209–216.

51. Park BJ, Stergachis A, Scholes D, Heidrich FE, Holmes KK, Stamm WE. Contraceptive methods and the risk of *Chlamydia trachomatis* infection in young women. Am J Epidemiol 1995;142:771–778.

52. Louv WC, Austin H, Perlman J, Alexander WJ Jr. Oral contraceptive use and risk of chlamydial and gonococcal infections. Am J Obstet Gynecol 1989;160:396–400.

53. Critchlow CW, Wölner Hanssen P, Eschenbach DA, Kiviat NV, Koutsky LA, Stevens CE, Holmes KK. Determinants of cervical ectopia and of cervicitis: Age, oral contraception, specific cervical infection, smoking, and douching. Am J Obstet Gynecol 1995;173:534–543.

54. Harrison HR, Costin M, Meder JB, et al. Cervical *Chlamydia trachomatis* infection in university women: Relationship to history, contraception, ectopy, and cervicitis. Am J Obstet Gynecol 1985;153:244–251.

55. Westrom L. Incidence, prevalence, and trends of acute pelvic inflammatory disease and its consequences in industrialized countries. Am J Obstet Gynecol 1980;138: 880–892.

56. Panser LA, Phipps WR. Type of oral contraceptive in relation to acute, initial episodes of pelvic inflammatory disease. Contraception 1991;93:91–99.

57. Rubin GL, Ory HW, Layde PM. Oral contraceptives and pelvic inflammatory disease. Am J Obstet Gynecol 1982;144:630–635.

58. Wölner-Hanssen P, Svensson L, Mårdh P-A, Westrom L. Laparoscopic findings and contraceptive use in women with signs and symptoms suggestive of acute salpingitis. Obstet Gynecol 1985;66:233–238.

59. Wölner-Hanssen P, Eschenbach DA, Paavonen J, et al. Decreased risk of symptomatic chlamydial pelvic inflammatory disease associated with oral contraceptive use. JAMA 1990;263:54–59.

60. Wölner-Hanssen P. Oral contraceptive use modifies the manifestations of pelvic inflammatory disease. Br J Obstet Gynaecol 1986;93:619–624.

61. Ness RB, Kader LM, Soper DE, et al. Oral contraception and the recognition of endometritis. Am J Obstet Gynecol 1997;176:580–585.

62. Cramer DW, Goldman MB, Schiff I, et al. The relationship of tubal infertility to barrier method and oral contraceptive use. JAMA 1987;257:2446–2450.

63. Westrom L. Chlamydia and its effect on reproduction. J Brit Fertil Soc 1996;1: 23–28.

64. Svensson L, Westrom L, Mårdh P-A. Contraceptives and acute salpingitis. JAMA 1984;251:2553–2555.

65. Soderstrom RM. Will progesterone save the IUD? J Reprod Med 1983;28: 305–308.

66. Patton DL, Sweeney YTC, Kuo C-C. Oral contraceptives do no alter the course of experimentally induced chlamydial salpingitis in monkeys. Sex Transm Dis 1994;21: 89–92.

67. Grossman C. Possible underlying mechanisms of sexual dimorphism in the immune response, fact and hypothesis. J Steroid Biochem 1989;34:241–251.

68. Hunter DJ, Mati JK. Contraception, family planning, and HIV. In: Chen L, Speulveda J, Segal S, eds. AIDS and Women's Health: Science for Policy and Action. New York: Plenum Press, 1992, pp. 235–242.

69. Taitel HF, Kafrissen ME. A review of oral contraceptive use and the risk of HIV-transmission. Br J Fam Plann 1995;20:112–116.

70. Plummer FA, Simonsen JN, Cameron DW, et al. Cofactors in male-female sexual transmission of human immunodeficiency virus type 1. J Infect Dis 1991;163: 233–239.

71. Plourde PJ, Pepin J, Agoki E, Ronald AR, Obette J, Tyndall M, Cheang M, Ndinya-Achola JO, D'Costa J, Plummer FA. Human immunodeficiency virus type 1 seroconversion in women with genital ulcers. J Infect Dis 1994;170:313–317.

72. Sinei SKA, Fortney JA, Kigondu CS, et al. Contraceptive use and HIV infection in Kenyan family planning clinic attenders. Int J STD AIDS 1996;7:65–70.

73. Nyange P, Martin H, Mandaliya K, Jackson D, et al. Cofactors for heterosexual transmission of HIV to prostitutes in Mombasa, Kenya [Abstract]. Presented at IX International Conference on AIDS and STD in Africa, 1995;106.

74. Marx PA, Gettie A, Dailey P, et al. Progesterone implants enhance SIV vaginal transmission and early virus load. Nat Med 1996;2:1084–1089.

75. Duerr A, Warren D, Smith D, et al. Contraceptives and HIV transmission [letter]. Nat Med 1997;3:124.

76. Edelman DA. The use of intrauterine contraceptive devices, pelvic inflammatory disease, and *Chlamydia trachomatis* infection. Am J Obstet Gynecol 1988;158: 956–959.

77. Rossing MA, Daling JR, Weiss NW, et al. Past use of an intrauterine device and risk of tubal pregnancy. Epidemiology 1993;4:245–251.

78. Avonts D, Sercu M, Heyerick P, Vandermeeren I, Meheus A, Piot P. Incidence of uncomplicated genital infections in women using oral contraception or an intrauterine device: A prospective study. Sex Transm Dis 1990;17:23–29.

79. Grimes DA. Intrauterine devices and pelvic inflammatory disease: Recent developments. Contraception 1987;36:97–109.

80. Senanayake P, Kramer DG. Contraception and the etiology of pelvic inflammatory disease: New perspectives. Am J Obstet Gynecol 1980;138:852–860.

81. Kahn JG, Walker CK, Washington AE, Landers DV, Sweet RL. Diagnosing pelvic inflammatory disease: A comprehensive analysis and new algorithm. JAMA 1991; 266:2594–2604.

82   Farley TMM, Rosenberg MJ, Rowe PJ, Chen J-H, Meirik O. Intrauterine devices and pelvic inflammatory disease: An international perspective. Lancet 1992;339: 785–788.

83. Sinei SKA, Schulz KF, Lamptey PR, et al. Preventing IUD-related pelvic infection: The efficacy of prophylactic doxycycline at insertion. Br J Obstet Gynaecol 1990; 97:412–419.

84. Ladipo OA, Farr G, Otolorin E, et al. Prevention of IUD-related pelvic infection: The efficacy of prophylactic doxycycline at IUD insertion. Adv Contracept 1991;7:43–54.

85. Walsh TL, Bernstein GS, Grimes DA, et al. Effect of prophylactic antibiotics on morbidity associated with IUD insertion: Results of a pilot randomized controlled trial. Contraception 1994;50:319–327.

86. Lee NC, Rubin GL, Ory HW, et al. Type of intrauterine device and the risk of pelvic inflammatory disease. Obstet Gynecol 1983;61:1–6.

87. Luukkainen T, Toivonen J. Levonorgestrel-releasing IUD as a method of contraception with therapeutic properties. Contraception 1995;52:269–276.

88. Vessey M, Huggins G, Lawless M, Yeates D, McPherson K. Tubal sterilization: Findings in a large prospective study. Br J Obstet Gynaecol 1983;90:203–209.

89. Burkman RT, Tonascia JA, Atienza M, King TM. Untreated endocervical gonorrhea and endometritis following elective abortion. Am J Obstet Gynecol 1976;126: 648–651.

90. Sawaya GF, Grady D, Kerlikowske K, Grimes DA. Antibiotics at the time of induced abortion: The case for universal prophylaxis based on a meta-analysis. Obstet Gynecol 1996;87:884–890.

91. The Alan Guttmacher Institute. Clandestine Abortion: A Latin American reality. New York: The Alan Guttmacher Institute, 1994.

92. Henshaw SK. Induced abortion: A world review, 1990. Fam Plann Perspect 1990;22:76–89.

93. Cates W Jr. Legal abortion: The public health record. Science 1982;215: 1586–1590.

94. Tinker A, Koblinsky MA. Making Motherhood Safe. World Bank Discussion Papers, No. 202. Washington, DC: World Bank, 1993.

95. Hanenberg RS, Rojanapithayakorn W, Kunasol P, et al. Impact of Thailand's HIV-control programme as indicated by the decline of sexually transmitted diseases. Lancet 1994;344:243–245.

96. Albert AE, Warner DL, Hatcher RA, Trussell J, Bennett C. Condom use among female commercial sex workers in Nevada's legal brothels. Am J Public Health 1995;85: 1514–1520.

97. World Health Organization. Global Estimates of Curable Sexually Transmitted Diseases. Geneva: World Health Organization, 1995.

98. Cates W Jr, Farley TMM, Rowe PJ, the WHO Task Force on Infertility. Worldwide patterns of infertility: Is Africa different? Lancet 1985;2:596–598.

99. WHO Task Force on Infertility. Infections, pregnancies and infertility: Perspectives on prevention. Fertil Steril 1987;47:964–968.

18

MATERNAL HEALTH EFFECTS OF PREGNANCY

Donna Kritz-Silverstein

This chapter focuses on the effects of pregnancy on women's long-term health and disease. It includes discussions of the association of reproductive history and cardiovascular disease as well as cardiovascular risk factors such as hypertension, diabetes, obesity, and lipid levels. Also included is a discussion of the relation between reproductive history and ovarian cancer.

Cardiovascular disease and ovarian cancer were chosen as endpoints for several reasons. First, they illustrate the fact that pregnancy can have opposing effects on women's health. Specifically, pregnancy increases the risk of cardiovascular disease but protects against ovarian cancer. Pregnancy can lead to hormonal or metabolic alterations as well as to changes in behaviors that increase the risk of disease. To an extent, both of the chosen endpoints may involve a genetic predisposition or susceptibility. However, the mediating influences for cardiovascular disease are more likely to be behavioral whereas for ovarian cancer they are more likely to be hormonal.

Although the long-term effects of childbearing on women's health have received relatively little study, there was interest in this issue as long ago as the 1930s. In the 1940s and 1950s several studies attempted to examine the long-term effects of pregnancy. However, these studies, which were generally case–control in design, used small samples of women and failed to adequately adjust for age. The associations observed in younger women may be different from those observed in older women because older women are within the age range when they develop heart disease and other disorders. More recent studies have overcome many of these limitations. Most have been adjusted for age as well as other potentially confounding covariates such as obesity and socioeconomic status. Several recent studies stratified results by age or menopausal status, permitting an examination of independent and synergistic effects of age and pregnancy on health. Therefore, although this chapter will include results of early studies, the discussion will center on the more recent studies. Throughout the chapter, the term "gravidity" will be used to refer to the number of pregnancies and the term "parity" will be used to refer to the number of births.

PREGNANCY AND CARDIOVASCULAR DISEASE

Cardiovascular disease is the most common cause of death in U.S. women.[1] It is biologically plausible that reproductive history is associated with cardiovascular disease risk. Levels of estrogen, progesterone, cortisol, and other steroid hormones during pregnancy increase to several hundred times their usual level.[2] The progestin components of both oral contraceptives and postmenopausal hormone replacement therapy (HRT) and corticosteriods produce elevations in low-density lipoprotein (LDL) cholesterol, decrements in high-density lipoprotein (HDL) cholesterol, and insulin resistance. Cortisol, unlike estradiol, continues to increase during labor,[3] but it is unknown whether this elevation persists after labor.[2] Cortisol levels during the perigestational period have been correlated with serum cholesterol values[3] and hypercortisolemia has been known to cause obesity and upper-body fat distribution. As suggested by Ness et al.,[2] the long-term hormonal fluctuations associated with multiparity may have latent effects by producing long-term alterations in cardiovascular risk factors.

There have been several studies that directly examined the association of reproductive history with cardiovascular disease. In two early case–control studies by Winkelstein and colleagues, there was a positive association between the number of pregnancies and risk of coronary artery disease as defined by nonfatal myocardial infarction[4] or by atherosclerotic heart disease.[5] In both of these studies, however, the association was primarily due to a higher rate of pregnancy loss (i.e., spontaneous abortions) among the cases than among controls.

Since these early studies, there have been numerous case–control and cross-sectional studies that yielded inconsistent results (see Table 18–1). For instance, Bengtsson,[6,7] who also included abortions in the definition of pregnancy, reported a significantly increased risk of nonfatal myocardial infarction among women with four or more pregnancies. In contrast, Abramov[8] reported a significantly lower risk of nonfatal myocardial infarction for women who had previously undergone induced abortions. Both Oliver[9] and La Vecchia et al.[10] found no associations between spontaneous abortion, stillbirths, or number of pregnancies and risk of heart disease.

The age of the women studied as well as the sample size can also affect the observed results. For instance, case–control studies that primarily included women younger than age 50 failed to show an increased risk of cardiovascular

Table 18–1. Case–Control and Cross-sectional Studies of Gravidity or Parity and Coronary Heart Disease

REFERENCE	STUDY GROUP	CONTROL GROUP	AGE (YEARS) AT ENDPOINT	FINDINGS IN CASES	COMMENTS
Winkelstein et al.[4]	Cases surviving myocardial infarction (n = 50)	Neighbors (n = 50) Population sample (n = 149)	Mean = 64	Parity increased. Abortions increased.* Gravidity increased.	Adjusted for age.
Winkelstein and Rekate[5]	Cases surviving atherosclerotic heart disease (n = 59)	Hospitalized women without CHD (n = 64)	50–80	Parity equal. Gravidity increased. Spontaneous abortions increased.	Most of the effect was seen in women with ≥5 pregnancies. Adjusted for age and diabetes mellitus.
Parrish et al.[16]	Cross-sectional autopsy study of cancer patients and accident patients (n = 352)		40–≥80	Reproductive index (1.5, twins; 1.0, singletons; 0.5, stillbirths; 0.25, abortions) equal for all grades of atherosclerosis.	Adjusted for age, race, hypertension, and being overweight.
Bengtsson et al.[7]	Myocardial infarction (n = 44) Angina (n = 29) ECG suggesting CHD (n = 23)	Population sample (n = 578)	Not given	Gravidity increased angina.* Parity increased I, angina,* ECG,* Abortions increased MI	
Oliver[9]	Cases surviving MI (n = 81) Cases with angina (n = 64)	General reference population of same age	Mean = 40	Parity equal. Spontaneous abortions equal.	Adjusted for age, marital status, and year of admission by matching.

Study	Cases	Controls	Age	Findings	Comments
Mann et al.[11]	Patients discharged with diagnosis of MI (n = 63)	Patients with acute medical surgical conditions (n = 189)	Mean = 40.1	Parity equal	Adjusted for age by matching.
Mann and Inman[12]	Cases who died from MI (n = 219) (reported on, n = 153) Cases with CHD (n = 169)	Patient from same general practice (n = 219) Women seeking medical care (n = 338)	<50, stratified	Parity equal.	
Beard et al.[14]	Cases with CHD (n = 169)	Women seeking medical care (n = 338)	<60	Parity increased (≥4 pregnancies). First pregnancy at age <20 years increased.*	Adjusted for age and year of diagnosis by matching.
La Vecchia et al.[10]	Cases surviving acute MI (n = 202)	Hospitalized women without CHD (n = 374)	Median, 47	Parity equal (≥3 pregnancies). Spontaneous abortions equal. First pregnancy at age <20 year increased.*	Adjusted for age. No trend was found with increasing number of births or abortions.
Croft and Hannaford[13]	Cases with first acute MI (n = 158)	Patients with no history of MI (n = 474)	Mean = 48	Parity equal.	Adjusted for smoking, social class, and use of OC. Matched for age. *(Continued)*

Table 18–1. Case–Control and Cross-sectional Studies of Gravidity or Parity and Coronary Heart Disease (*Continued*)

REFERENCE	STUDY GROUP	CONTROL GROUP	AGE (YEARS) AT ENDPOINT	FINDINGS IN CASES	COMMENTS
Palmer et al.[15]	Cases with first acute MI (*n* = 858)	Community controls with no history of MI (*n* = 858)	45–67	Parity increased* (≥5 births). First pregnancy at age <20 years increased.*	Adjusted for age, smoking, hypertension, cholesterol, diabetes, family history, physical activity, BMI, alcohol, education, and occupation.
Beral[17]	CHD and IHD deaths in parous women during three time periods	CHD and IHD deaths in nulliparous women (*n* = 120, *n* = 543)	45–74	Parity equal 1938–1949 Parity increased* 1950–1960 Parity increased* 1959–1960	Proportionate mortality ratios were calculated for parous women vs. nulliparous women.

CHD, coronary heart disease; MI, myocardial infarction; ECG, electrocardiogram; OC, oral contraceptives; BMI, body mass index; IHD, ischemic heart disease. P <0.05.
[Reprinted with permission from Ness, et al., Reproductive history and coronary heart disease in women, Epidemiologic Reviews, Vol. 16., pages 298–314, 1994]

disease with increasing numbers of pregnancies or births.[11-13] However, case–control studies that included large samples of women over the age of 50 did reveal an increased risk of heart disease after four or more[14] or five or more pregnancies.[15] Furthermore, both of these studies[14,15] adjusted for multiple confounders, including age, smoking, hypertension, cholesterol, diabetes, and obesity, that might otherwise obscure associations.

In addition, three case–control studies[10,14,15] examined the association of having a first birth before 20 years of age with heart disease risk, and all showed a significant association. Results of Palmer et al.[15] suggest that parity and early age at first birth are independent risk factors for coronary heart disease, and that women with both of these reproductive characteristics have over twice the risk of myocardial infarction compared with women having neither of these characteristics.

Other studies focused on mortality from cardiovascular disease as an outcome. Parrish et al.[16] used autopsy records from women who had died from cancer or accidents to examine the relation between pregnancy and atherosclerosis. After adjustment for age, race, and year of birth, there was no significant association in degree of atherosclerosis and reproductive rate.[16] However, two large case–control and cross-sectional studies (that used census data for all ever-married women in England and Wales who died between 1938 and 1960[17] and between 1971 and 1981[18]) found that among parous women, there were higher rates of mortality from many diseases including ischemic and degenerative heart disease, cerebrovascular disease, hypertension, and diabetes mellitus. Likewise, a prospective study of 63,090 Norwegian women reported a positive trend of increasing mortality from ischemic heart disease with increasing parity.[19]

These results can be contrasted with three retrospective case–control studies in which sudden cardiac death was examined.[20-22] Sudden cardiac death can be defined as a death occuring within 24 hours of onset in an individual with no previous clinical history of heart disease who died outside the hospital. Coroner's reports and death certificates were used to ascertain these cases. Next-of-kin interviews were obtained and age-matched neighborhood controls were used as comparison groups. In all three of these studies, parity was protective against this sudden cardiac death; there were fewer children among the cases than among the controls.[20-22] However, as Ness et al.[2] note in their comprehensive review of the literature, it is difficult to compare the results of studies of sudden cardiac death with studies addressing coronary heart disease specifically, since sudden death is typically the immediate consequence of cardiac arrhythmia, which may result from coronary heart disease or a variety of other underlying causes.

The majority of prospective, population-based investigations that used representative or unselected samples reported a positive association between parity and coronary heart disease, with a few exceptions. For instance, in separate analyses, Ness et al.[23] examined data from 2,357 women aged 35 to 68 years who were followed for 28 years through the Framingham Heart Study, and 2,533 women aged 45 to 74 years at baseline who were followed for at least 12 years through the First National Health and Nutrition Examination Survey National Epidemiologic Follow-up Study (NHEFS). In both of these cohorts, the rates of coronary heart disease were significantly higher among multigravid women than among women who had never been pregnant. However, differences were statistically significant only in women with six or more pregnancies. The rate ratio (RR) after adjustment for age and educational level for women with six or more pregnancies compared with those with no pregnancies was 1.6 (95% confidence interval [CI] 1.1.–2.2) in the Framingham cohort, and 1.5 (95% CI 1.1–1.9) in the NHEFS cohort. Adjustment for other cardiovascular risk factors, such as weight, blood pressure, cigarette smoking, and cholesterol level, did not materially alter these results.[23] Additionally, among a subset of Framingham women aged 45 to 64 years, those who were parous, worked outside the home (generally in clerical jobs), and had raised three or more children were found to have higher rates of coronary heart disease than both employed women without children and nulliparous homemakers.[24] Finally, a 28-year prospective study of 1,200 married Dutch civil servants aged 40–65 years at enrollment reported that the relative mortality rate among women with four or more children was 2.5 times greater than that of women with no children (95% CI 1.0–5.8).[25]

In contrast, other prospective studies, mainly those of selected populations, failed to find an association between parity and heart disease. For instance, among 119,963 women aged 30 to 55 years who were enrolled in the Nurse's Health Study and followed between 1976 and 1982, there were no statistically significant differences between parous and nulliparous women in rate of coronary heart disease.[26] Analyses restricted to parous women also found no differences between those in the highest parity group (five or more births) compared with those in the median parity group (three births).[26] Likewise, a 1976 report from the Framingham Study found no association between parity and cardiovascular disease in women aged 40–54 who were followed for 20 years and had a total of only 90 cardiovascular events.[27] However, both of these studies examined young women who would likely have a relatively low rate of coronary heart disease which could mask a real association between gravidity or parity and coronary heart disease.[2] A recent analysis of data from 585,445 women enrolled in the American Cancer Society Cancer Prevention Survey II (CPS II)[28] reported a significantly increased risk in heart disease mortality for women with six or more live births after adjustment for age (RR = 1.18, 95% CI = 1.04–1.34), but not after adjustment for multiple cardiovascular disease risk factors. Because the cohorts of women in the Nurses Health Study and the CPS II are highly educated and more economically homogeneous, Steenland et al.[28]

suggested that the positive association of parity and heart disease observed in studies of cohorts representative of the general population may be due in part to confounding by uncontrolled variables related to socioeconomic status. However, a re-analysis of data from the representative sample of women in NHANES I[24] yielded significant associations similar to those previously reported by Ness et al.[23] after adjustment for both age and multiple risk factors.

Several influences, in addition to socioeconomic status, may also mediate the observed relation between pregnancy and heart disease. As suggested by Ness et al.,[2] hormonal alterations occurring during pregnancy combined with stress occurring during childbearing might result in early coronary heart disease death. For this to be the case, one would have to posit that the acute effects of pregnancy persist (e.g., that hormone levels are persistently elevated or that continued stress leads to irreversible consequences).[2] However, a study of recently postmenopausal women[29] reported that increased levels of parity and gravidity were only associated with increased estradiol; no effects in other sex hormones were observed. Furthermore, among this postmenopausal sample, there was no evidence that pregnancy permanently reset baseline ovarian function[29] although others reported a persistent alteration of hormone levels (i.e., lowered estrogen levels and increased sex hormone–binding globulin) in parous, premenopausal women.[30] As reviewed by Ness et al.,[2] caring for young children resembles a stressful occupational situation in that it is very demanding with few opportunities for control. The stress experienced during child-rearing may be associated with anatomic changes in coronary arteries that do not present as clinical disease until later in life when compounded with the effects of aging.[2] However, stress is difficult to measure and has generally not been studied in relation to parity and heart disease.[28] Pre-eclampsia has been associated with increases in coagulation factors known to predict cardiovascular events[31] and an increased death rate from ischemic heart disease.[32] Thus, it is possible that the observed parity–heart disease association may be the persistent effects of stress or pre-eclampsia. Finally, differences in behaviors that increase cardiovascular risk, such as a more sedentary lifestyle and the consumption of a high-fat diet, may be associated with child-rearing but have been little investigated.[2]

In sum, there is inconsistency in the literature;[2] whereas previous case–control studies that failed to show a relation between pregnancy and heart disease included predominantly women who were aged 60 years or younger, an age range in which few women develop heart disease, studies that found a positive association included women of all ages. Most case–control studies did not adjust for multiple confounders of cardiovascular risk such as obesity, cholesterol, and hypertension, which may vary with increasing numbers of pregnancies.[2] However, prospective studies of representative samples of the general population, as well as the larger case–control or cross-sectional studies that examined older women and adjusted for potential cardiovascular risk factors, did show a modest but increased risk of heart disease among women with more and/or earlier reproductive events.[2]

PREGNANCY, OBESITY AND FAT DISTRIBUTION

Obesity, whether assessed by weight alone or by body mass index (weight in kg/height in m[2]), and upper-body fat distribution, typically assessed by the ratio of waist circumference to hip circumference (waist/hip ratio), have been associated with increased risk of cardiovascular disease, hypertension, diabetes, and mortality in both women and men.[33–40] During pregnancy, an average of 3.5 to 4 kg of maternal fat tissue is accumulated, preferentially in the femoral area.[2] It has been widely believed that pregnancy is associated with weight gain and abdominal or central adiposity,[41–43] although it is not clear whether it is the weight cycling associated with multiple pregnancies[44] or childbearing per se that is the cause.

There have been numerous studies that examined the association of pregnancy and childbearing with obesity and fat distribution. Although a few studies reported no association of pregnancy with weight gain or maximum lifetime weight,[45,46] (see Table 18–2)[47–58], most previous studies reported increases in various measures of obesity, including weight, body mass index, and waist/hip ratio, with increasing numbers of pregnancies and births.[2] More recent studies have also shown that increases in weight,[59] prevalence of being overweight,[60] and upper-body fat distribution as assessed by waist/hip ratio[44,61,62] are associated with pregnancy and childbearing.

Numerous studies have reported that obesity and central adiposity increase with age and menopause.[34,59,63–65] In all previous reviewed studies of pregnancy and obesity[2] as well as in the more recent studies,[44,59–63] age was the factor most strongly related to obesity and fat distribution. The effects of pregnancy and childbearing on measures of obesity and fat distribution may, in fact, be relatively weak. In a study of 41,184 postmenopausal women, Brown and colleagues[64] reported that between the ages of 18 and 50, parity was associated with an increase in body weight of 0.55 kg per live birth and that women with a lifetime parity of one or two live births had a lower mean body weight, lower mean body mass index, and a lower proportion of overweight than either nulliparous women or women with three or more lifetime births.

Several studies have reported mean weight gains for women with two or more pregnancies of only 0.5 to 2.3 kg above age-related increases.[66–70] For example, Ohlin and Rosner[69] followed 1,423 pregnant Swedish women and found that by 1 year postpartum, they weighed an average of only 1.5 kg more than their prepregnancy weight. These authors estimated that a 0.18 kg gain would have occurred from age alone, and that an additional correction for inaccurate estimation of prepregnancy weight (which was based on self-reports) would yield an average weight gain of only 0.53 kg. Schauberger et al.[70] reported that by 6 months postpartum, the average weight of 795 white U.S. women was only 1.4 kg above their initial weight obtained at their first prenatal visit. In a recent review, Lederman[71] reported that average weight increments are generally less than 1.5 kg during a single reproductive cycle (i.e., from before pregnancy to 1 year postpartum).

As suggested by Ness et al.,[2] an important limitation of studies of older women is that body composition was not measured until near the end or after the end of the participants' reproductive period. Thus, in studies that are not adjusted for age, one cannot be certain whether pregnancy among high-parity women is a causal factor for elevated body mass or waist/hip ratio or merely a correlate. However, the association of pregnancy with obesity and upper-body fat distribution has been observed in studies statistically adjusted for age, which indicates that there is an effect, possibly small, of pregnancy that is independent of age.

There may also be a synergistic effect of age and pregnancy on obesity such that women with several pregnancies are at greater risk of becoming obese later in life. Ohlin and Rossner[69] reported that at 1 year postpartum, women who had children after age 35 had greater increases in weight than younger women. In this study, women of all parities aged 26 to 35 at delivery were 1.4 kg heavier at 1 year postpartum than they were prior to pregnancy. However, women over the age of 35 with similar parities had larger weight increases. This was particularly true for women having their first birth after age 35, who were 2.9 kg heavier at 1 year postpartum.[69]

Correlational analyses are often used to examine the association between pregnancy and obesity. However, because the significance of a correlation is partly determined by sample size, it is also important to examine the strength of observed associations. One measure of the strength of an association can be calculated by squaring the correlation between the dependent and independent variables of interest. The resultant r^2 shows the proportion of variance (or the amount of variability) in the outcome (in this instance, obesity, weight, or waist/hip ratio) that can be accounted for by a particular independent variable (in this instance, number of pregnancies or births). In the few studies where the r^2 is either given or can be calculated, the proportion of variance in measures of obesity that is accounted for by numbers of pregnancies or births is low. For instance, both Lanska et al.,[72] in a study of over 53,000 U.S. members of a weight reduction organization, and Kritz-Silverstein et al.,[73] in a subsample of over 1,000 postmenopausal women from the Rancho Bernardo (California) cohort, reported that although statistically significant associations were observed, the number of pregnancies accounted for less than 1% of the variability in body mass index. Similarly, correlational data from the Nurses Health Study also suggest that parity explained less than 1% of the variability in body mass index,

Table 18–2. Selected Studies of Gravidity or Parity and Body Weight

REFERENCE	STUDY DESIGN	NO. OF SUBJECTS	ADIPOSITY MEASUREMENT DATA COLLECTED	CHANGES OCCURRING WITH INCREASED PARITY/GRAVIDITY	COMMENTS
Lowe and Gibson[47]	Retrospective employment record review, women aged 20–59 years	5,081	Weight and height	Weight increased within all 5-year age-groups.	
McKeown and Record[48]	Cohort	>1,000	Weight of 124 days' gestation and 3, 12, and 24 months postpartum	Weight gain increased with years postpartum with higher parity.	
Cederlof and Kaij[49]	Retrospective, monozygotic twins; one twin with ≥1 children, cotwin childless	378 pairs	Questionnaire items included number of children and weight at the time of the investigation.	Weight increased.*	
Garn et al.[50]	Cohort of women with ≥2 pregnancies	>6,000	Prepregnancy weight for three consecutive pregnancies	Weight increased in non-smoking women.	
Noppa and Bengtsson[51]	Cross-sectional, women in five age strata	1,462	WI (weight (kg)/(height(cm) −100)) × 100	WI increased.*	Adjusted for age, social class, age of husband, educational level, and husband's income.

Study	Design	N	Measure	Result	Adjustment
Heliovarra and Aromaa[52]	Cross-sectional, non-pregnant women	17,688	Quetelet index equal (weight (kg)/height (m)^2)	Quetelet index increased; % obese increased.	Adjusted for geographic area, region, occupation, smoking, and marital status.
Rona and Morris[53]	Cohort of English (E) and Scottish (S) couples	E = 5,470[a] S = 1,543[a]	Self-reported height and weight. W:H equal (log (weight/height −20))	W:H increased* in English mothers. W:H equal in Scottish mothers.	Adjusted for husband's social class and employment status, parents' age, and husband's weight.
Baecke et al.[54]	Cross-sectional, women aged 19–31 years	2,092	Weight, height, and BMI−equal (kg)/height (m)^2	Weight increased* in married women with ≥2 births.	Adjusted for age marital status, education, occupation, urbanization, religion, and church attendance.
Forster et al.[55]	Cross-sectional, black (B) and white (W) women	W = 884 B = 289	BMI (weight (kg)/height (m)^2)	BMI increased in blacks and whites.*	Analysis of covariance. Adjusted for age, education, and family income.
Greene et al.[56]	Prospective, women with two pregnancies in 6 years	7,116	Interpregnancy weight gain; prepregnancy weight self-reported	Weight increased.*	Adjusted for race, smoking, complications, marital status, interpregnancy interval, breast feeding, and % of ideal body weight.

(Continued)

Table 18–2. Selected Studies of Gravidity or Parity and Body Weight (*Continued*)

REFERENCE	STUDY DESIGN	NO. OF SUBJECTS	ADIPOSITY MEASUREMENT DATA COLLECTED	CHANGES OCCURRING WITH INCREASED PARITY/GRAVIDITY	COMMENTS
Ohlin and Rossner[69]	Historical cohort of pregnant and post-partum women	2,295	Weight before (self-reported) and during pregnancy and 2.5, 6, and 12 months postpartum	Weight gain increased ($n = 1,432$); prepregnancy BMI increased* ($n = 2,295$).	Adjusted for age and smoking.
Rissanen et al.[57]	Prospective, 4- to 7-year follow-up	6,165	Mean weight change by number of pregnancies between two surveys	Weight increased.*	Adjusted for education, marital status, smoking, alcohol, coffee, health status, and physical activity.
Brown et al.[58]	Cross-sectional, Iowa women.	41,184	BMI at ages 18, 30, 40, and 50 years	BMI increased.*	Adjusted for education, marital status, and smoking. Strong association seen between aging and weight gain. Weak association between parity and both weight gain and being overweight.

WI, weight index; W:H, mean weight:height index; BMI, body mass index. [a]No. of couples. *$p < 0.05$.

[Reprinted with permission from Ness, et al., Reproductive history and coronary heart disease in women, Epidemiologic Reviews, Vol. 16., pages 298–314, 1994[2]] waist circumference, hip circumference, and waist/hip ratio.[62] The proportion of variance in waist/hip ratio accounted for by parity is greater than 1% in only one recent study[44] where after adjustment for age and body mass index, a correlation of .24 was observed, indicating that parity accounted for slightly more than 4% of the variance in the ratio of fat distribution. In all of these studies, current age accounted for the largest proportion of variance in obesity and fat distribution.

Other psychological and physical factors associated with increased obesity and upper-body fat distribution may be misattributed to pregnancy. For instance, because of a greater tendency to underestimate their previous weight, obese women may appear to be gaining more weight during pregnancy and retaining more weight postpartum than are nonobese women with the same weight gain and retention.[71] Lanska et al.[72] suggested that increases in waist circumference following multiple pregnancies may be due to an increase in laxity and stretching of abdominal wall musculature following pregnancy. Ness et al.[2] suggested that the association between waist/hip ratio and pregnancy may reflect an increase in overall, rather than site-specific, adiposity. However, investigators using magnetic resonance imaging (MRI) during and after pregnancy concluded that adipose tissue remaining more than 1 year after delivery actually does tend to be localized in the trunk.[74]

Other behavioral and lifestyle changes that result in increased weight gain during pregnancy or a failure to lose weight during the postpartum period may also be misattributed to pregnancy. Women often stop smoking while pregnant and smoking cessation often results in weight gain. Ohlin and Rossner[69] found that smokers who stopped smoking early in pregnancy gained more weight during pregnancy than either non-smokers or persistent smokers (weight gains = 16.1 kg vs. 13.9 kg and 13.8 kg, respectively). As reviewed by Lederman,[71] lifestyle changes following childbearing (such as a decrease in exercise and general activity, a relaxation of attitudes about weight gain, or the increased access to food throughout the day that may accompany a delay in return to work or unemployment) may all contribute to a failure to lose weight during the postpartum period.

In sum, results of these studies indicate that there are strong age-related effects for obesity and fat distribution. These studies also indicate that the effects of other physical, psychological, and lifestyle changes that accompany pregnancy cannot be discounted. However, these studies have shown that there are consistent, (although relatively small), long-term changes in obesity and fat distribution that may be attributed independently to pregnancy.

PREGNANCY AND LIPID AND LIPOPROTEIN LEVELS

High-density lipoprotein (HDL) cholesterol has a strong inverse relation to coronary heart disease in women.[75-78] In the Framingham study, a 1 mg/dl in-

Table 18–3. Studies of Gravidity or Parity and Serum Lipids

REFERENCE	STUDY DESIGN	NO. OF SUBJECTS	FOLLOW-UP TIME
Potter and Nestel[79]	Prospective; women <8 weeks gravid through pregnancy compared with other non-pregnant women	43	12 months post-partum
Fahraeus et al.[80]	Prospective; same women from before conception, every 6–8 weeks through pregnancy	19	8 weeks postpartum
DeSoye et al.[81]	Prospective; women 10 weeks gravid through pregnancy compared with other non-pregnant women	25	6–8 weeks postpartum
Hubert et al.[86]	Prospective; women aged 20–29 years at baseline; multivariate-controlled[b,c]	497	8 years
van Stiphout et al.[83]	Prospective; *(1)* same women with levels 1 year before, during, and after pregnancy *(2)* women ever vs. never pregnant	22	±3 years
Knopp et al.[82]	Prospective; same women 10 weeks gravid through pregnancy	8–20	6 weeks postpartum
Deslypere et al.[84]	Cross-sectional; women 48 hours postpartum with various reproductive histories	510	None
Flegal et al.[90]	Cross-sectional; NHANES II white women aged 20–74 years; multivariate-controlled[b,d]	1,781 pre-menopausal; 2,374 post-menopausal	None
Kritz-Silverstein et al.[88]	Cross-sectional; women aged 50–89 years recalling number of pregnancies; multivariate-controlled[b]	1,275	None
Haertel et al.[85]	Prospective; women aged 24–64 years at baseline; multivariate-controlled[e]	1,998	3 years

[a]LDL, low density lipoprotein; HDL, high density lipoprotein; NHANES II, Second National Health and Nutritional Examination Survey. [a]+, above baseline; 2, below baseline; =, at baseline.

[b]Controlled for age, body mass index, alcohol consumption, cigarette use, oral contraception or estrogen use, education.

[c]Also controlled for occupation, martial status, and Type A personality.

Table 18–3. Studies of Gravidity or Parity and Serum Lipids *(Continued)*

TRIMESTER			ASSOCIATIONS WITH HIGHER PARITY	
1	2	3		
			6 weeks	*12 months*
+ Total cholesterol	+ Total cholesterol	+ Total cholesterol	+ Total cholesterol	= Total cholesterol
+ LDL cholesterol	+ LDL cholesterol	+ LDL cholesterol	+ LDL cholesterol	+ LDL cholesterol
+ HDL cholesterol	+ HDL cholesterol	+ HDL cholesterol	= HDL cholesterol	− HDL cholesterol
			8 weeks	
+ Total cholesterol	+ Total cholesterol	+ Total cholesterol	+ Total cholesterol	
= LDL cholesterol	+ LDL cholesterol	+ LDL cholesterol	+ LDL cholesterol	
+ HDL cholesterol	+ HDL cholesterol	− HDL cholesterol	= HDL cholesterol	
			6 weeks	
	+ Total cholesterol	+ Total cholesterol	+ Total cholesterol	
	+ LDL cholesterol	+ LDL cholesterol	+ LDL cholesterol	
	+ HDL cholesterol	− HDL cholesterol	= or + HDL cholesterol	
			− Total cholesterol	
			= LDL cholesterol	
			− HDL cholesterol	
			12 months	*Ever*
	+ Total cholesterol	+ Total cholesterol	= Total cholesterol	= Total cholesterol
	+ HDL cholesterol	= HDL cholesterol	− HDL cholesterol	− HDL cholesterol
			6 weeks	
	+ LDL cholesterol	+ LDL cholesterol	+ LDL cholesterol	
	+ HDL cholesterol	− HDL cholesterol	= HDL cholesterol	
		+ Total cholesterol		
		+ LDL cholesterol		
		− HDL cholesterol		
		− Total cholesterol		
		= LDL cholesterol		
		− HDL cholesterol		
		= Total cholesterol		
		= LDL cholesterol		
		− HDL cholesterol		
		− HDL cholesterol		

[d]Also controlled for menopausal status, income and triceps and subscapular skinfold sum/ratio.

[e]Controlled for employment, body mass index, and alcohol consumption.

[Reprinted with permission from Ness, et al., Reproductive history and coronary heart disease in women, Epidemiologic Reviews, Vol. 16., pages 298–314, 1994[2]] crease in HDL cholesterol was related to a significant 3% decrease in coronary hear disease risk.[73] In the Lipid Research Clinics Study,[78] a 1 mg/dl increment was associated with a 4.7% decrement in cardiovascular mortality rates. One possible mechanism by which pregnancy could be related to the subsequent development of cardiovascular disease is through the alteration of lipid levels. Although there are inconsistencies about the associations of gravidity and parity with total cholesterol, low density lipoprotein (LDL) cholesterol, and triglycerides, most studies have shown that pregnancy and childbearing are associated with decreased HDL levels (see Table 18–3).[79–86]

Van Stiphout et al.[83] reported that during pregnancy women have higher total and HDL cholesterol levels, but 1 year later, their levels drop below prepregnancy concentrations. Women who have ever been pregnant had lower HDL levels than those who have never been pregnant.[83] In a study of 516 women, Deslypere et al.[84] found that 48 hours after giving birth, the ratio of HDL cholesterol to total cholesterol (HDLC/TC) was significantly lower among women who had five or more pregnancies compared with those who had given birth for the first time.

Large prospective studies that followed women for longer periods of time have also been consistent in finding an inverse association between pregnancy and HDL cholesterol level. The MONICA (Monitoring of Trends and Determinants in Cardiovascular Disease) Augsburg Survey in Germany[81] followed 1,998 women aged 25–64 years for up to 3 years and found that women who had a pregnancy during the follow-up period had HDL cholesterol levels that were on average 2.4 mg/dl lower than those who had not been pregnant during follow-up. Similarly, in a prospective study of Framingham offspring, Hubert et al.[86] found that number of live births was significantly associated with reduced levels of HDL cholesterol levels in premenopausal women; the follow-up was 8 years but the interval since the last pregnancy was not given. Lewis et al.[87] analyzed data from over 2,000 women enrolled in the CARDIA (Coronary Artery Risk Development in Young Adults) Study in 1985–86 who participated in two repeat evaluations in 1987–88 and 1990–91. At both follow-ups, the change in HDL cholesterol level was significantly different among the parity groups. High density lipoprotein cholesterol levels decreased significantly more in women who had their first pregnancy of at least 28 weeks duration during follow-up (mean = −3.5 the first follow-up interval and −5.2 for the second follow-up interval) compared with nulliparous women and parous women who did not have any further pregnancies. Adjusting for potential confounders such as age, obesity, education, race, socioeconomic status, physical activity, cigarette smoking, and alcohol use did not materially alter the results.[87]

Two studies showed a long-term effect of pregnancy for lipid and lipoprotein levels by cross-sectionally examining these associations in large samples of older women. Using data from a sample of 1,275 postmenopausal women aged

50–89 who were participants in Rancho Bernardo Study, Kritz-Silverstein et al.,[88] reported that multiparity (as measured by five or more pregnancies or live births) was associated with significantly lower HDL levels. After adjustment for age, obesity, cigarette smoking, alcohol use, exercise, diabetes, estrogen replacement therapy, and age at menopause, women who had five or more pregnancies had HDL cholesterol levels that were 4.9 mg/dl lower than those of women with four or fewer pregnancies, a difference that is of clinical and statistical significance. Women in the Rancho Bernardo cohort are on average leaner than other U.S. women.[89] In populations that are less lean than the Rancho Bernardo cohort, the association between parity and HDL level might be noted with fewer pregnancies. For example, using a representative sample of the U.S. population from the Second National Health and Nutrition Examination Survey (NHANES II), Flegal et al.[90] found a significant negative and more linear association between parity and HDL level.

It is unclear whether the observed differences in HDL levels reflect a long-term effect of pregnancy or some psychosocial or behavioral aspect of parenthood. If differences in HDL cholesterol level reflect a psychosocial or behavioral effect of parenthood, then one would expect to observe similar differences in men. A recent study by Kritz-Silverstein et al.[91] addressed this issue by examining the association between the number of children men had and their lipid and lipoprotein levels. Men with five or more biological children were significantly more obese than men without biological children. However, after adjustment for age and obesity, there were no statistically significant differences in any of the lipid or lipoprotein levels based on number of children. Although one cannot completely discount an effect of stress from child-rearing that is unique to women, these data support the view that the relations observed between parity and HDL levels in women are long-term biological consequences of pregnancy.[91]

PREGNANCY AND GLUCOSE TOLERANCE AND NONINSULIN DEPENDENT DIABETES MELLITUS

It is biologically plausible that pregnancy is diabetogenic, not only during pregnancy but later as well. It is well known that women who have had gestational diabetes are at increased risk of having noninsulin-dependent diabetes mellitus (NIDDM) in later life.[92,93] Pregnancy has profound effects on glucose, insulin, and carbohydrate metabolism.[94–99] During early pregnancy, insulin action is enhanced by estrogen and progesterone, leading to a decrease in glucose levels.[100] However, as pregnancy progresses, basal insulin and stimulated insulin secretion increase, leading to a state of insulin resistance in the mother.[101–104] Exposure to multiple pregnancies, with the repeated demand for flexible insulin, may increase the risk of permanent glucose intolerance and hyperinsulinemia to the degree that is characteristic of NIDDM, and the number of times a woman is pregnant may determine this risk.[100]

Studies have examined the association between pregnancy and diabetes with conflicting results. As early as the 1930s, there were reports that death from diabetes was more common among married or widowed women than single women, suggesting an association between parity and diabetes.[105,106] In a more recent study based on death certificates previously described, Beral[17] found that parous women were more likely than nulliparous women to die of diabetes mellitus. In another early study, Pyke,[107] noted that the incidence of diabetes diagnosed in middle and later life increased with parity. However, in a 1978 review of the literature, West[108] found 9 studies that showed an increasing risk of diabetes with increasing parity, 14 studies that showed no association between diabetes and parity, and 2 cross-cultural studies that found a relation in some cultures but not in others. West[108] suggested that the association between diabetes and parity observed in some populations might not be a direct cause-and-effect relation but could be mediated by other factors such as obesity. However, more recent, cross-sectional studies, which have adjusted for potentially confounding or mediating variables such as age and obesity have also yielded inconsistent results.

Kritz-Silverstein et al.[109] examined the independent relation of parity with NIDDM and impaired glucose tolerance (IGT) in a sample of 1,186 middle- to upper-middle-class white women aged 40 to 89 who were participants in the Rancho Bernardo Study. All participants had an oral glucose tolerance test with a 75-g glucose load after an overnight fast. On the basis of World Health Organization criteria,[110] women were classified as those with normal glucose tolerance ($n = 714$), impaired glucose tolerance ($n = 326$), and NIDDM ($n = 146$). After adjustment for age, obesity, and family history diabetes, increased parity was positively associated with small but significantly increased risks of both NIDDM (odds ratio [OR] = 1.16, 95% CI 1.04–1.29, per pregnancy) and impaired glucose tolerance (OR = 1.10, 95% CI 1.01–1.19, per pregnancy). Women who had more pregnancies also had an earlier onset of diabetes.[109] Although abnormal glucose tolerance (defined as having either NIDDM or impaired glucose tolerance) increased with increasing pregnancy, the effects of parity specifically on NIDDM and IGT may not be linear. There was a greater increase in the prevalence of NIDDM observed among women who had five or more pregnancies, but a concomitant decrease in the prevalence of impaired glucose tolerance.[109,111] Because impaired glucose tolerance precedes the development of NIDDM, the amount of either at any given time probably depends on pressures such as age, obesity, and multiparity, with lesser pressures leading to impaired glucose tolerance and greater pressures to NIDDM. Thus, the exact risk of NIDDM or IGT per pregnancy depends on a number of variables and may vary from cohort to cohort.[109,112]

Other large studies of U.S. women, including the nationally representative sample of NHANES II[113] and the Nurse's Health Study,[114] failed to find a significant association between parity and diabetes after adjusting for the confounding effects of age, obesity, and education. However, women in both of these studies were younger on average than women in the Rancho Bernardo cohort[109,113,114] and thus at a lower risk of diabetes. Women were classified on the basis of self-report in the Nurses Health Study[114] and by a supplemental questionnaire given only to those who responded affirmatively to a question about diagnosis of diabetes mellitus on a previous survey. Thus, women with undiagnosed NIDDM would have been missed, which could potentially obscure an association between parity and NIDDM.

Studies of women in populations outside the U.S. have failed to find significant associations between parity and diabetes after adjusting for potentially confounding covariates. These studies included South Asian and European women,[115] as well as women from Pacific Island populations,[116,117] where there are large numbers of women at higher parity levels.[117] However, a recent study of 666 Latino women[118] reported that a single additional pregnancy in women with previous gestational diabetes independently increased the rate ratio of NIDDM to 3.34 (95% CI 1.80–6.19) compared with women without an additional pregnancy. This implies that episodes of insulin resistance may contribute to the decline in β cell function that leads to NIDDM in high-risk women.

Only two studies directly tested the notion that the number of pregnancies would be associated with a reduced sensitivity to insulin and hyperinsulinemia. In 764 nondiabetic, relatively lean, postmenopausal white women from the previously described Rancho Bernardo cohort, an increased number of pregnancies was significantly associated with increased fasting insulin and decreased insulin sensitivity.[119] These associations, although small, were independent of obesity and were present even when analyses were restricted to only normoglycemic women.[119] Postchallenge insulin was unrelated to pregnancy history. Among 735 Hispanic and non-Hispanic white control subjects aged 20–74 years from the San Luis Valley Diabetes Study,[120] an increasing number of live births was related to significantly lower C-peptide and insulin levels. However, analyses including the 196 cases as well as the controls indicated that after adjustment for obesity, there was no significant increase in risk of NIDDM or impaired glucose tolerance with increased childbearing among these women.[120]

Although it is biologically plausible that multigravidity might alter glucose regulation, long-term studies of the association of pregnancy with diabetes and glucose intolerance are inconsistent and inconclusive. It is possible that gravidity is related to hyperglycemia independent of obesity within certain subgroups (e.g., older women and those from high-risk ethnic groups). However, even where an association exists, the effect is very small and should not be used as a determinant of family planning decisions.

PREGNANCY AND HYPERTENSION

Reports of the relation between pregnancy and subsequent hypertension in women are not consistent. Of the studies conducted since 1945, approximately half found either that there is an inverse association between reproductive history and blood pressure or that blood pressure tends to be lowest in women with two to five children and rises in women with six or more children.[121–128] The remaining studies showed no association between reproductive history and blood pressure or hypertension.[73,129–133]

Most of these studies examined the effects of number of pregnancies or births on blood pressure only among women less that 45 years of age. Studies of older women also yielded inconsistent results.[73,121,124,126,131] Only four studies adjusted for the effects of age and obesity,[73,128,131,132] and only two studies[73,128] adjusted for the effects of other confounders, such as cigarette smoking, alcohol consumption, exercise, estrogen use, education, or social class, that may affect blood pressure.[134–137]

In one study, Kritz-Silverstein et al.[73] used data from 1,093 postmenopausal women in the Rancho Bernardo cohort aged 50 and older and found that hypertensive women reported fewer pregnancies and live births than normotensive women (means = 1.9 vs. 2.4 pregnancies, respectively; means = 1.5 and 2.0 live births, respectively, P <0.001). But after adjustment for age, there were no differences between hypertensive and normotensive women for either pregnancies (means = 2.2 for both groups) or live births (means = 1.8 for both groups). In unadjusted data using blood pressure as a continuous variable, it appeared that women with six or more pregnancies had lower blood pressure than women with 0, 1, 2, or 3 pregnancies (means = 130.5 vs. 143.7, 143.1, 139.8 and 137.2, for systolic blood pressures, respectively). After adjustment for age, however, these differences were no longer significant. Multiple regression analyses that adjusted for age, obesity, cigarette smoking, alcohol consumption, and postmenopausal estrogen use also indicated that neither pregnancy nor live births were significantly associated with systolic and diastolic blood pressure; age and obesity explained most of the variability.[73]

In another large, well-controlled study, Ness et al.[128] examined the relationship of gravidity to blood pressure and hypertension in 4,626 women aged 20 to 74 years who were examined in the Second National Health and Nutrition Examination Survey (NHANES II). In unadjusted comparisons of women within each 10-year age-group, a greater number of pregnancies was not associated with higher mean systolic or diastolic blood pressure levels or a higher risk of hypertension. However, regression models that adjusted for the effects of potentially confounding variables showed that for both premenopausal and postmenopausal women, gravidity had small, negative associations with systolic and diastolic blood pressure levels. The change in systolic blood pressure with each additional pregnancy was -0.5 mmHg for premenopausal women and -0.4 mmHg for postmenopausal women. Among premenopausal (but not post-menopausal) women, there was a significant interaction between age and gravidity such that the observed effect was greater for younger premenopausal women. Change in diastolic blood pressure with increasing parity was smaller but followed a similar trend. Ness et al.[128] also found that gravidity had a small but significant association with a decreased risk of hypertension in both pre- and postmenopausal women. However, the estimated effect of each additional pregnancy on decreasing the odds of hypertension was stronger for pre-menopausal women (OR = 0.90; 95% CI 0.81–0.99) than for postmenopausal women (OR = 0.95; 95% CI 0.92–0.98).[128]

Changes in blood pressure can occur during pregnancy.[138,139] It is also pos-sible that the relation of number of pregnancies to blood pressure and hyperten-sion may be different for women of younger ages who are temporally closer to childbearing or who are still coping with small children. Results of studies of older women suggest that reproductive history exerts at most only a small, long-term effect on blood pressure or risk of hypertension.

SUMMARY

Previous studies on the whole have suggested small but adverse effects of parity and gravidity on subsequent cardiovascular disease that may not become appar-ent until older ages. The observed associations may reflect the direct biological effects of pregnancy and/or indirect effects through other metabolic and physio-logic changes (e.g., lowered HDL levels, weight cycling) that increase the risk of cardiovascular disease. Ness et al.[2] have proposed alternative explanations for the association of parity with cardiovascular disease, including the possibil-ity that pregnancy or child-rearing could cause increased stress or changes in other lifestyle factors (e.g., diet, exercise), which are in turn associated with in-creased risk of cardiovascular disease. Finally, it is also possible that part or all of the observed associations are due to confounding by unmeasured variables or residual confounding from poorly controlled factors such as socioeconomic sta-tus.[2,19] Regardless of the mechanism, and although the evidence of an associa-tion is far from conclusive, previous research points to the need for additional care and consideration in monitoring older, multiparous women for heart dis-ease and its risk factors.

PREGNANCY AND OVARIAN CANCER

Ovarian cancer is the fourth leading cause of cancer deaths among U.S. women; each year, over 20,000 women develop ovarian cancer and over 12,000 die of the disease.[140,141] Ovarian cancer incidence rates increase with age and are highest among older women, but they increase with age less rapidly after menopause than before it.[142]

There are two major hypotheses about the pathogenesis of ovarian cancer.[143,144] According to the ovulation hypothesis, ovulation increases ovarian cancer risk by subjecting the surface epithelium to repeated minor trauma, increased cellular proliferation,[145,146] and exposure to hormone-rich follicular fluid.[147] Thus, any factor that reduces the cumulative frequency of ovulation should reduce the risk of ovarian cancer. The ovulation hypothesis is supported by the observed protective effects of pregnancy, breast-feeding, and oral contraceptive use, all of which suppress ovulation,[144] and by the reported increased risk of ovarian cancer from infertility drugs that stimulate ovulation.[144] Pike[148] further proposed that ovarian cancer rates are proportional to ovarian "tissue age," measured in units of cellular mitoses, and that the observed flattening of the incidence rates of ovarian cancer after menopause reflects the decreased rate of mitotic activity after cessation of ovulation. Although some studies have reported a positive association between the number of years of ovulation and cancer risk,[146,149,150] analyses of the effect of ages at menarche and menopause on ovarian cancer risk have been inconsistent.[142,144]

Other observations refute the ovulation hypothesis. For instance, according to the ovulation hypothesis, a month of anovulation, regardless of the reason, should confer equal protection against ovarian cancer. However, a month of pregnancy is more protective than a month of lactation or a month of oral contraceptive use.[144,151] Furthermore, oral contraceptive use appears to be more protective for older than younger women, which suggests that the high-dose formulations used by older women protect more against ovarian cancer.[142] This would argue against the ovulation hypothesis, as all dosages similarly suppress ovulation.[142] One study also suggested that the effect of each pregnancy is not equivalent, that first pregnancies are more protective than later ones.[152] Finally, hysterectomy without bilateral oophorectomy (which should have no effect the cumulative frequency of ovulation) has been reported to reduce the risk of ovarian cancer in most studies.[153–157]

The alternative hypothesis is that high circulating levels of pituitary gonadotrophins which stimulate the ovary have a pathogenic role in ovarian cancer separate from the mechanical damage of ovulation itself.[144,158,159] According to this hypothesis, any factor associated with suppression of pituitary gonadotrophin secretion, such as pregnancy and oral contraceptive use, would reduce the risk of ovarian cancer. Because this hypothesis allows protection to vary with different causes of anovulation it can explain the variability in level of protection or risk associated with different factors.[144] Thus, the earlier, high-dose oral contraceptives afford a greater reduction in risk of ovarian cancer because they are more effective at reducing gonadotrophin levels.[160,161] Late age at menopause, which postpones exposure to high postmenopausal gonadotrophin levels, may also reduce ovarian risk.[162] The observed increase in ovarian cancer risk with use of fertility drugs (which increase gonadotrophin levels) or by a diet high in galactose (which is thought to cause ovarian damage and consequently increased gonadotrophin secretion) can both be explained by the hypotheses.[144,163] However, this hypothesis cannot explain the reported lack of protection[142] or the increased risk of ovarian cancer with use of postmenopausal estrogen.[156]

Numerous epidemiological studies, most of which were case–control, have examined the association of reproductive factors with ovarian cancer and have consistently reported an inverse association between ovarian cancer risk and parity. Parous women are at a significantly lower risk than nulliparous women, and risk decreases with increasing parity.[19,142,149,153,155–157,162,164–172] There is some controversy however, about the linearity of the decrease in risk. Although some studies have indicated that the greatest reduction in risk of ovarian cancer occurred after the first pregnancy, and smaller reductions in risk were associated with subsequent pregnancies,[169,170] others have reported an incremental reduction in ovarian cancer risk that was similar for every pregnancy.[142,162] For instance, a recent collaborative analysis of 12 case–control studies conducted in the U.S. between 1956 and 1986[142] showed that the risk of ovarian cancer among parous women relative to nulliparous women was 0.76 (95% CI 0.63–0.93) for the six hospital-based studies and 0.47 (95% CI 0.40–0.56) for the six population-based studies. Risk decreased monotonically with increasing parity.[142] Similarly, an inverse association was found between parity and ovarian cancer risk during 12 years of follow-up in the Nurses' Health Study[162]; in statistical models with number of births as a continuous variable, each birth was associated with a 16% decrease in risk after adjustment for multiple confounders. Overall, parous women had a 45% reduction in risk of ovarian cancer relative to nulliparous women (age-adjusted RR = 0.55; 95% CI 0.38–0.80). Comparisons of women by categorical numbers of births (1, 2, 3, 4, 5, and ≥6 vs. 0) indicated that there was a small, nonsignificant decrease in risk associated with one birth, but the risk continued to consistently decrease with each additional birth such that, in comparison to nulliparous women, those with 6 or more pregnancies had a multivariate adjusted risk of 0.39 (95% CI 0.20–0.74).[162] Other studies have estimated that ovarian cancer risk declines by approximately 15% for each additional pregnancy or birth.[164,165]

There is also some controversy over the effects of incomplete or failed pregnancies (defined as miscarriages, abortions, ectopic pregnancies, or stillbirths) on ovarian cancer risk. Whittemore[142] reported that risk of ovarian cancer decreased monotonically with increasing numbers of failed pregnancies. Likewise, others have reported that incomplete pregnancies reduce risk to the same degree as full-term pregnancies.[19,164,172,173] However, some studies have shown no effects of incomplete pregnancies on ovarian cancer risk,[156,157,165] nor have they shown an increase in risk.[173]

Findings on the relation between age at first birth and ovarian cancer risk have also been inconsistent.[142,162,169,170,174] For instance, in Whittmore's[142] collaborative analysis and the prospective study of nurses[162] as well as in other studies,[153,157,175] no clear trends in risk of epithelial ovarian cancer were seen with age at first live birth. However, Adami et al.[174] reported a decreasing risk with late age at first birth whereas others reported that late age at first pregnancy was positively associated with ovarian cancer.[156,164] In studies indicating a positive association, the relation was most evident in comparisons of women with an age at first birth of less than 20 years to those with an age at first birth of 34 years or older. As Hankinson et al.[162] conclude, overall, there is little evidence of an independent effect of age at first birth within the range of 22 to 30 years, but an independent effect at younger versus older ages may exist.

Ovarian cancer incidence rates flatten out after 55 years of age.[142] Therefore, it is conceivable that a woman's status with regard to menopause would influence the observed association between parity and ovarian cancer. Results of studies examining this issue are nonetheless inconclusive. In the collaborative analysis of U.S. case–control studies, the absolute decrease in incidence of ovarian cancer was greater among older than among younger women but the percentage of risk reduction due to parity decreased, suggesting that high parity would prevent a smaller percentage of ovarian cancer in older than in younger women.[142] In contrast, a study of 172 cases and 441 controls from Mexico City found a decrease in risk with increasing parity only among postmenopausal women.[173] Similarly, a 15-year prospective study of Norweigan women reported that although the observed mortality rates for ovarian cancer decreased with increasing parity for all women, stratified analyses indicated a protective effect of childbearing only among women aged 45–54 years (i.e., postmenopausal) at the start of follow-up.[152] In comparison to nulliparous women, postmenopausal women with 8–11 children had a relative risk of 0.30 (95% CI 0.17–0.54). The percent reduction in mortality from ovarian cancer among postmenopausal women was 13.6% (95% CI 11.1–15.9) with each additional child. This reduction was not materially altered by adjustment for age at first birth or social class in analyses.[152]

Rates and risks of ovarian cancer may differ and be modified by other important risk factors, such as family history of ovarian cancer and use of oral contraceptives, thus different subgroups of women may have different risks. Hartge et al.[176] reported that at birth, the estimated risk of developing ovarian cancer before age 65 is 0.08% for the total population. The risks for different subgroups may vary 15-fold, from 0.3 (for women with no family history of ovarian cancer, three or more pregnancies, and four or more years of oral contraceptive use) to 4.4% (for women with a positive family history of ovarian cancer, no pregnancies, and no use of oral contraceptives).[176] Infertility may also confound the observed parity–ovarian cancer relation. However, distinguishing the effects of infertility and its treatment from the effects of low parity on ovarian cancer risk is difficult; the few studies that have attempted this have yielded inconsistent results. Although several cohort studies of infertile women reported no increase in risk,[177–179] one showed an increased risk of ovarian cancer among infertile women who had used clomiphene to induce ovulation for 12 or more cycles.[180] Additionally, a meta-analysis of U.S. case–control studies of infertile women reported an increased ovarian cancer risk (RR = 27.0) only among those who used fertility drugs.[169] However, the meaning of this result is controversial because the relative risk was based on only 12 exposed cases and one exposed control, the treatments used were not identified or verified, and the timing of these treatments preceded the introduction of any of the fertility drugs in current use.[144,181–183]

Finally, most epidemiologic investigations of parity and risk of epithelial ovarian cancer group together a variety of different histological (cell) types that occur under this designation. The few studies that evaluated the association of parity with ovarian cancer risk according to specific histologic subtypes reported protective associations for nonmucinous tumors but not for mucinous tumors.[184–187] On the basis of these studies, Risch et al.[187] have suggested that mucinous ovarian tumors may be etiologically unrelated to other types of epithelial ovarian tumors and should be considered separately in studies of ovarian cancer, including those examining the associations between pregnancy and related variables.

One of the most consistent findings in the literature about the long-term effects of childbearing is the protective effect of parity against ovarian cancer. Parous women have a lower risk of ovarian cancer than nulliparous women. It is still unclear, however, whether this decrease is the same for subsequent births as it is for the first birth and whether incomplete pregnancies confer the same degree of protection as term pregnancies. There is also controversy over the effects of age at first pregnancy and whether the risk reduction is greater for postmenopausal women who have a higher incidence of ovarian cancer than for premenopausal women. Finally, the protective effects of parity may be moderated by family history of ovarian cancer, use of oral contraceptives, and histological type of ovarian cancer.

CONCLUSION

Overall, the available literature suggests that there may be residual and cumulative effects of pregnancy and childbearing that exert a long-term influence on women's health and disease. These effects may be negative, as in the case of cardiovascular disease and its comorbidities such as obesity, lipoprotein levels, diabetes, and hypertension, or the effects may be positive, as in the case of ovarian cancer. There may be a delayed or synergistic effect with age such that the effects of pregnancy are not apparent until older ages when there is an increased risk or susceptibility to these diseases. Genetics as well other behavioral and lifestyle factors, such as stress (from parenthood or other sources), cigarette smoking, diet, or use of oral contraceptives, may also interact with the effects of pregnancy to influence the incidence of disease. Most of the long-term effects of pregnancy are relatively small; certainly they are not large enough to warrant counseling women for or against having children. Clinicians nonetheless need to be aware of these potential effects and view pregnancy history as a potential additional risk factor for health and disease.

REFERENCES

1. National Center for Health Statistics. Vital Statistics of the United States, 1986, Vol 2. Mortality. Part A. Washington, DC: U.S. Government Printing Office, 1988, DHHS pub. no. (PHS) 88–1122.

2. Ness RB, Schotland HM, Flegal KM, Shofer FS. Reproductive history and coronary heart disease risk in women. Epidemiol Rev 1994;16:298–314.

3. Schwertner HA, Torres L, Jackson WG. Cortisol and the hypercholesterolemia of pregnancy and labor. Atherosclerosis 1987;67:237–244.

4. Winkelstein W, Stenchever MA, Lilienfeld AM. Occurrence of pregnancy, abortion, and artificial menopause among women with coronary artery disease: A preliminary study. J Chronic Dis 1958;7:273–286.

5. Winkelstein W, Rekate AC. Age trend of mortality from coronary artery disease in women and observations on the reproductive patterns of those affected. Am Heart J 1964;67:481–488.

6. Bengtsson C. Ischemic heart disease in women: A study based on a randomized population sample of women with myocardial infarction in Goteberg, Sweden. Acta Med Scand 1973;549:1–128.

7. Bengtsson C, Rybo G, Westerberg H. Number of pregnancies, use of oral contraceptives and menopausal age in women with ischemic heart disease, compared to a population sample of women. Acta Med Scand 1973;549(suppl):75–81.

8. Abramov LA. Sexual life and sexual frigidity among women developing acute myocardial infarction. Psychosom Med 1976;38:418–425.

9. Oliver MF. Ischemic heart disease in young women. Br Med J 1974;2:253–259.

10. La Vecchia C, DeCarli A, Franceschi S, et al. Menstrual and reproductive factors and risk of myocardial infarction in women under fifty-five years of age. Am J Obstet Gynecol 1987;157:1108–1112.

11. Mann JI, Vessey MP, Thorogood M, et al. Myocardial infarction in young women with special reference to contraceptive practice. Br Med J 1975;2:241–245.

12. Mann JI, Inman WHW. Oral contraceptives and death from myocardial infarction. Br Med J 1975;2:245–248.

13. Croft P, Hannaford PC. Risk factors for acute myocardial infarction in women: Evidence from the Royal College of General Practitioners' oral contraception study. BMJ 1989;298:165–168.

14. Beard CM, Fuster V, Annegers JF. Reproductive history in women with coronary heart disease: A case control study. Am J Epidemiol 1984;120:108–114.

15. Palmer JR, Rosenberg L, Shapiro S. Reproductive factors and risk of myocardial infarction. Am J Epidemiol 1992;136:408–416.

16. Parrish HM, Carr C, Silberg SL, King TM. Relationship of pregnancy to coronary atherosclerosis. Am J Obstet Gynecol 1967;97:1087–1091.

17. Beral V. Long term effects of childbearing on health. J Epidemiol Community Health 1985;39:343–346.

18. Green A, Beral V, Moser K. Mortality in women in relation to their childbearing history. BMJ 1988;297:391–395.

19. Kvale G, Heuch I, Nilssen S. Parity in relation to mortality and cancer incidence: A prospective study of Norwegian women. Int J Epidemiol 1994;23:691–699.

20. Talbot E, Kuller LE, Detre K, et al. Biologic and psychosocial risk factors of sudden death from coronary disease in white women. Am J Cardiol 1977;39:858–864.

21. Talbot E, Kuller LE, Perper J, et al. Sudden and unexpected death in women: Biological and psychosocial origins. Am J Epidemiol 1981;114:671–682.

22. Talbot E, Kuller LE, Detre K, et al. Reproductive history of women dying of sudden cardiac death: A case control study. Int J Epidemiol 1989;18:589–594.

23. Ness RB, Harris T, Cobb J et al. Number of pregnancies and the subsequent risk of cardiovascular disease. N Engl J Med 1993;328:1528–1533.

24. Haynes SG, Feinleib M. Women, work and coronary heart disease: Prospective findings from the Framingham Heart Study. Am J Public Health 1980;70:133–141.

25. Dekker JM, Schouten EG. Number of pregnancies and risk of cardiovascular disease [Letter]. N Engl J Med 1993;329:1893–1894.

26. Kannel WB, Hjortland MC, McNamara PM, et al. Menopause and the risk of cardiovascular disease: The Framingham Study. Ann Int Med 1976;85:447–452.

27. Colditz GA, Willett WC, Stampfer MJ, et al. A prospective study of age at menarche, parity, age at first birth, and coronary heart disease in women. Am J Epidemiol 1987;126:861–870.

28. Steenland K, Lally C, Thun M. Parity and coronary heart disease among women in the American Cancer Society CPS II population. Epidemiology 1996;7: 641–643.

29. Ness RB, Connors-Beatty DJ, Kuller LH. Reproductive history in relation to plasma hormone levels in healthy post-menopausal women. (In press).

30. Bernstien L, Pike MC, Ross RK, Judd HL, Brown JB, Henderson BE. Estrogen and sex hormone-binding globulin levels in nulliparous and parous women. J Natl Cancer Inst 1985;74(4):741–745.

31. Bremme K, Blomback M. Hemostatic abnormalities may predict chronic hypertension after preeclampsia. Gynecol Obstet Invest 1996;41:20–26.

32. Jonsdottir LS, Arngrimsson R, Geirsson RT, Sigvaldason H, Sigfusson N. Death rates from ischemic heart disease in women with a history of hypertension in pregnancy. Acta Obstet Gynecol Scand 1995;74:772–776.

33. Lapidus L, Bengtsson C, Larsson B, Pennert K, Rybo E, Sjostrom L. Distribution of adipose tissue and risk of cardiovascular disease and death: A 12-year follow-up of participants in the population study of women in Gothenburg, Sweden. Br Med J 1984;289:1261–1663.

34. Peiris AN, Sothmann MS, Hoffmann RG, et al. Adiposity, fat distribution, and cardiovascular risk. Ann Int Med 1989;110:867–872.

35. Bjorntorp P. Obesity and the risk of cardiovascular disease. Ann Clin Res 1985;17:3–9.

36. Larsson B, Svardsudd K, Welin L, Wilhelmsen L, Bjorntorp P, Tibblin G. Abdominal adipose tissue distribution, obesity, and risk of cardiovascular disease and
death: A 13-year follow-up of participants in the study of men born in 1913. Br Med J
1984;288:1401–1404.

37. Stern M, Haffner S. Body fat distribution and hyperinsulinemia as risk factors
for diabetes and cardiovascular disease. Arteriosclerosis 1986;6:123–130.

38. Lundgren H, Bengtsson C, Blohme G, Lapidus L, Sjostrom L. Adiposity and
adipose tissue distribution in relation to incidence of diabetes in women: Results from a
prospective population study in Gothenburg, Sweden. Int J Obes 1989:13:413–423.

39. Campaigne BN. Body fat distribution in females: Metabolic complications and
implications for weight loss. Med Sci Sports Exercise 1990;22:291–297.

40. Folsom AR, Kaye SA, Sellers TA, et al. Body fat distribution and 5-year risk
of death in older women. JAMA 1993;289:483–487.

41. Bradley PJ. Conditions recalled to have been associated with weight gain in
adulthood. Appetite 1985;6:235–241.

42. Pitkin RM, Kaminetzky HA, Newton M, Pritchard JA. Maternal nutrition. A
selective review of clinical topics. Obstet Gynecol 1972;40:773–785.

43. Parham ES, Astrom MF, King SK. The association of pregnancy weight gain
with the mother's postpartum weight. J Am Diet Assoc 1990;90:550–554.

44. Rodin J, Radke-Sharpe N, Rebuffe-Scrive M, Greenwood MRC. Weight cycling and fat distribution. Int J Obes 1990;14:303–310.

45. Rookus MA, Rokebrand P, Burema J, Durenberg P. The effect of pregnancy on
the body mass index nine months postpartum in 49 women. Int J Obes 1987;11:609–618.

46. Kritz-Silverstein D, Barrett-Connor E, Wingard DL. The effects of parity on
the later development of non-insulin-dependent diabetes mellitus or impaired glucose
tolerance. N Engl J Med 1989;321:1214–1219.

47. Lowe CR, Gibson JR. Changes in body weight associated with age and marital
status. Br Med J 1955;1006–1008.

48. McKeown T, Record RG. The influence of reproduction on body weight in
women. J Endocrinol 1957;15:393–409.

49. Cederlof R, Kaij L. The effect of childbearing on body weight: A twin control
study. Acta Psychiatr Scand 1970;219(suppl):47–49.

50. Garn SM, Shaw HA, McCabe KD. Effect of maternal smoking on weight and
weight gain between pregnancies. Am J Clin Nutr 1978;31:1302–1303.

51. Noppa H, Bengtsson C. Obesity in relation to socioeconomic status: A population study of women in Goteborg, Sweden. J Epidemiol Community Health 1980;34:
139–142.

52. Heliovaara M, Aromaa A. Parity and obesity. J Epidemiol Community Health
1981;35:197–199.

53. Rona RJ, Morris RW. National study of health and growth: Social and family
factors and overweight in English and Scottish parents. Ann Hum Biol 1982;9:147–156.

54. Baecke JAH, Burema J, Frijters JER, et al. Obesity in young Dutch adults. I.
Sociodemographic variables and body mass index. Int J Obes 1983;7:1–12.

55. Forster JL, Bloom E, Sorensen G, et al. Reproductive history and body mass
index in black and white women. Prev Med 1986;15:685–691.

56. Greene GW, Smiciklas-Wright H, Scholl TO, et al. Post-partum weight
change: How much of the weight gained in pregnancy will be lost after delivery? Obstet
Gynecol 1988;71:701–707.

57. Rissanen AM, Heliovaara M, Knekt P, et al. Determinants of weight again and
overweight in adult Finns. Eur J Clin Nutr 1991;45:419–430.

58. Brown JE, Kaye SA, Folsom AR. Parity-related weight change in women. Int J Obes 1992;16:627–631.

59. Bjorkelund C, Lissner L, Anderson S, Lapidus L, Bengtsson C. Reproduction history in relation to relative weight and fat distribution. Int J Obes 1996;20:213–219.

60. Arroyo P, Avila-Rosas H, Fernandez V, Casanueva E, Galvan D. Parity and the prevalence of overweight. Int J Gynecol Obstet 1995;48:269–272.

61. den Tonkelaar I, Seidell JC, van Noord PAH, Baaanders-van Halewijn EA, Ouwehand IJ. Fat distribution in relation to age, degree of obesity, smoking habits, parity, estrogen use: A cross-sectional study in 11,825 Dutch women participating in the DOM-Project. Int J Obes 1990;14:753–761.

62. Troisi RJ, Wolf AM, Manson JE, Klinker KM, Colditz GA. Relation of body fat distribution to reproductive factors in pre-and postmenopausal women. Obes Res 1995;3:143–151.

63. Wang Q, Hassager C, Ravn P, Wang S, Christainsen C. Total and regional body-composition changes in early postmenopausal women: Age-related or menopause-related? Am J Clin Nutr 1994;60:843–848.

64. Brown JE, Kaye SA, Folsom AR. Parity-related weight change in women. Int J Obes 1992;16:627–631.

65. Kritz-Silverstein D, Barrett-Connor E. Long-term postmenopausal hormone use, obesity, and fat distribution in older women. JAMA 1996;275:46–49.

66. Billewicz WZ, Thompson AM. Body weight in parous women. Br J Prev Soc Med 1970;24:97–104.

67. Forsum E, Sadurski A, Wager J. Resting metabolic rate and body composition of healthy Swedish women during pregnancy. Am J Clin Nutr 1988;47:942–947.

68. Weiss W, Jackson EC, Niswander K, Eastman NJ. The influence on birth weight of change in maternal weight gain in successive pregnancies in the same woman. Int J Gynecol Obstet 1969;7:210–233.

69. Ohlin A, Rossner S. Maternal body weight development after pregnancy. Int J Obes 1990;14:159–173.

70. Schauberger CW, Rooney BL, Brimer LM. Factors that influence weight loss in the puerperium. Obstet Gynecol 1992;79:424–429.

71. Lederman SA. The effect of pregnancy weight gain on later obesity. Obstet Gynecol 1993;82:148–155.

72. Lanska DJ, Lanska MJ, Hartz AJ, Rimm AA. Factors influencing anatomic location of fat tissue in 52,953 women. Int J Obes 1985;9:29–38.

73. Kritz-Silverstein D, Wingard DL, Barrett-Connor E. The relation of reproductive history and parenthood to subsequent hypertension. Am J Epidemiol 1989;130: 399–403.

74. Sohlstrom A, Forsum E. Changes in adipose tissue volume and distribution during reproduction in Swedish women as assessed by magnetic resonance imaging. Am J Clin Nutr 1995;61:287–295.

75. Miller VT. Dylipoproteinemia in women. Endocrinol Metab Clin North Am 1990;19:381–398.

76. Kannel WB, Castelli WP, Gordon T. Cholesterol in the prediction of athero-sclerotic disease. Ann Int Med 1979;80:85–91.

77. Lerner DJ, Kannel WB. Patterns of coronary heart disease morbidity and mortality in the sexes: A 26-year follow-up of the Framingham population. Am Heart J 1986; 111:383–390.

78. Gordon DJ, Probstfield JL, Garrison RJ, et al. High density lipoprotein cholesterol and cardiovascular disease: Four prospective American studies. Circulation 1989; 79:8–15.

79. Potter JM. Nestel PJ. The hyperlipidemia of pregnancy in normal and complicated pregnancies. Am J Obstet Gynecol 1979;133:165–170.

80. Fahraeus L, Larsson-Cohn U, Wallentin L. Plasma lipoproteins including high density lipoprotein subfractions during normal pregnancy. Obstet Gynecol 1985;66: 468–477.

81. Desoye G, Schweditsch MO, Pfeiffer KP, et al. Correlation of hormones with lipid and lipoprotein levels during normal pregnancy and postpartum. J Clin Endocrinol Metab 1987;64:704–712.

82. Knopp RH, Montes A, Childs M, et al. Metabolic adjustments in normal and diabetic pregnancy. Clin Obstet Gynecol 1981;24:21–39.

83. Van Stiphout WAHJ, Hofman A, De Bruijn AM. Serum lipids in young women before, during, and after pregnancy. Am J Epidemiol 1987;126:922–928.

84. Deslypere JP, Van Trappen Y, Thiery M. Influence of parity on plasma lipid levels. Eur J Obstet Gynecol Reprod Biol 1990;35:1–6.

85. Haertel U, Heiss G, Filipiak B, Doering A. Cross-sectional and longitudinal associations between high density lipoprotein cholesterol and women's employment. Am J Epidemiol 1992;135:68–78.

86. Hubert HB, Eaker ED, Garrison RJ, et al. Lifestyle correlates of risk factor change in young adults: An eight-year study of coronary heart disease risk factors in the Framingham offspring. Am J Epidemiol 1987;125:812–831.

87. Lewis CE, Funkhouser E, Raczynski JM, Sidney S, Bild DE, Howard BV. Adverse effect of pregnancy on high density lipoprotein (HDL) cholesterol in young adult women. The CARDIA Study. Am J Epidemiol 1996;144:247–254.

88. Kritz-Silverstein D, Barrett-connor E, Wingard DL. The relationship between multiparity and lipoprotein levels in older women. J Clin Epidemiol 1992;45: 761–767.

89. Barrett-Connor E. The prevalence of diabetes mellitus in an adult community as determined by history of fasting hyperglycemia. Am J Epidemiol 1980;111:705–712.

90. Flegal KM, Ness RB, Kramer RA. Parity and high density lipoportein (HDL) cholesterol levels in white women from the Second National Health and Nutrition Examination Survey (NHANES II). Am J Epidemiol 1990;132:766A.

91. Kritz-Silverstein D, Barrett-Connor E, Friedlander NJ. Parenthood and lipid and lipoprotein levels in older men. Ann Epidemiol 1997;7:275–279.

92. O'Sullivan JB. Body weight and subsequent diabetes mellitus. JAMA 1982; 248:949–952.

93. Mestman JH, Anderson GV, Guadalupe V. Follow-up study of 360 subjects with abnormal carbohydrate metabolism during pregnancy. Obstet Gynecol 1972;39: 421–425.

94. Kuhl C. Glucose metabolism during and after pregnancy in normal and gestational diabetic women. I. Influence of normal pregnancy on serum glucose and insulin concentration during basal fasting conditions and after a challenge with glucose. Acta Endocrinol (Copenh) 1975;79:709–719.

95. Spellacy WN, Goetz FC, Greenberg BZ, Ells J. Plasma insulin in normal "early" pregnancy. Obstet Gynecol 1965;25:862–865.

96. Kuhl C. Serum insulin and plasma glucagon in human pregnancy on the pathogenesis of gestational diabetes. A review. Acta Diabetologica Latina 1977;14:1–8.

97. Bleicher SJ, O'Sullivan JB, Freinkel N. Carbohydrate metabolism in pregnancy. V. The interrelations of glucose, insulin and free fatty acids in late pregnancy and postpartum. N Engl J Med 1964;271:866–872.

98. Lind T, Billewicz WZ, Brown G. A serial study of changes occurring in the oral glucose tolerance test during pregnancy. J Obstet Gynaecol Br Commonw 1973;80: 1033–1039.

99. Van Assche FA, Aerts L, De Prins F. A morphological study of the endocrine pancreas in human pregnancy. Br J Obstet Gynaecol 1978;85:818–820.

100. Kalkhoff R, Schlach DS, Walker JL, Beck P, Kipnis DM, Daughaday WH. Diabetogenic factors associated with pregnancy. Trans Assoc Am Physicians 1964;77: 270–280.

101. Moore P, Kolterman O, Weyant J, Olefsky JM. Insulin binding in human pregnancy: Comparisons to the postpartum, luteal, and follicular states. J Clin Endocrinol Metab 1981;52:937–941.

102. Tsibris JC, Rayno LO, Buhi WC, Buggie J, Spellacy WN. Insulin receptors to circulating erythrocytes and monocytes from women on oral contraceptives or pregnant women near term. J Endocrinol Metab 1980;51:711–717.

103. Phelps RL, Metzger BE, Freinkel N. Carbohydrate metabolism in pregnancy. XVII. Diurnal profiles of plasma glucose, insulin, free fatty acids, triglycerides, cholesterol, and individual amino acids in late normal pregnancy. Am J Obstet Gynecol 1981; 140:730–736.

104. Freinkel N. Of pregnancy and progeny. Diabetes 1980;29:1023–1035.

105. Mosenthal HO, Bolduan C. Diabetes mellitus—problems of present-day treatment. Am J Med Sci 1933;186:605.

106. Joslin EP, Dublin LI, Marks HH. Studies in diabetes mellitus. IV. Etiology. Am J Med Sci 1936;191:759–775.

107. Pyke DA. Parity and the incidence of diabetes. Lancet 1956;270:818–821.

108. West KM. Epidemiology of Diabetes and its Vascular Lesions. New York: Elsevier, 1978, pp. 221–224.

109. Kritz-Silverstein D, Barrett-Connor E, Wingard DL. The effect of parity on the later development of non-insulin dependent diabetes mellitus or impaired glucose tolerance. N Engl J Med 1989;321:1214–1219.

110. Diabetes mellitus: Report of a WHO Study Group. WHO. Tech Rep Ser 1985; 727:1–113.

111. Boyko EJ. The effect of parity on the later development of diabetes [Letter]. N Engl J Med 1990;322:1320.

112. Kritz-Silverstein D, Barrett-Connor E, Wingard DL. The effect of parity on the later development of diabetes—reply [Letter]. New Engl J Med 1990;322:1320.

113. Boyko EJ, Alderman BW, Keane EM, et al. Effects of childbearing on glucose tolerance and NIDDM prevalence. Diabetes Care 1990;13:848–854.

114. Manson JE, Rimm EB, Colditz GA, et al. Parity and Incidence of non-insulin-dependent diabetes mellitus. Am J Med 1992;93:13–18.

115. Simmons D. Parity, ethnic group and the prevalence of type 2 diabetes: The coventry diabetes study. Diabetic Med 1992;9:706–709.

116. Sicree RA, Hoet JJ, Zimmet P, King HOM, Coventry JS. The association of non-insulin-dependent diabetes with parity and still-birth occurrence amongst five Pacific population. Diabetes Res Clin Pract 1986;2:113–122.

117. Collins VR, Dowse GK, Zimmet P. Evidence an association between parity and NIDDM from five population groups. Diabetes Care 1991;14:975–981.

118. Peters RK, Kjos SL, Xiang A, Buchanan TA. Long-term diabetogenic effect of single pregnancy in women with previous gestational diabetes mellitus. Lancet 1986; 347:227–230.

119. Kritz-Silverstein D, Barrett-Connor E, Wingard DL, Friedlander NJ. Relation of pregnancy history to insulin levels in older, nondiabetic women. Am J Epidemiol 1994;140:375–382.

120. Alderman BW, Marshall JA, Boyko EJ, Markham KA, Baxter J, Hamman RF. Reproductive history, glucose tolerance, and NIDDM in Hispanic and non-Hispanic white women. The San Luis Valley Diabetes Study. Diabetes Care 1993;16:1557–1664.

121. Miall WE, Oldham PD. Factors influencing arterial blood pressure in the general population. Clin Sci 1958;17:409–444.

122. Miall WE. Follow-up study of arterial pressure in the population of Welsh mining valley. Br Med J 1959;2:1204–1210.

123. Schenckloth RE, Corcoran AC, Stuart KL, et al. Arterial pressure and hypertensive disease in a West Indian Negro population: Report of a survey in St. Kitts, West Indies. Am Heart J 1962;63:607–628.

124. Parry EHO. Ethiopian cardiovascular studies III. The casual blood pressure in Ethiopian highlanders in Addis Ababa. East Afr Med J 1969;46:246–256.

125. Humerfelt S, Wedervang F. A study of the influence upon blood pressure of marital status, number of children, and occupation. Acta Med Scand 1957;159:489–497.

126. Miall WE, Kass EH, Ling J, et al. Factors influencing arterial pressure in the general population in Jamaica. Br Med J 1969;2:497–506.

127. Ree GH. Arterial pressures in a West African (Gambian) rural population. J Trop Med Hyg 1973;76:65–70.

128. Ness RB, Kramer RA, Flegal KM. Gravidity, blood pressure and hypertension among white women in the Second National Health and Nutrition Examination Survey. Epidemiology 1993;4:303–309.

129. Barnes J, Browne FJ. Blood pressure and the incidence of hypertension in nulliparous and parous women in remote prognosis of the toxemia of pregnancy. J Obstet Gynecol Br Emp 1954;52:1–12.

130. Johnson BC, Remington RD. A sampling study of blood pressure levels in white and Negro residents of Nassau, Bahamas. J Chronic Dis 1961;13:39–51.

131. Baird JT, Quinlivan LG. Parity and hypertension. National Center for Health Statistics. Vital Health Stat [11] 1972;38 (DHEW pub. no. (HSM)72–1024).

132. Akinkugbe A. Arterial pressures in nonpregnant women of childbearing age in Ile-Ife, Nigeria. Br J Obstet Gynaecol 1976;83:545–549.

133. Lee-Feldstein A, Harburg E, Hauenstein L. Parity and blood pressure among four race-stress groups of females in Detroit. Am J Epidemiol 1980;111:356–366.

134. Rose G. Review of primary prevention trials. Am Heart J 1987;114: 1013–1017.

135. Lang T. Degoulet P, Aime F, et al. Relationship between alcohol consumption and hypertension prevalence and control in a French population. J Chronic Dis 1987;40: 713–720.

136. Liao Y, Emidy LA, Gosch FC, et al. Cardiovascular responses to exercise of participants in a trial on the primary prevention of hypertension. J Hypertens 1987;5: 317–321.

137. Maschak CA, Lobo RA. Estrogen replacement therapy and hypertension. J Reprod Med 1985;30(suppl):805–810.

138. Davey DA, MacGillivray I. The classification and definition of the hypertensive disorders of pregnancy. Am J Obstet Gynecol 1988;158:892–898.

139. Ferris TF. Toxemia and hypertension. In: Burrow GN, Ferris TF, eds. Medical Complications During Pregnancy, 3rd ed. Philadelphia: W.B. Saunders, 1988, pp. 1–38.

140. Frey CM. Ovary. In: Miller BA, Reis LAG, Hankey BF, Cosary CL, Edward BK, eds. Cancer Statistics Review 1973–1989. NIH pub. no. 92–2789. Bethesda, MD: National Cancer Institute, 1992, pp. 1–7.

141. Cancer Statistics Review 1973–87. NIH pub. no. 90-2789:128. Bethesda, MD: U.S. Department of Health and Human Services, National Institutes of Health, 1990.

142. Whittemore AS. Personal characteristics relating to risk of invasive epithelial ovarian cancer in older women in the United States. Cancer 1993;71:558–565.

143. Whittemore AS, Harris R, Intyre J, Halpern J, and the Collaborative Ovarian Cancer Group. Characteristics relating to ovarian-cancer risk: Collaborative analysis of 12 US case-control studies. IV The pathogenesis of epithelial ovarian cancer. Am J Epidemiol 1992;132:1212–1220.

144. Westhoff C, Ovarian Cancer. Ann Rev Public Health 1996;17:85–96.

145. Fathalla MF. Incessant ovulation—a factor in ovarian neoplasia? Lancet 1971; 2:163.

146. Cassagrande JT, Louis EW, Pike MC, et al. "Incessant ovulation" and ovarian cancer. Lancet 1979;2:170–173.

147. Whittemore AS, Wu ML, Paffenbarger RS, et al. Personal and environmental characteristics related to epithelial ovarian cancer. II. Exposures to talcum powder, tobacco, alcohol, and coffee. Am J Epidemiol 1988;128:1228–1240.

148. Pike MC. Age-related factors in cancers of the breast epithelium. J Chronic Dis 1987;40(suppl 2):59s–69s.

149. Hildreth HG, Kelsey JL, LiVolsi VA, Fischer DB, Holford TR, Mostow ED, et al. An epidemiological study of epithelial carcinoma of the ovary. Am J Epidem 1981; 114:398–405.

150. Franchesi S, la Veechia C, Helmreich SP, et al. Risk Factors epithelial ovarian cancer in Italy. Am J Epidemiol 1982;115:714–719.

151. Gwinn ML, Lee NL, Rhodes PH, Layde PM, Rubin GL. Pregnancy and breast-feeding, and oral contraceptives and the risk of epithelial ovarian cancer. J Clin Epidemiol 1990;43:559–568.

152. Lund E. Mortality from ovarian cancer among women with many children. Int J Epidemiol 1992;21:872–876.

153. Cramer DW, Hutchinson GB, Welch WR, Scully RE, Ryan KJ. Determinants of ovarian cancer risk. I. reproductive experiences and family history. J Natl Cancer Inst 1983;711–716.

154. Irwin KL, Weiss NS, Lee NC, Peterson NB, Tubal sterilization, hysterectomy, and subsequent occurrence of epithelial ovarian cancer: Am J Epidemiol 1991;134: 362–369.

155. John EM, Whittemore AS, Harris R, Itnyre J, Collaborative Ovarian Cancer Group. Characteristics relating to ovarian cancer risk: Collaborative analysis of seven U.S. case–control studies. Epithelial ovarian cancer risk in Black women. J Natl Cancer Inst 1993;85:142–146.

156. Polychronopoulou A, Tzonou A, Hsieh C-C, Kapromos G, Rebelakos A, Toupadaki N, et al. Reproductive variables, tobacco, ethane, coffee, and somatometry as risk factors for ovarian cancer. Int J Cancer 1993;55:402–407.

157. Risch HA, Marrett LD, Howe GR. Parity, contraception, infertility, and the risk of epithelial ovarian cancer. Am J Epidemiol 1994;140:585–597.

158. Stadel BV. The etiology and prevention of ovarian cancer. Am J Obstet Gynecol 1975;123:772–774.

159. Cramer DW, Welch WR. Determinants of ovarian cancer risk. II. inferences regarding pathogenesis. J Natl Cancer Inst 1983:839–845.

160. Scott JZ, Kletzky OA, Brenner PF, Mischell DR Jr. Comparison of the effects of contraceptive steroid formulations containing two doses of estrogen on pituitary function. Fertil Steril 1978;30:141–145

161. Spellacy WN, Kalra PS, Buhi WC, Birk SA. Pituitary and ovarian responsiveness to a graded gonadotrophin releasing factor simulation test in women using a low estrogen or regular type of oral contraceptive. Ann J Obstet Gynecol 1980;137:109–115.

162. Hankinson SE, Colditz GA, Hunter MB, et al. A prospective study of reproductive factors and risk of epithelial ovarian cancer. Cancer 1995;76:284–290.

163. Cramer DW, Xu H, Sahi T. Adult hypolactasia, milk consumption, and age-specific fertility. Am J Epidemiol 1994;139:282–289.

164. Booth M, Beral V, Smith P. Risk factors for ovarian cancer: A case control study. Br J Cancer 1989;60:592–598.

165. Hartge P, Schiffman MH, Hoover R, McGowan L, Lesher L, Norris HJ. A case control study of epithelial ovarian cancer. Am J Obstet Gynecol 1989;161:10–16.

166. Nasca PC, Greenwald P, Chorost S, Richart R, Caputo T. An epidemiologic case–control study of ovarian cancer and reproductive factors. Am J Epidemiol 1984; 119:705–713.

167. Shu XO, Brinton LA, Fao YT, Yuan JM. Population-based case–control study of ovarian cancer in Shanghai. Cancer Res 1989;49:3670–3674.

168. Chen Y, Wu PC, Lang JH, Ge WJ, Hartge P, Brinton LA. Risk factors for epithelial ovarian cancer in Bejing, China. Int J Epidemiol 1992;21:23–29.

169. Whittemore AS, Harris R, Itnyre J, Collaborative Ovarian Cancer Group. Characteristics relating to ovarian cancer risk: Collaborative analysis of 12 U.S. case–control studies. II. Invasive epithelial ovarian cancers in white women. Am J Epidemiol 1992;136:1184–1203.

170. Negri E, Franceschi S, Tzonous A, et al. Pooled analysis of 3 European case–control studies: I. reproductive factors and risk of epithelial ovarian cancer. Int J Cancer 1991;49:50–56.

171. Purdie D, Green A, Bain C, Siskind V, Ward B, Hacker N, et al. Reproductive and other factors and risk of ovarian cancer: An Australian case–control study. Int J Cancer 1995;62:678–684.

172. La Vecchia C, Neori E, Franceschi S, Parazzini F. Long-term impact of reproductive factors on cancer risk. Int J Cancer 1993;53:215–219.

173. Bernal A, Mendez-Moran L, Fajardo-Gutieeres A, Gonzalez-Lira G, Escudero P, Ortiz H. Univariate and multipvariate analysis of risk factors for ovarian cancer: Case–control study, Mexico City. Arch Med Res 1995;26:245–249.

174. Adami HO, Hsieh C, Lambe M, Trichopoulos D, Leon D, Persson I, et al. Parity, age at first childbirth, and risk of ovarian cancer. Lancet 1994;344:1250–1254.

175. Kelsey JL, Hildreth NG. Breast and Gynecologic cancer epidemiology. Boca Raton, FL: CRC Press, 1983, pp. 93–115.

176. Hartge P, Whittemore AS, Itnyre J, McGowan L, Cramer D, and the Collaborative Ovarian Cancer Group. Rates and risks of ovarian cancer in subgroups of white women in the United States. Obstet Gynecol 1994;84:760–764.

177. Brinton LA, Melton LJ, Malkasian GD, Bond A, Hoover R. Cancer risk after evaluation for infertility. Am J Epidemiol 1989;129:712–722.

178. Coulam CB, Annegers JF, Kranz JS. Chronic anovulation syndrome and associated neoplasia. Obstet Gynecol 1983;61:403–407.

179. Ron E, Lunenfield B, Menczer J, et al. Cancer incidence in a cohort of infertile women. Am J Epidemiol 1987;125:780–790.

180. Rossing MA, Daling JR, Weiss NS, Moore DE, Self SG. Ovarian tumors in a cohort of infertile women. N Engl J Med 1994;771–776.

181. Balasch J, Barri PN. Follicular stimulation and ovarian cancer. Hum Reprod 1993;8:990–996.

182. International Federation of Fertility Societies. Fertility drugs and ovarian cancer. Fertil Steril 1993;60:406–408.

183. Kaufman SC, Spiritas R, Alexander NJ. Do fertility drugs cause ovarian tumors? J Womens Health 1995;4:247–259.

184. Cramer DW, Hutchinson GB, Welsh WR, et al. Factors affecting the association of oral contraceptives and ovarian cancer. N Engl J Med 1982;307:1047–1051.

185. Kvale G, Heuch I, Nilssen S, et al. Reproductive factors and risk of ovarian cancer: A prospective study. Int J Cancer 1988;42:246–251.

186. WHO Collaborative Study of Neoplasia and Steroid Contraceptives. Epithelial ovarian cancer and combined oral contraceptives. Int J Epidemiol 1989;18:538–545.

187. Risch HA, Marrett LD, Jain M, Howe GR. Differences in risk factors for epithelial ovarian cancer by histological type. Results of a case-control study. Am J Epidemiol 1996;144:363–372.

INDEX